Phytochemicals in Nutrition and Health

Phytochemicals in Nutrition and Health

Editor: Josie Sparks

STATES
ACADEMIC PRESS
www.statesacademicpress.com

States Academic Press,
109 South 5th Street,
Brooklyn, NY 11249, USA

Visit us on the World Wide Web at:
www.statesacademicpress.com

ISBN: 978-1-63989-417-8 (Hardback)

Cataloging-in-Publication Data

Phytochemicals in nutrition and health / edited by Josie Sparks.
p. cm.
Includes bibliographical references and index.
ISBN 978-1-63989-417-8
1. Phytochemicals--Physiological effect. 2. Phytochemicals--Therapeutic use.
3. Nutrition. 4. Health. 5. Alternative medicine. I. Sparks, Josie.

QP144.V44 P49 2022
613.2--dc23

Table of Contents

Preface

Every book is a source of knowledge and this one is no exception. The idea that led to the conceptualization of this book was the fact that the world is advancing rapidly; which makes it crucial to document the progress in every field. I am aware that a lot of data is already available, yet, there is a lot more to learn. Hence, I accepted the responsibility of editing this book and contributing my knowledge to the community.

Chemicals of plants origin are defined as phytochemicals. These are produced by plants to help them resist against bacteria, fungi, virus, insects and other pathogens. Phytochemicals are produced by primary or secondary metabolism. They are classified into cartenoids, flavonoids, phenolic acids and lignans. Flavonoids are further divided into flavones, flavonones, anthocyanin, and flavanols. Phytochemicals are found in colorful parts of plants, fruits, legumes and vegetables. They have been found to be effective in preventing cancer, diabetes and cardiovascular diseases. Some common examples of phytochemicals include vitamin A, vitamin C and dietary fiber. This book includes some of the vital pieces of work being conducted across the world, on various topics related to phytochemicals. The various studies that are constantly contributing towards advancing technologies and evolution of this field are examined in detail. This book is a vital tool for all researching or studying phytochemicals as it gives incredible insights into emerging trends and concepts.

While editing this book, I had multiple visions for it. Then I finally narrowed down to make every chapter a sole standing text explaining a particular topic, so that they can be used independently. However, the umbrella subject sinews them into a common theme. This makes the book a unique platform of knowledge.

I would like to give the major credit of this book to the experts from every corner of the world, who took the time to share their expertise with us. Also, I owe the completion of this book to the never-ending support of my family, who supported me throughout the project.

Editor

1

Role of Flavonoids as Wound Healing Agent

Muhammad Shahzad Aslam,
Muhammad Syarhabil Ahmad, Humayun Riaz,
Syed Atif Raza, Shahzad Hussain,
Omer Salman Qureshi, Povydysh Maria,
Zainab Hamzah and Osama Javed

Abstract

Flavonoids are found as the most abundant bioactive compounds all around the world. It is found in a number of medicinal plants that are used as wound healing agents in traditional medicinal uses such as *Buddleja globosa, Moringa oleifera*, Lam, *Butea monosperma, Parapiptadenia rigida* and *Ononis spinosa*. Flavonoids nowadays are being used in different formulation and wound healing dressings. Inflammation, proliferation and reepithelialization are involved in wound healing. Most of the wound healing medicinal plants possess multiple flavonoids that act as synergistic effect or combined effect. This chapter briefly reviews the role of flavonoids as wound healing agent in traditional and modern medicine.

Keywords: medicinal plants, flavonoids, wound healing, mechanism of flavonoids in wound healing

1. Introduction

The care of acute and chronic wound is the biggest challenges worldwide [1]. There are different kind of wounds, among them burns remain a major public health problem in developing countries [2]. There are different ways to heal the wound such as nano dressing [3], negative pressure [4], medicinal plants [5], synthetic polymers [6], gene therapy [7], stem cell [8], growth factors [9] and Functionalized Silk Biomaterials [10]. Flavonoids is one of an important bioactive source from medicinal plants that possess different pharmacological activities such as antioxidant, free radical scavenging capacity, coronary heart disease prevention, hepatoprotective, anti-inflammatory, anticancer activities, growth regulators [11]. Wound results in edema, redness followed by pain. Inflammation is the major characteristics as a result of wound due to the release of eicosanoids, prostaglandins, leukotrienes and reactive oxygen species. By controlling all these factors will result in healing the wound faster. Recent students on Buddleja species and three Ghanaian species *Spathodea campanulata, Commelina diffusa* and *Secamone afzelii* showed antioxidant and anti-inflammatory properties. These anti-oxidant and anti-inflammatory properties were due to the presence of flavonoids and other bioactive compounds that works in combination to heal the wound [12]. The chapter deals with the study of role of flavonoids, mechanism of action that involves in healing the wound.

2. Wound healing medicinal plants

Healing the wound with medicinal plants is an alternative method of treatment used by traditional wound healer. The most commonly used plants all over the world is *Curcuma longa.* In Malaysia, there are few more species that act as wound healing such as *Elephantopus scaber, Centella asiatica, Clinacanthus nutans* and *Aloe barbadensis.* List of famous medicinal plants that plays an important role in wound healing is mentioned in **Table 1**.

Medicinal plants	Pharmacological uses	Reference
Aloe barbadensis miller	Anti-oxidant, anti-inflammatory, wound healing, antimicrobial	[13–16]
Azadirachta indica	Anti-malarial, wound healing, antiseptic, febrifuge, antihelminthic, anti-microbial	[17, 18]
Curcuma longa Linn.	Hepatoprotective, nephroprotective, anticoagulant, wound healing, anti-HIV to combat AIDS, anti-microbial	[19, 20]
Clinacanthus nutans	Anti-papillomavirus infectivity, anti-viral activity on varicella-zoster virus, anti-inflammatory activity, anti-herpes simplex virus type 1 and type 2 activity, anti-oxidant and protective effect against oxidative induced hemolysis	[21]
Chromolaena odorata	Wound healing, analgesic, anti-inflammatory and antipyretic activities	[22, 23]
Centella asiatica	Antimicrobial activity, anticancer activity, wound healing activity, neuroprotective activity, immunomodulatory activity, anti-inflammatory activity, hepatoprotective activity, insecticidal activity, and antioxidant activity	[24, 25]
Elephantopus scaber	Antimicrobial, hepatoprotective, antioxidant, antidiabetic, anti-inflammatory, analgesic, antiasthmatic, antiplatelet, and wound healing	[26]
Euphorbia neriifolia	Analgesic, hepatoprotective, immunostimulant, anti-inflammatory, mild CNS depressant, wound healing, radioprotective	[27, 28]
Lantana camara	Anticancer activity, wound healing, anti-inflammatory activity, antidiabetic activity, anthelmintic, antibacterial activity, antifungal activity, hepatoprotective activity, antioxidant activity, larvicidal activity	[29, 30]
Tridax procumbens	Hepatoprotective activity, anti-inflammatory, wound healing, antidiabetic activity, hypotensive effect, immunomodulating property, bronchial catarrh, dysentery, diarrhea and to prevent falling of hair promotes the growth of hair, and antimicrobial activity	[31]

Table 1. List of medicinal plants in healing the wound.

3. What is the role of flavonoids on human health?

Flavonoids are phenolic substances isolated from a wide range of vascular plants, with over 8000 individual compounds known [32]. They possess wide variety of activities such as anti-microbial [33], anti-oxidant [34], anti-cancer [35], anti-inflammatory [36] and wound healing [37]. Among all flavonoids there are some flavonoids such as flavan-3-ols and flavonols, possess a wide spectrum due to suppress a number of microbial virulence factors and show synergism with antibiotics [38]. While there has been a major focus on the antioxidant properties, there is an emerging view that flavonoids, and their in vivo metabolites, do not act as conventional hydrogen-donating antioxidants but may exert modulatory actions in cells through actions at protein kinase and lipid kinase signaling pathways. Flavonoids, and more recently their metabolites, have been reported to act at phosphoinositide 3-kinase (PI 3-kinase), Akt/protein kinase B (Akt/PKB), tyrosine kinases, protein kinase C (PKC), and mitogen activated protein kinase (MAP kinase) signaling cascades. Inhibitory or stimulatory actions at these pathways are likely to affect cellular function profoundly by altering the phosphorylation state of target molecules and by modulating gene expression [39]. In many molecular mechanisms of action for prevention against cancer, flavonoids play a major role by interacting between different types of genes and enzymes. Many mechanisms of action have been identified, including carcinogen inactivation, antiproliferation, cell cycle arrest, induction of apoptosis, inhibition of angiogenesis, antioxidation, and reversal of multidrug resistance or a combination of these mechanisms [40].

4. Flavonoids and wound healing

Catechins are one of the most widely tested classes of flavonoids for their wound healing modulation [41]. Lastly, considering that the delay in wound healing is due to insufficient or excessive fibroblast activity, some authors suggest that inhibition of fibroblast growth by flavonoids such as apigenin is beneficial for the treatment of skin injuries. Luteolin is another famous flavonoid present in medicinal plants, vegetables and fruits. It was also found as wound healing agent in different wound models [42]. Rutin which is found in many medicinal

Medicinal plants	Flavonoids isolated	Wound healing model	Reference
Buddleja globosa	Linarin (acacetin-7-O-rutinoside), luteolin and 6-hydroxyluteolin	Fibroblast growth stimulation	[44]
Moringa oleifera Lam	Vicenin-2, kaempferol and quercetin	Cell viability, proliferation, and wound scratch test assays.	[45]
Butea monosperma	Genistein and prunetine	Excision wound model, Incision wound model, Dead space wound model	[46]
Parapiptadenia rigida	Catechin	Fibroblast proliferation assay	[41]
Ononis spinosa L	Ononin, sativanone-7-O-glucoside	Linear incision and circular excision wound models and hydroxyproline estimation assay	[47]

Table 2. List of medicinal plants possessing flavonoids in healing the wound.

plants also possess wound healing activities [43]. List of medicinal plants possessing flavonoids in healing the wound is mentioned in **Table 2**.

5. Flavonoids in fruits and vegetables

Flavonoids found in number of fruits and vegetable. A study indicates a number of vegetable (28) and fruits (9) that possess anti-carcinogenic flavonoids [48]. Fruits such as apple, berries, and onions possess cardioprotective properties and bring a positive impact on blood pressure, vascular function and serum lipid levels [49].

6. Conclusion

Flavonoids is an essential bioactive compounds found in our daily life in the form of fruits and vegetable. It possesses wound healing properties. There are number of research that showed the importance of flavonoids as wound healing agent. For example the flowers of *Ipomoea carnea* belong to family Convolvulaceae. The isolated bioactive compounds such as Kaempferol, Kaempferol-3-O-β-D-glucoside confirm the wound healing activities on all animal models [50]. There is yet to explore its structure activity relationship on different wound models. Furthermore, there is little knowledge about mechanism involve in wound healing. Optimization use of flavonoids and their dosage as wound healing is another aspect that yet to explore.

Author details

Muhammad Shahzad Aslam[1*], Muhammad Syarhabil Ahmad[2], Humayun Riaz[1], Syed Atif Raza[3], Shahzad Hussain[4], Omer Salman Qureshi[5], Povydysh Maria[6], Zainab Hamzah[7] and Osama Javed[3]

*Address all correspondence to: aslammuhammadshahzad@gmail.com

1 Rashid Latif College of Pharmacy, Lahore, Pakistan

2 School of Bioprocess Engineering, Universiti Malaysia Perlis, Arau, Perlis, Malaysia

3 University College of Pharmacy, University of the Punjab, Lahore, Pakistan

4 National Institute of Health, Islamabad, Pakistan

5 Department of Pharmacy, University of the Lahore, Pakistan

6 Saint-Petersburg State Chemical-Pharmaceutical Academy, Ministry of Healthcare of the Russian Federation, St. Petersburg, Russia

7 Department Chemical Engineering, Faculty of Engineering Technology (FETech), Universiti Malaysia Perlis, Padang Besar, Perlis, Malaysia

References

[1] Serena TE. A global perspective on wound care. Advances in Wound Care. 2014;**3**(8): 548-552

[2] Gupta VK, Pathak SS, Jain MK. Evaluation of burn wound healing property of ocimum sanctum by monitoring of period of re-epithelization in rabbits. International Journal of Basic & Clinical Pharmacology Research. 2016;**5**(1):146-148

[3] Archana D, Dutta J, Dutta PK. Evaluation of chitosan nano dressing for wound healing: Characterization, in vitro and in vivo studies. International Journal of Biological Macromolecules. 2013;**57**:193-203

[4] Huang C, Leavitt T, Bayer LR, Orgill DP. Effect of negative pressure wound therapy on wound healing. Current Problems in Surgery. 2014;**51**(7):301-331

[5] Jivad N, Bahmani M, Asadi-Samani M. A review of the most important medicinal plants effective on wound healing on ethnobotany evidence of Iran. Der Pharmacia Lettre. 2016;**8**(2):353-357

[6] Moura LIF, Dias AMA, Carvalho E, De Sousa HC. Recent advances on the development of wound dressings for diabetic foot ulcer treatment—A review. Acta Biomaterialia. 2013;**9**(7):7093-7114

[7] Cheng CF et al. A fragment of secreted Hsp90α carries properties that enable it to accelerate effectively both acute and diabetic wound healing in mice. The Journal of Clinical Investigation. 2011;**121**(11):4348-4361

[8] Asai J et al. Topical application of ex vivo expanded endothelial progenitor cells promotes vascularisation and wound healing in diabetic mice. International Wound Journal. 2013;**10**(5):527-533

[9] Barrientos S, Brem H, Stojadinovic O, Tomic-Canic M. Clinical application of growth factors and cytokines in wound healing. Wound Repair and Regeneration. 2014;**22**(5):569-578

[10] Gil ES, Panilaitis B, Bellas E, Kaplan DL. Functionalized silk biomaterials for wound healing. Advanced Healthcare Materials. 2013;**2**(1):206-217

[11] Kumar S, Pandey AK. Chemistry and Biological Activities of Flavonoids: An Overview. The Scientific World Journal. 2013;**2013**(162750):16. https://doi.org/10.1155/2013/162750

[12] Houghton PJ, Hylands PJ, Mensah AY, Hensel A, Deters AM. In vitro tests and ethnopharmacological investigations: Wound healing as an example. Journal of Ethnopharmacology. 2005;**100**:100-107

[13] Surjushe A, Vasani R, Saple DG. Aloe vera: A short review. Indian Journal of Dermatology. 2008;**53**(4):163-166

[14] Hu Y, Xu J, Hu Q. Evaluation of antioxidant potential of Aloe vera (*Aloe barbadensis Miller*) extracts. Journal of Agricultural and Food Chemistry. 2003;**51**(26):7788-7791

[15] Hutter JA et al. Antiinflammatory C-glucosyl chromone from Aloe barbadensis. Journal of Natural Products. 1996;**59**(5):541-543

[16] Irshad S, Butt M, Younus H. In-vitro antibacterial activity of *Aloe barbadensis Miller* (Aloe vera). International Research Journal. 2011;**1**(2):59-64

[17] Hashmat I, Azad H, Ahmed A. Neem (*Azadirachta indica A.* Juss)—A Nature's drugstore : An overview. International Research Journal of Biological Sciences. 2012;**1**(6):76-79

[18] Koul O, Isman MB, Ketkar CM. Properties and uses of neem, *Azadirachta indica*. Canadian Journal of Botany. 1990;**68**(1):1-11

[19] Krup V, Prakash LH, Harini A. Pharmacological activities of turmeric (*Curcuma longa* Linn): A review. Journal of Homeopathy & Ayurvedic Medicine. 2013;**2**(4):133. DOI: 10.4172/2167-1206.1000133

[20] Rafieian-Kopaei M, Nasri H, Sahinfard N, Rafieian M, Rafieian S, Shirzad M. Turmeric: A spice with multifunctional medicinal properties. Journal of Herbmed Pharmacology. 2014;**3**(1):5-8

[21] Aslam MS, Ahmad MS, Mamat AS. A review on phytochemical constituents and pharmacological activities of *Clinacanthus nutans*. International Journal of Pharmacy and Pharmaceutical Sciences. 2015;**7**(2):30-33

[22] Ayyanar M, Ignacimuthu S. Herbal medicines for wound healing among tribal people in southern India: Ethnobotanical and scientific evidences. International Journal of Applied Research in Natural Products. 2009;**2**(3):29-42

[23] Owoyele BV, Oguntoye SO, Dare K, Ogunbiyi BA, Aruboula EA, Soladoye AO. Analgesic, anti-inflammatory and antipyretic activities from flavonoid fractions of *Chromolaena odorata*. Journal of Medicinal Plants Research. 2008;**2**(9):219-225

[24] Orhan IE. *Centella asiatica* (L.) Urban: From traditional medicine to modern medicine with neuroprotective potential. Evidence-based Complementary and Alternative Medicine. 2012;**2012**(946259):8. https://doi.org/10.1155/2012/946259

[25] Dipankar CR, Barman SK, Shaik MM. Current updates on *Centella asiatica*: Phytochemistry, pharmacology and traditional uses. Journal of Medicinal Plants Research. 2013;**3**(4):20-36

[26] Hiradeve SM, Rangari VD. *Elephantopus scaber* Linn.: A review on its ethnomedical, phytochemical and pharmacological profile. Journal of Applied Biomedicine. 2014;**12**(2):49-61

[27] Papiya B, Rana C. A comprehensive phyto-pharmacological review of *Euphorbia neriifolia* Linn. Pharmacognosy Reviews. 2008;**2**(4):57-66

[28] Ahmed SA, Nazim S, Siraj S, Siddik PM, Wahid CA. *Euphorbia neriifolia* Linn: A phytopharmacological review. International Research Journal of Pharmacy. 2011;**2**(5):41-48

[29] Saxena J, Khare S. A brief review on: Therapeutical values of *Lantana camara* plant. International Journal of Pharmacy and Life Sciences. 2012;**3**(3):1551-1554

[30] Kalita S, Kumar G, Karthik L, Rao KVB. A review on medicinal properties of *Lantana camara* Linn. Research Journal of Pharmacy and Technology. 2012;**5**(6):711-715

[31] Mundada S, Shivhare R. Pharmacology of *Tridax procumbens* a weed: Review. International Journal of PharmTech Research. 2010;**2**(2):1391-1394

[32] Pietta PG. Flavonoids as antioxidants. Journal of Natural Products. 2000;**63**(7):1035-1042

[33] Cushnie TPT, Lamb AJ. Antimicrobial activity of flavonoids. International Journal of Antimicrobial Agents. 2005;**26**(5):343-356

[34] Procházková D, Boušová I, Wilhelmová N. Antioxidant and prooxidant properties of flavonoids. Fitoterapia. 2011;**82**(4):513-523

[35] Ren W, Qiao Z, Wang H, Zhu L, Zhang L. Flavonoids: Promising anticancer agents. Medicinal Research Reviews. 2003;**23**(4):519-534

[36] Kim HP, Son KH, Chang HW, Kang SS. Anti-inflammatory plant flavonoids and cellular action mechanisms. Journal of Pharmacological Sciences. 2004;**96**(3):229-245

[37] Chirumbolo S. Flavonoids in propolis acting on mast cell-mediated wound healing. Inflammopharmacology. 2012;**20**(2):99-102

[38] Daglia M. Polyphenols as antimicrobial agents. Current Opinion in Biotechnology. 2012; **23**(2):174-181

[39] Williams RJ, Spencer JP, Rice-Evans C. Flavonoids: Antioxidants or signalling molecules? Free Radical Biology & Medicine. Apr. 2004;**36**(7):838-849

[40] Sharma N, Dobhal M, Joshi Y, Chahar M. Flavonoids: A versatile source of anticancer drugs. Pharmacognosy Reviews. 2011;**5**(9):1

[41] Schmidt CA et al. Catechin derivatives from *Parapiptadenia rigida* with in vitro wound-healing properties. Journal of Natural Products. 2010;**73**(12):2035-2041

[42] Ozay Y et al. Evaluation of the wound healing properties of luteolin ointments on excision and incision wound models in diabetic and non-diabetic rats. Records of Natural Products. 2018;**12**(4):350-366

[43] Tran NQ, Joung YK, Lih E, Park KD. In situ forming and rutin-releasing chitosan hydrogels as injectable dressings for dermal wound healing. Biomacromolecules. 2011;**12**(8): 2872-2880

[44] Mensah AY et al. Effects of *Buddleja globosa* leaf and its constituents relevant to wound healing. Journal of Ethnopharmacology. 2001;**77**(2-3):219-226

[45] Muhammad AA, Pauzi NAS, Arulselvan P, Abas F, Fakurazi S. In vitro wound healing potential and identification of bioactive compounds from *Moringa oleifera* Lam. BioMed Research International. 2013;**2013**

[46] Muralidhar A, Sudhakar Babu K, Sankar TR, Reddanna P, Latha J. Wound healing activity of flavonoid fraction isolated from the stem bark of *Butea monosperma* (Lam) in albino wistar rats. European Journal of Experimental Biology. 2013;**3**(6):1-6

[47] Ergene Öz B, Saltan İşcan G, Küpeli Akkol E, Süntar İ, Bahadır Acıkara Ö. Isoflavonoids as wound healing agents from Ononidis Radix. Journal of Ethnopharmacology. 2018; **211**:384-393

[48] Hertog MGL, Hollman PCH, Hertog MGL, Katan MB. Content of potentially anticarcinogenic flavonoids of 28 vegetables and 9 fruits commonly consumed in the Netherlands. Journal of Agricultural and Food Chemistry. 1992;**40**(12):2379-2383

[49] Toh JY, Tan VMH, Lim PCY, Lim ST, Chong MFF. Flavonoids from fruit and vegetables: A focus on cardiovascular risk factors. Current Atherosclerosis Reports. Dec. 2013;**15**(12):368

[50] Ambiga S, Narayanan R, Gowri D, Sukumar D, Madhavan S. Evaluation of wound healing activity of flavonoids from *Ipomoea carnea* Jacq. Ancient Science of Life. Jan. 2007; **26**(3):45-51

2

Potential Adverse Effects of Alteration of Phytochemical Accumulation in Fruits and Vegetables

Sechene Stanley Gololo

Abstract

Alterations in the accumulation of phytochemicals in fruits and vegetables may have adverse effects on the health benefits emanating from their consumption. Plants parts possess secondary metabolites in addition to their primary metabolites. Plants secondary metabolites possess many inherent biological activities that include antimicrobial, anti-inflammatory, and enzyme inhibitory properties, which are health benefits to humans. Accumulation of phytochemicals in plants is reportedly influenced by environmental factors or growth conditions such as lack of nutrients, pathogens attack, competitive co-habitation plant species, insect predation, and herbivorous attack. Human interventions such as agricultural practices may affect biochemical processes in plants or crops in a manner that may limitations or alterations in the accumulation of phytochemicals. The limitation of phytochemicals accumulation in fruits and vegetables may have the adverse effect on their health benefits in humans that may explain the high prevalence of life style diseases such as diabetes and cancer experienced in today's world. The proper assessment of the influence on phytochemical responses in crops, fruits, and vegetables by modern agricultural practices such as weeding methods, herbicides, insecticides, fertilizer application, crop rotation, and co-habitation needs to be carried out. Such assessment is important since while crop production may be improved, caution should be exercised not to erode, or negatively alter phytochemical biosynthesis in crops.

Keywords: plant metabolites, phytochemicals, biological activities, phytochemical accumulation, environmental conditions, weeding methods, herbicides, insecticides, fertilizer application, crop rotation, crop co-habitation

1. Introduction

The purpose of this chapter is to highlight the potential adverse effects of phytochemical accumulation alterations in fruits and vegetables on the well-being of people. The chapter deals with the introduction of plant metabolites with the distinguishing between primary and secondary metabolites based on their roles in plants. The chapter also deals with the biosynthesis and accumulation of phytochemicals in plants that are based on the effects of different environmental factors on phytochemical compositions in plants. This includes the review of the effect of pesticides on phytochemicals in agricultural products through comparison on products produced by organic farming and conventional farming. The potential adverse effect of phytochemical accumulation limitation in fruits and vegetables on the well-being of people is also highlighted through the discussion of the health benefits of the actions of phytochemicals in prevention and treatment of diabetes and cancer.

2. Plant metabolites

In addition to nutritional value, consumption of fruits and vegetables also provide health benefits to humans due to the nature of their secondary metabolites [1]. Plants of all kinds, including fruits and vegetables, possess two types of metabolites with distinct roles known as primary and secondary metabolites as shown in **Figure 1**. Primary metabolites, generally possessed by all plants, are metabolites that contribute to the plants' growth [2]. Primary plant metabolites include carbohydrates, lipids, proteins, and nucleic acids. Secondary metabolites, sometimes found in specific plants or plants parts, are for the performance of protection

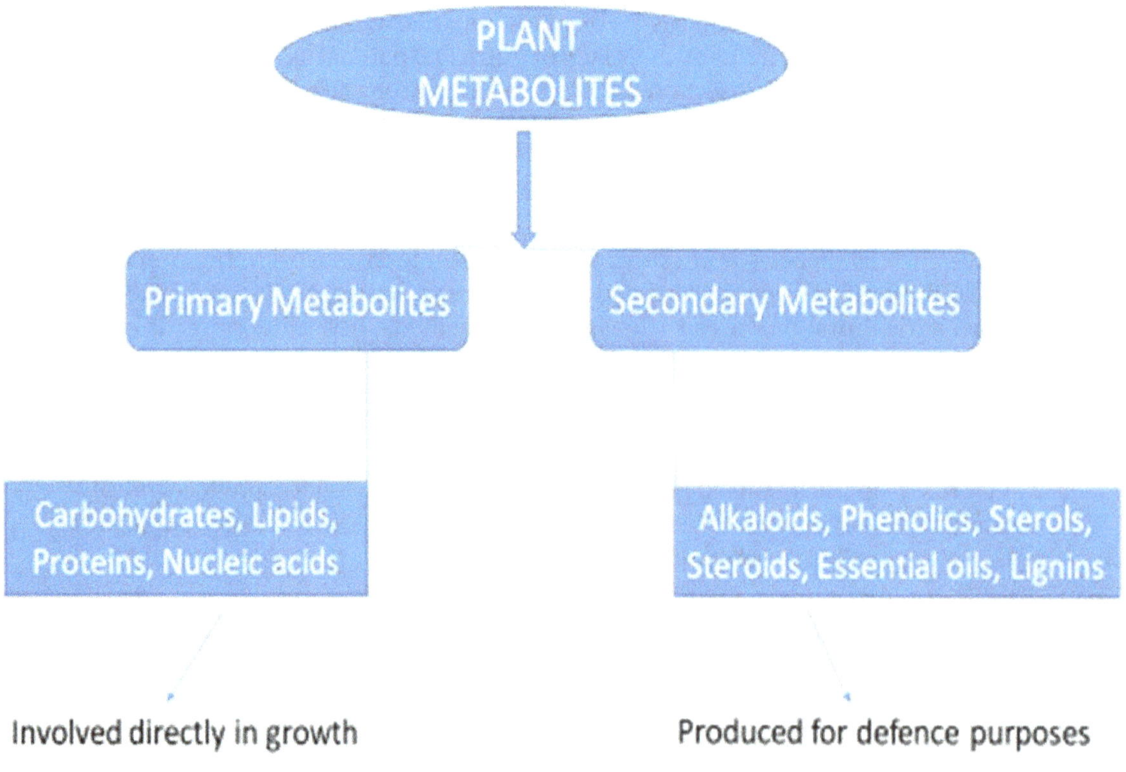

Figure 1. Plant metabolites and their different roles in plants.

functions from threats that emanate mainly from external factors [3]. Secondary plant metabolites include alkaloids, phenolic compounds, sterols, steroids, essential oils and lignins, and are commonly known or referred to as phytochemicals.

3. Biosynthesis and accumulation of phytochemicals in plants

The biosynthesis of phytochemicals in plants is mainly achieved through the Shikimate and the Acetate-Mevalonate pathways [4], as shown in **Figure 2**. Most end-products of the catabolic metabolism of primary metabolites serve as precursors for the biosynthesis of a range of secondary metabolites that are commonly referred to as phytochemicals. Aromatic amino acids enter secondary metabolite biosynthesis via the Shikimate pathway. The Shikimate pathway leads to the production of simple compounds such as gallic acid and *p*-coumaric acid that are precursors to complex products like tannins and nitrogen-containing phytochemicals [5]. Acetyl-CoA, an end-product of carbohydrate metabolism, leads to the biosynthesis of terpenes and steroids through the Acetate-Mevalonate pathway [6].

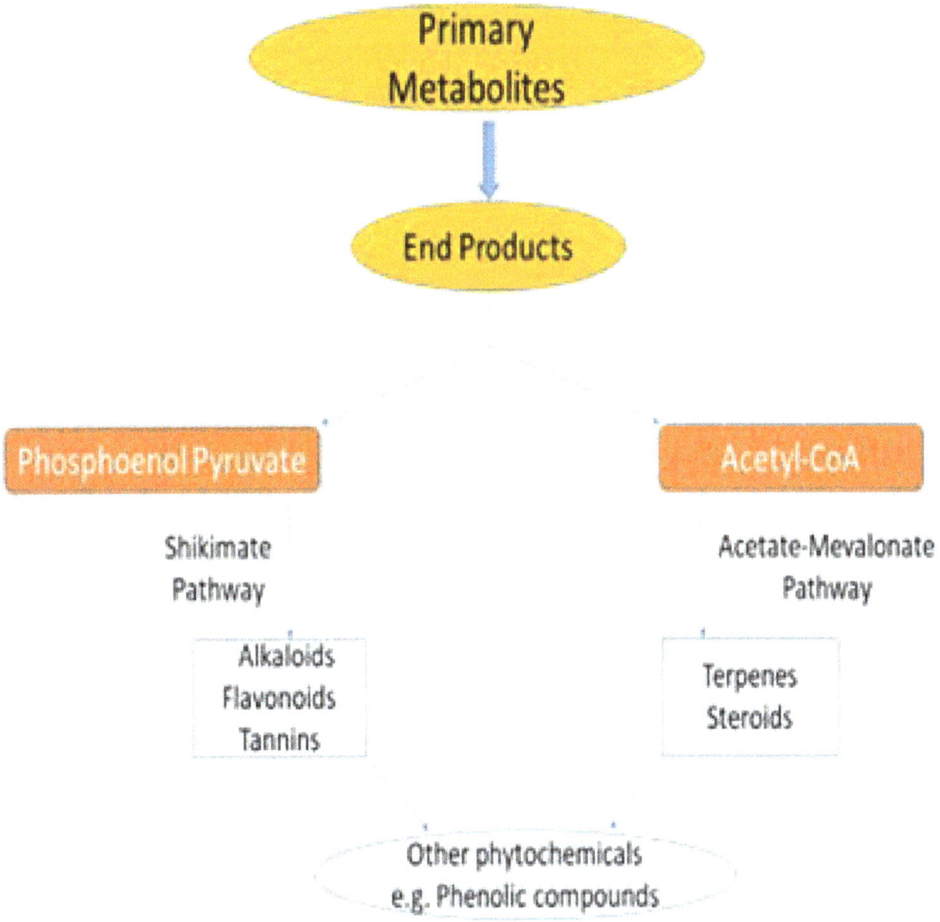

Figure 2. Biosynthesis of phytochemicals.

The biosynthesis of phytochemicals in plants, as described above, is reported to be also induced by external stimuli [7]. As such, phytochemical compositions of plants are mostly found to differ both qualitatively and quantitatively depending on the exposure or susceptibility to the stimuli [8]. The external stimuli that induce phytochemical biosynthesis in plants may be summed up through environmental factors under which plants grow. Environmental factors under, which plants grow and affect their phytochemical compositions may include geographical location parameters such as altitudes and soil types, seasonal variations, and exposure to pollution [9]. In the case of fruits and vegetables, such environmental factors may also include agricultural practices such as the use of insecticides and herbicides. Some findings on the effects of certain agricultural practices on the presence and accumulation of phytochemicals in fruits and vegetables, as well as their implications on people's health are discussed below.

3.1. Effects of agricultural practices on phytochemicals in fruits and vegetables

Undisputedly, the introduction of pesticides (synthetic) like insecticides and herbicides in the period between 1970 and 1980 contributed to increased agricultural productions. However, this intervention in agriculture has had some unintended results toward human life. The criticism of the usage of pesticides is mainly based on their direct cause of fatal health challenges and chronic diseases due to their poisonous effect upon exposure [10]. However, in addition, the potential consequences of the limitations in the phytochemical accumulations by agricultural plant products are not being given adequate attention or canvassing in the public discourse.

The effect of pesticide application on the phytochemical accumulation in fruits and vegetables could be assessed through the comparison of phytochemical quantities between crop products produced through organic farming, which does not involve the use of synthetic pesticides, and those produced through conventional farming that uses synthetic pesticides. In this regard, organic farming was reported to have been given yield to sweet pepper (*Capsicum annum*) of higher intensities in color (both red and yellow); higher mineral contents and higher total carotenoids than those produced through conventional farming [11]. In addition, the same study reported that highest antioxidant activity was found in red peppers produced through organic farming. In a separate study, a higher ratio of reducing sugars/organic acids, as well as high amounts of total sugars, vitamin C, and total flavonoids were recorded in tomato fruits produced by organic farming compared to those of conventional farming practice [12]. According to Oliveira et al. [13], the accumulation of more phytochemicals such as phenolics and vitamin C in tomato fruits from organic farming was a result of the stressing conditions associated with the farming system. It thus follows that conventional farming practice reduces or remove stressful growing conditions that then limit the accumulation of important phytochemicals in crops. The demonstration through some studies that the production of food products through conventional farming methods with the excessive use of insecticides and herbicides may limit the accumulation of phytochemicals in fruits and vegetables necessitate the assessment of potential implications of such limitations on people's health.

The quality and quantity of phytochemicals in plants depend on a number of factors that include the growing environment. Organic farming inherently provides a different growing environment compared to conventional farming, which relies heavily on inputs such as pesticides, synthetic fertilizers, and excessive irrigation. The growing environment in organic farming exposes plants and crops to biotic stress due to pests and diseases [14]. Herbivore and pathogen attack lead to enhanced biosynthesis and accumulation of defense-related phytochemicals in fruits and vegetables [15]. Deficiency of nitrogen, phosphate, and iron that emanate from non-application of synthetic fertilizers in organic farming contribute to the accumulation of phenolic compounds in fruits and vegetables [15]. Drought or less irrigation associated with organic farming also induce accumulation of polyphenols and total tannins in crops through the activation of the phenylalanine ammonia-lyase enzyme that is involved in the biosynthesis of phytochemicals in plants [16].

3.2. Potential adverse effects of phytochemical accumulation alterations in plant products

In Africa, people have relied on consumption of fruits and vegetables for many years with no profound problems of life style diseases. Fruits and vegetables are known to possess phytochemical compounds with biological activities that have the ability to prevent and reverse the development of chronic diseases such as diabetes and cancer [17, 18]. Therefore, a question arises as to how come the world, Africa in particular, is today burdened with the advent of life style diseases such as diabetes and cancer in the midst of massive agricultural production of fruits and vegetables. The answer to this imminent question may lie in the understanding of the possession or the presence of plant metabolites in fruits and vegetables, more especially the accumulation of secondary metabolites that are commonly referred to as phytochemicals.

The secondary metabolites found in different plants parts; including fruits and vegetables, possess many biological activities. Amongst the biological activities exerted by different phytochemicals are the enzyme inhibitory properties. There are two enzymes that are reported to contribute to the fast postprandial release of glucose from a carbohydrate-rich meal, namely the alpha-amylase and alpha-glucosidase. Inhibitory actions of these enzymes that are inherent in some phytochemicals present in plant products such as fruits and leafy vegetables contribute to the regulation of blood glucose levels as the slow release of glucose from diet sources may afford its proper metabolism, which mitigate against the development of diabetes mellitus [19]. Carbohydrates are of course important dietary requirements to supply living organisms with the necessary energy for growth. However, malfunctioning or poorly regulated carbohydrate metabolism may lead to the rapid postprandial release of glucose into the bloodstream with potential discrepancies in its further breakdown. The advent of discrepancies in the breakdown of glucose may result in its accumulation in blood, which gives rise to the potential development of diabetes mellitus [20].

In addition, the enzyme inhibitory properties inherent in some phytochemicals may affect kinases that are involved in cell cycle progression, which may contribute to the mitigation against the development of cancer. Cancer is a disease of uncontrolled cell growth, which is propelled through up-normal continuous cell division cycle [21]. Cell division cycle progression is regulated through the activity of phosphorylation enzymes known as kinases [22]. Cell division cycle progression is also depended on the intactness of the DNA that is safeguarded by the action of tumor suppressor genes. Tumor suppressor genes act by way of effecting cell division cycle arrest in case of DNA damage that affords DNA repair or cell death. One of the major causes of DNA damage is oxidative stress that emanates from the imbalances between reactive oxygen species (ROSs), known as free radicals and antioxidants. In the case, where DNA damage results in the malfunctioning of tumor suppressor genes, cell division cycle continues even in situations, where it should not of which the result is uncontrolled cell growth. Oxidative DNA damage may also affect metabolism regulatory genes that may lead to inadequate or impaired insulin. As such, oxidative DNA damage may culminate in the development of diseases such as cancer and diabetes mellitus [23]. The continuous supplementing of the human body with antioxidants is an important intervention that contributes immensely to the attainment of a balance between ROSs and antioxidants, which reduces oxidative stress. Consumption of fruits and vegetables contribute to the replenishing of the body with antioxidant as they are sources of phytochemicals with antioxidant properties [24].

Explanation of the molecular basis of diseases such as diabetes and cancer brings forth the understanding that adequate consumption of fruits and vegetables may result in the prevention and reversal of these conditions [18]. In the case of diabetes, high blood glucose levels, complications arise from the accumulation of glycated proteins known as advanced glycation end-products (AGEs). Antioxidation, one of the known major biological activities of phytochemicals is reported to contribute to the prevention of the formations of AGEs [25], as well as having protective effects against AGEs induced in stem cells [26]. As such, the immediate question is what contributes to the escalation of the prevalence of these diseases as well as escalated fatalities they cause, in the midst of massive production of fruits and vegetables that is taking place. The answer to this question may lie in understanding the biosynthesis and accumulation of phytochemicals in fruits and vegetables. The accumulation of phytochemicals in plants parts are reported to be for plants survival or defense mechanism in response to adverse environmental influences. Such environmental influences may include pathogens attacks, competitive co-habitation plant species, insect predation, and herbivorous attack. This exposure to hostile environmental settings mainly occurs in wild set-ups. Plants have been shown to have both qualitative and quantitative differences in their phytochemical compositions when growing under varying conditions [27]. In today's world, crops and plantations are shielded from hostile environmental conditions due to modern agricultural practices that also include the use of insecticides and chemical weed removals (herbicides). While production targets may be improved and attained [10], these modern agricultural practices may lead to the alteration of phytochemical compositions accumulation in agricultural products such as fruits and vegetables. Phytochemical accumulation alterations in plants may creep in since the threat that induces biosynthesis of phytochemicals would have been removed. This alteration in the accumulation of phytochemicals in fruits and vegetables may have adverse effects on human health such as inadequate availability of phytochemicals with antidiabetic and anticancer properties. As such, while production could be optimized through modern agricultural practices the quality of the agricultural produce may be negatively affected in terms of their phytochemical compositions. Thus, caution should be exercised not to erode or negatively alter the phytochemical biosynthesis patterns in fruits and vegetables in pursuit of massive production. Alternatively, agricultural practices could include the creation of conditions that will induce bioaccumulation of phytochemicals in fruits and vegetables.

4. Conclusion

Plants products, including fruits and vegetables, generally possess two types of chemicals that play different roles known as primary and secondary metabolites. Secondary metabolites are produced for defense purposes in plants in response to detrimental environmental stimuli and contribute to the well-being of humans upon consumption due to their disease prevention and reversal properties. However, modern agricultural methods, although with improved production yields, may give rise to phytochemical accumulation alterations in agricultural products such as fruits and vegetables that eventually have negative effects on their health benefits in human beings. The extent, to which modern agricultural practices may affect the accumulation of important phytochemicals in fruits and vegetables still needs to be fully determined, which presents scope for future research.

Acknowledgements

The author would like to acknowledge the Sefako Makgatho Health Sciences University for the conducive scholarly environment that enabled completion of this Book Chapter.

Conflict of interest

The author declares no conflict of interest.

Author details

Sechene Stanley Gololo

Address all correspondence to: stanley.gololo@smu.ac.za

Department of Biochemistry, School of Science and Technology, Sefako Makgatho Health Sciences University, Pretoria, South Africa

References

[1] Slavin JL, Lloyd B. Health benefits of fruits and vegetables. Advances in Nutrition. 2012;**3**(4):506-516. DOI: 10.3945/an.112.002154

[2] Sharma A, Batra A. Primary metabolite profiling of *Tinospora cordifolia*. Natural Products Chemistry and Research. 2016;**4**(4):1-7. DOI: 10.4172/2329-6836.1000221

[3] Wink M. Modes of action of herbal medicines and plant secondary metabolites. Medicines (Basel). 2015;**2**(3):251-286. DOI: 10.3390/medicines2030251

[4] Ncube B, Van Staden J. Tilting plant metabolism for improved metabolite biosynthesis and enhanced human benefit. Molecules. 2015;**20**:12698-12731. DOI: 10.3390/molecules200712698

[5] Montes-Ávila J, López-Angulo G, Delgado-Vargas F. Tannins in fruits and vegetables: Chemistry and biological functions. In: Yahia EM, editor. Fruit and Vegetable Phytochemicals: Chemistry and Human Health. 2nd ed. Chichester: John Wiley & Sons, Ltd; 2017. pp. 221-268. DOI: 10.1002/9781119158042.ch13

[6] Vickery ML, Vickery B. The acetate-mevalonate pathway. In: Secondary Plant Metabolism. London: Palgrave; 1981. DOI: 10.1007/978-1-349-86109-5_5

[7] Hasan M, Bae H. An overview of stress-induced resveratrol synthesis in grapes: Perspectives for resveratrol-enriched grape products. Molecules. 2017;**22**(2):1-18. DOI: 10.3390/molecules22020294

[8] Liu W, Yin D, Li N, Hou X, Wang D, Li D, Liu J. Influence of environmental factors on the active substance production and antioxidant activity in *Potentilla fruticosa* L. and its quality assessment. Scientific Reports. 2016;**6**:1-18. DOI: 10.1038/srep28591

[9] Liu W, Liu J, Yin D, Zhao X. Influence of ecological factors on the production of active substances in the anti-cancer plant *Sinopodophyllum hexandrum* (Royle) T.S. Ying. PLoS One. 2015;**10**(4):1-22. DOI: 10.1371/journal.pone.0122981

[10] Aktar MW, Sengupta D, Chowdhury A. Impact of pesticides use in agriculture: Their benefits and hazards. Interdisciplinary Toxicology. 2009;**2**(1):1-12. DOI: 10.2478/v10102-009-0001-7

[11] Pérez-López AJ, López-Nicolas JM, Núñez-Delicado E, del Amor FM, Carbonell-Barachina AA. Effects of agricultural practices on color, carotenoids composition, and minerals contents of sweet peppers, cv. Almuden. Journal of Agricultural and Food Chemistry. 2007;**55**:8158-8164. DOI: 10.1021/jf071534n

[12] Hallmann E. The influence of organic and conventional cultivation systems on the nutritional value and content of bioactive compounds in selected tomato types. Journal of the Science of Food and Agriculture. 2012;**92**:2840-2848. DOI: 10.1002/jsfa.5617

[13] Oliveira AB, Moura CFH, Gomes-Filho E, Marco CA, Urban L, Miranda MRA. The impact of organic farming on quality of tomatoes is associated to increased oxidative stress during fruit development. PLoS ONE. 2013;**8**(2):e56354. DOI: org/10.1371/journal.pone.0056354

[14] Zhao X, Carey EE, Wang W, Rajashekar CB. Does organic production enhance phytochemical content of fruits and vegetables? Current knowledge and prospects for research. HortTechnology. 2006;**16**(3):449-456

[15] Dixon RA, Paiva NL. Stress-induced phenylpropanoid metabolism. The Plant Cell. 1995;**7**:1085-1097. DOI: 10.1105/tpc.7.7.1085

[16] Tovar MJ, Romero MP, Girona J, Motilva MJ. L-phenylalanine ammonia-lyase activity and concentration of phenolics in developing olive (*Olea curopaca* L. cv. Arbequina) fruit grown under different irrigation regimes. Journal of Science, Food and Agriculture. 2002;**82**:892-898. DOI: 10.1002/jsfa.1122

[17] Babu PVA, Liu D, Gilbert ER. Recent advances in understanding the anti-diabetic actions of dietary flavonoids. Journal of Nutritional Biochemistry. 2013;**24**:1777-1789. DOI: 10.1016/j.jnutbio.2013.06.003

[18] Chen AY, Chen YC. A review of the dietary flavonoid, kaempferol on human health and cancer chemoprevention. Food Chemistry. 2013;**138**:2099-2107. DOI: 10.1016/j.foodchem.2012.11.139

[19] Zengin G, Guler GO, Aktumsek A, Ceylan R, Picot CMN, Mahomoodally MF. Enzyme inhibitory properties, antioxidant activities, and phytochemical profile of three medicinal plants from Turkey. Advances in Pharmacological Sciences. 2015;**410675**. DOI: 10.1155/2015/410675

[20] Chiu HK, Tsai EC, Juneja R, Stoever J, Brooks-Worrel B, Goel A, Palmer JP. Equivalent insulin resistance. Diabetes Research and Clinical Practice. 2007;**77**(2):237-244. DOI: 10.1016/j.diabres.2006.12.013

[21] Collins K, Jacks T, Pavletich NP. The cell cycle and cancer. Proceedings of the National Academy of Sciences of the United States of America. 1997;**94**:2776-2778. DOI: 0027-8424/97/942776-3$2.00/0

[22] Alberts B, Johnson A, Lewis J, Raff M, Roberts K, Walter P. Molecular Biology of the Cell. 4th ed. New York: Garlan Science; 2002. p. 1616. DOI: 10.1093/aob/mcg023

[23] Wright E, Scism-Bacon J, Glass L. Oxidative stress in type 2 diabetes: The role of fasting and postprandial glycaemia. International Journal of Clinical Practice. 2006;**60**(3):308-314. DOI: 10.1111/j.1368-5031.2006.00825.x

[24] Van Duyn MAS, Pivonka E. Overview of the health benefits of fruits and vegetables consumption for the dietetics professional: Selected literature. Journal of the American Dietetic Association. 2000;**100**(12):1511-1521. DOI: 10.1016/S0002-8223(00)00420-X

[25] Grzegorczyk-Karolak I, Gołąb K, Gburek J, Wysokińska H, Matkowski A. Inhibition of advanced glycation end-product formation and antioxidant activity by extracts and polyphenols from *Scutellaria alpina* L. and *S. altissima* L. Molecules. 2016;**21**(6):E739. DOI: 10.3390/molecules21060739

[26] Wang Z, Li H, Guo R, Wang Q, Zhang D. Antioxidants inhibit advanced glycosylation end-product-induced apoptosis by downregulation of miR-223 in human adipose tissue-derived stem cells. Scientific Reports. 2016;**6**:23021. DOI: 10.1038/srep23021

[27] Iriti M, Faoro F. Chemical diversity and defence metabolism: How plants cope with pathogens and ozone pollution. International Journal of Molecular Sciences. 2009;**10**(8):3371-3399. DOI: 10.3390/ijms10083371

3

Plant Extracts, Energy, and Immune Modulation in Broilers

Vasil Pirgozliev, Stephen C. Mansbridge,
Paul Rose and David Bravo

Abstract

This chapter presents information obtained from experiments involving male Ross 308 broiler chickens on the effects of a standardised combination of plant extracts (PE) including carvacrol, cinnamaldehyde and capsicum oleoresin, on bird performance, hepatic antioxidant concentration and immunomodulation. Birds were reared under industry-recognised environments and were fed one of four diets. There were two control diets based on either wheat or maize, formulated to be iso-energetic and iso-nitrogenic. The other two diets were the control diets supplemented with 100 g per tonne of PE, respectively. Feeding PE improved dietary feed efficiency, dietary net energy and hepatic antioxidant contents of the birds, but did not change dietary metabolisable energy (ME). Overall, feeding PE reduced the mRNA transcript levels of three cytokines (IL-12B, IFN-G, and IL-6) and the marker CD 40 LG in caecal tonsils. Dietary PE may maximise the nutritional value of feed through improving gut health by reducing intestinal inflammation. Their mode of action is associated with improved dietary energy availability, immune status and hepatic antioxidant contents of the birds. However, studies that have focused solely on the effect of PE on ME alone may not have detected their full benefit to improve the efficiency of broiler meat production.

Keywords: plant extracts, essential oils, broiler chickens, immunity, available energy

1. Introduction

Phytogenics, also referred to as plant secondary metabolites, phytochemicals, phytobiotics, or botanicals, are plant-derived products/extracts (PE) and include a wide range of substances. These include those derived from herbs and spices such as essential oils and oleoresins, reported to exhibit growth promoting and/or therapeutic properties [1, 2]. Initially, PE were extensively studied because of the adverse effects they have when ingested by animals [3]. However, the use of PE as an alternative to in-feed antibiotics to prevent the risk of developing pathogens resistant to antibiotics and to satisfy consumer demand for a poultry food chain free of drug residues has gained recent interest [4]. Antibiotics have been added to poultry diets to maintain health and production efficiency in the last few decades [5]. The withdrawal of in-feed antibiotics as growth promoters have increased the risk of bacterial disease, especially in growing poultry [6]. The ability of PE to contribute to the health of the host is well documented [1]; however, the exact mechanisms by which PE exerts its effects remain speculative. As documented, PE are composed of a diverse group of natural products [7]. However, while some are nutritionally valuable, others have no nutritional value or even possess antinutritional properties. This is likely due to PE varying widely in their chemical structures [3]. Since the effects of PE depend to a great extent on the chemistry of the compounds, it is impossible to have a uniform explanation of their mode of action. This chapter provides a brief overview of the main benefits of adding selective PE to poultry diets. Specifically, it describes the mode of action of carvacrol, cinnamaldehyde and capsaicin when fed to broiler chickens as a standardised commercial mix.

2. Effects of dietary plant extracts when fed to poultry

2.1. Bird growth performance and dietary available energy

It has been hypothesised that PE additives may stabilise overall digestive functions in the gastrointestinal tract of poultry, however, the available literature does not provide a consistent picture. Numerous feeding trials involving dietary supplementation with various PE have been reviewed [1, 6]. Regarding growth performance (assessed primarily as feed efficiency) and nutrient digestibility, the effect of added PE was beneficial in 11 of the studies; no effects were observed in 17 and there was a detrimental effect in 18 of the reviewed studies.

The information on the effect of PE on dietary metabolisable energy (ME) is also inconsistent. Some authors found an increase in dietary ME in response to PE [8, 9], others [10, 11] did not. There is also a discrepancy in the published data in the differences in ME and growth performance of birds fed dietary PE. Recent studies [10, 11, 8] found an improvement in bird growth performance but not in dietary ME when various PE were fed to poultry. It has been reported [9] that there is a parallel improvement in dietary ME and feed efficiency when feeding a standardised commercial mix of carvacrol, cinnamaldehyde and capsaicin to broiler chickens.

2.2. Antioxidant status

Due to the general consumer rejection of synthetic food additives there is a growing interest in studies of natural additives as potential antioxidants. Research on the antioxidative properties of herbs and spices showed that they are effective in retarding the process of lipid peroxidation in oils and fatty foods (summarised by [12]). Herbal phenolic compounds also improved the oxidative stability of animal derived products such as poultry meat, pork, rabbit meat and eggs (reviewed by [1]). Furthermore, research with rats [13] and poultry [14] suggested that dietary phytogenic supplements may improve the antioxidative status of the animals, reducing intestinal cell damage and sustaining the integrity of the intestinal mucosal layer. These supplements acted as effective free radical scavengers and also influenced the *in vivo* antioxidant defence systems in the animal. In addition, diets supplemented with turmeric, curcumin, green tea, grape seed proanthocyanidins and society garlic, which all possess antioxidative properties, reduced small intestinal lesion scores, lowered oxidative stress and improved weight gains during coccidial infection (summarised by [6]). All these compounds may exert their anticoccidial activity by protecting infected tissues from oxidative damage and therefore reducing the severity of coccidiosis.

2.3. Immune status

Immunomodulation is described as a change of the indicators of cellular and humoral immunity and nonspecific defence factors [15]. Immunomodulation can present as immunosuppression (substances that inhibit the immune system) or immunostimulation (substances that activate or induce the mediators or components of the immune system), thus regulating or altering the scope, type, duration or competency of the immune response [16, 17].

It has been speculated that the benefit of using PE in animal diets is associated with reduced intestinal inflammation in part from a reduction of proinflammatory cytokines. One study [18] reported that cinnamaldehyde suppressed the lipopolysaccharide-induced production of tumour necrosis factor (TNF), interleukin 6 (IL-6) and IL-1, thus suggesting that the inclusion of cinnamaldehyde could show suppressive effects on the production of various types of inflammatory cytokines. Similarly, [19] also found that a mixture of capsicum and turmeric oleoresins was an effective phytonutrient against clinical signs of experimental avian necrotic enteritis when supplied in dietary form. Research by Lee et al. [20] suggested that immunomodulatory effects are responsible for improved weight gain, oocyst shedding, increased interferon gamma (IFN-γ) and IL-15, when powder from oriental plum (a plant rich in phenolic compounds) was fed to coccidia challenged birds. Furthermore, supplementation with Chinese mushroom and herb extracts resulted in enhancement of both cellular and humoral immune responses in *Eimeria tenella* infected chickens [21].

There is strong evidence that PE have antimicrobial properties, being able to reduce the proliferation of pathogenic organisms at minimal inhibitory concentrations of 0.05–5 microliters per millilitre *in vitro*, and at higher concentrations (0.5–20 microliters per gram) in food [22]. While these levels are unlikely to be met in animal feedstuffs, and therefore not the primary use of PE in feed, there is evidence that PE have effective antimicrobial action against pathogens common in poultry production. These include *Escherichia coli* and *Clostridium perfringens* [23–25]. Pathogenic microorganisms in the gut are able to trigger immune responses in the gastrointestinal tract. This results in inflammation of the intestine contributing to poor gut health. In addition to reducing pathogenic challenge, PE may also possess direct immunomodulation properties. For example, it is known that cinnamaldehyde in particular is involved in gene regulation, including antigen presentation, humoral immune response and inflammatory disease [26].

2.4. Chemical structure and properties of carvacrol, cinnamaldehyde and capsaicin

Carvacrol ($C_{10}H_{14}O$) is a chemical (see **Figure 1**) found in several plants including: wild bergamot, thyme and pepperwort, but it is most abundant in oregano (*Origanum vulgare*) oil [27]. Carvacrol gives oregano a slightly spicy flavour, is colourless, and has a distinct warm odour. Overall, carvacrol has a promising antibacterial, antiviral, antioxidant, and antifungal impact. Carvacrol also demonstrated significant anti-cancer effects when tested against breast cancer, prostate, lung and mouth cancer cells [28].

Cinnamaldehyde (C_9H_8O) is a chemical (see **Figure 1**) that naturally occurs in the inner bark of several tree species from the genus Cinnamomum. Cinnamaldehyde, the principal component of the essential oil of cinnamon bark, gives the cinnamish odour responsible for the characteristic taste and odour of cinnamon spice. Cinnamaldehyde has strong antimicrobial, antifungal and anticorrosion properties [29].

Capsaicinoids ($C_{18}H_{27}NO_3$) are produced by peppers as a protection against certain mammals and fungi (see **Figure 1**). They have no flavour or odour, but act directly on the pain receptors in the mouth and throat. Capsaicin, the most common capsaicinoid, is an irritant for most mammals, including humans, and produces a sensation of burning in any tissue with which it comes into contact [30]. However, birds are not sensitive to the capsaicin [31] and can benefit from the nutritional value of the chilli peppers. Capsicum oleoresin (active ingredient capsaicin) is found in pepper fruits and has antifungal and antibacterial activity [32].

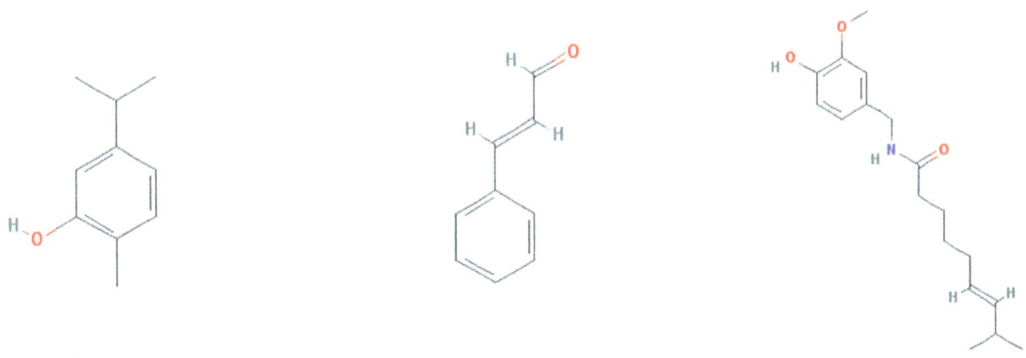

Figure 1. Chemical structure (2-D) of (left to right) carvacrol, cinnamaldehyde and capsaicin.

3. Poultry experiments (methodology)

The experiments described in this chapter followed internationally recognised guidelines for work with poultry. All birds were cared for according to laws and regulations detailed in UK guidelines. Data from four experiments performed under similar environmental and dietary conditions were used in this chapter.

3.1. Dietary formulation, husbandry and sample collection

The four experiments employed the same dietary formulations (**Table 1**). Birds were fed one of four diets. There were two control diets based on either wheat (WC) or maize (MC) which were formulated to be iso-energetic (12.13 MJ/kg AME) and iso-nitrogenic (215 g/kg CP).

Dietary ingredients	Wheat-based diet	Maize-based diet
	kg/100 kg	kg/100 kg
Maize	—	52.86
Wheat	54.68	—
Soybean meal (48)	27.49	31.30
Vegetable oil	3.50	1.00
Barley	5.84	6.33
Rye	5.00	5.00
Monodicalcium phosphate	1.43	1.43
Limestone	1.15	1.15
NaCl	0.27	0.33
Lysine	0.15	0.15
Methionine	0.39	0.35
Vitamin mineral premix[1]	0.10	0.10
	100	100
Calculated analysis (as fed)		
Crude Protein, g/kg	215	215
ME, MJ/kg	12.12	12.13
Crude Fat, g/kg	47	34
Ca, g/kg	8.4	8.3
Available P, g/kg	4.5	4.4
Lysine, g/kg	12.3	12.3
Methionine + Cysteine, g/kg	9.5	9.5

ME = metabolisable energy.

[1]The Vitamin and mineral premix contained vitamins and trace elements to meet the requirements specified by the National research Council (1994). The premix provided (units/kg diet): retinol, 12,000 IU; cholecalciferol, 5000 IU; α-tocopherol, 34 mg; menadione, 3 mg; thiamine, 2 mg; riboflavin, 7 mg; pyridoxine, 5 mg; cobalamin, 15 μg; nicotinic acid, 50 mg; pantothenic acid, 15 mg; folic acid, 1 mg; biotin, 200 μg; 80 mg iron as iron sulphate (30%); 10 mg copper as a copper sulphate (25%); 100 mg manganese as manganous oxide (62%); 80 mg zinc as zinc oxide (72%); 1 mg iodine as calcium iodate (52%); 0.2 mg selenium as sodium selenite (4.5%); 0.5 mg molybdenum as sodium molybdate (40%).

Table 1. Composition of the control diets.

The other two diets were the control diets supplemented with a standardised combination of PE (XTRACT 6930; Pancosma S.A., Geneva, Switzerland) including 5% carvacrol, 3% cinnamaldehyde and 2% capsicum oleoresin (100 grams per tonne, respectively, i.e. WC + PE; MC + PE). The PE was added in powder form to the diets and all diets were fed as mash. The diets did not contain any coccidiostat or antimicrobial growth promoters, prophylactic or other similar additives.

Day old male Ross 308 broiler chickens were purchased from a commercial hatchery and reared in floor pens littered with wood shavings. The temperatures were kept at 32°C during the first 2 days on birds arrival and were gradually reduced to 20°C by 21 days of age. A standard lighting programme following breeder's recommendations (Aviagen Ltd., Edinburgh, UK) for broilers was used. Access to the feed and the water was *ad libitum*. At 17 days of age, two birds from each pen were transferred to a pen with wire mesh floor and excreta samples were collected for four consecutive days from each pen, immediately dried at 60°C and then milled for further analyses. The birds were weighed on a per-pen basis and the average bird feed intake (FI), weight gain (WG) and gain: feed ratio (GF) were determined.

In the experiments where dietary net energy (NE) was determined, at the end of the study, all chickens were killed by cervical dislocation and the carcass of the birds, including intestine, blood and feather, from each pen were frozen and then minced, thoroughly mixed and sampled, and used for following analysis and calculations.

In the experiments where the hepatic antioxidant content was determined, at 21 days of age, one bird from each pen was randomly selected, stunned/killed and the liver was collected and stored at –20°C prior to analysis of antioxidant contents.

In the experiments where the gene expression was measured, at 21 days of age one bird from each pen was randomly selected, stunned/killed and the left caecal tonsil was collected and stored in RNAlater® (Sigma-Aldrich, USA) at −70°C prior to analysis of the relative expression of selected genes.

3.2. Chemical analysis of diets and excreta

The experimental diets and the excreta were milled (0.75 mm mesh) and analysed further. Dry matter (DM) was determined by drying samples in a forced draft oven at 105°C to a constant weight. Crude protein (6.25 × N) in samples was determined by dry combustion method [33] using a LECO (FP-528 N, Leco Corp., St. Joseph, MI). Oil (as ether extract) was extracted with diethyl ether by the ether extraction method [33], using a Soxtec system (Foss UK Ltd.). The GE value of the samples was determined in a bomb calorimeter (model 6200; Parr Instrument Co., Moline, IL), using benzoic acid as the standard.

3.3. Dietary available energy determination

The N-corrected apparent metabolisable energy (AMEn) of the diets was calculated as described by [34].

A comparative slaughter technique [35] was used to determine the energy retained in the carcase of birds. In brief, dietary NE was calculated using the following equation:

$$NE\ (MJ/kg) = (REc + FHP)/FI.$$

Where: FI is the dry matter (kg) consumed for the experimental period. REc is the total energy retained in the carcass (see [50]).

The fasting heat production (FHP MJ/bird) was estimated to be 0.450 MJ/d per kg of metabolic body weight $(BW)^{0.70}$ per day, which correspond to the asymptotic heat production at zero activity (as proposed by [36]).

3.4. Determination of hepatic antioxidant concentration

Concentration of antioxidants in liver was determined by high-performance liquid chromatography (HPLC) [37, 38]. In brief: approximately 300 mg of liver samples were mixed in 0.7 ml 5% sodium chloride solution, then 1 ml ethanol was added and samples homogenised. During homogenisation, 2 ml hexane was added. Then samples were centrifuged and the hexane phase, containing the vitamin E and coenzyme Q_{10} were collected. Extraction with hexane was performed twice, and the combined phase was evaporated under nitrogen and re-dissolved in a mixture of dichloromethane–methanol (1:1, v/v).

Vitamin E (α-, γ- and δ-tocopherols) was determined as previously described [39] using an HPLC system (Shimadzu Liquid Chromatograph, LC-10 AD, Japan Spectroscopic Co Ltd., with a Jasco Intelligent Spectrofluorometer 821-FP) fitted with a Spherisorb, type S30DS2, 3 mm C18 reverse phase HPLC column, 15 cm × 4.6 mm (Phase Separations Limited, UK). Chromatography was performed using a mobile phase of methanol–water (97:3, v/v) at a flow rate of 1.05 ml/min. Fluorescence detection of tocopherols and tocotrienols involved excitation and emission wavelengths of 295 and 330 nm, respectively. Standard solutions of tocopherols in methanol were used for instrument calibration and tocol was used as an internal standard.

Coenzyme Q_{10} was analysed in the same extract by injecting 50 ml into the same HPLC system, but using a Vidac 201TP54 column (5 μm, 25 cm × 4.6 mm) and mobile phase ethanol–methanol–2-propanol (70:15:15, v/v) and flow rate of 1.5 ml/min with a diode array detection at 275 nm [40]. Coenzyme Q_{10} (Sigma, Poole, UK) standard was used for calibration.

3.5. Gene expression analysis

The analyses of relative expression of genes of interest (GOI) in the caecal tonsils were performed by qStandard (Middlesex, UK).

3.5.1. Total RNA extraction and reverse transcription

Approximately 30 mg of macro-dissected caecal tonsil tissue per sample (previously submerged in RNAlater® (Sigma-Aldrich, USA) and stored frozen at -80°C) was homogenised in 500 uL

QIAzol lysis reagent for 10 min at 30 Hz in a Tissuelyzer LT (Qiagen, UK). Lysates were mixed with 100 μL chloroform, transferred to pegGold PhaseTrap tubes (PeqLab, UK) and centrifuged for 5 mins at room temperature. The aqueous phase was poured into fresh tubes, mixed with 1.5 volumes of ethanol and applied to Qiagen RNeasy columns (Qiagen, UK). RNA was purified according to the manufacturer's instructions (Qiagen, UK). RNA integrity was assessed using an Agilent Bioanalyzer and RIN was >8 for all samples. Purity and quantity were measured using a NanoDrop spectrophotometer; for all samples the absorbance peak was at 260 nm, A260/280 > 2 and A260/230 > 1. About 800 ng of RNA were reverse transcribed using a Quantitect reverse transcription kit (Qiagen, UK) in a 10 μL reaction according to the manufacturer's instructions. This RT kit includes a mandatory gDNA wipe out step. The completed reaction was diluted 10-fold with 5 μg/mL tRNA in water.

3.5.2. *Quantitative real-time PCR*

Two microlitres of cDNA were amplified in a 10 μL reaction using Agilent Brilliant III SYBR Ultra-Fast SYBR Green mix with each primer at a final concentration of 500 nmol/L. The no-template control reaction contained 2 μL of tRNA (0.5 μg/mL). DNA standards (10^7–10^1 copies/rxn) for each gene were included in each run. Reactions were pipetted robotically using a Qiagility (Qiagen, UK). Amplification parameters were: 95°C for 3 min followed by 40 cycles of 95°C for 5 sec, 57°C for 1 sec in a Rotor-Gene 6000. Melt curves were checked

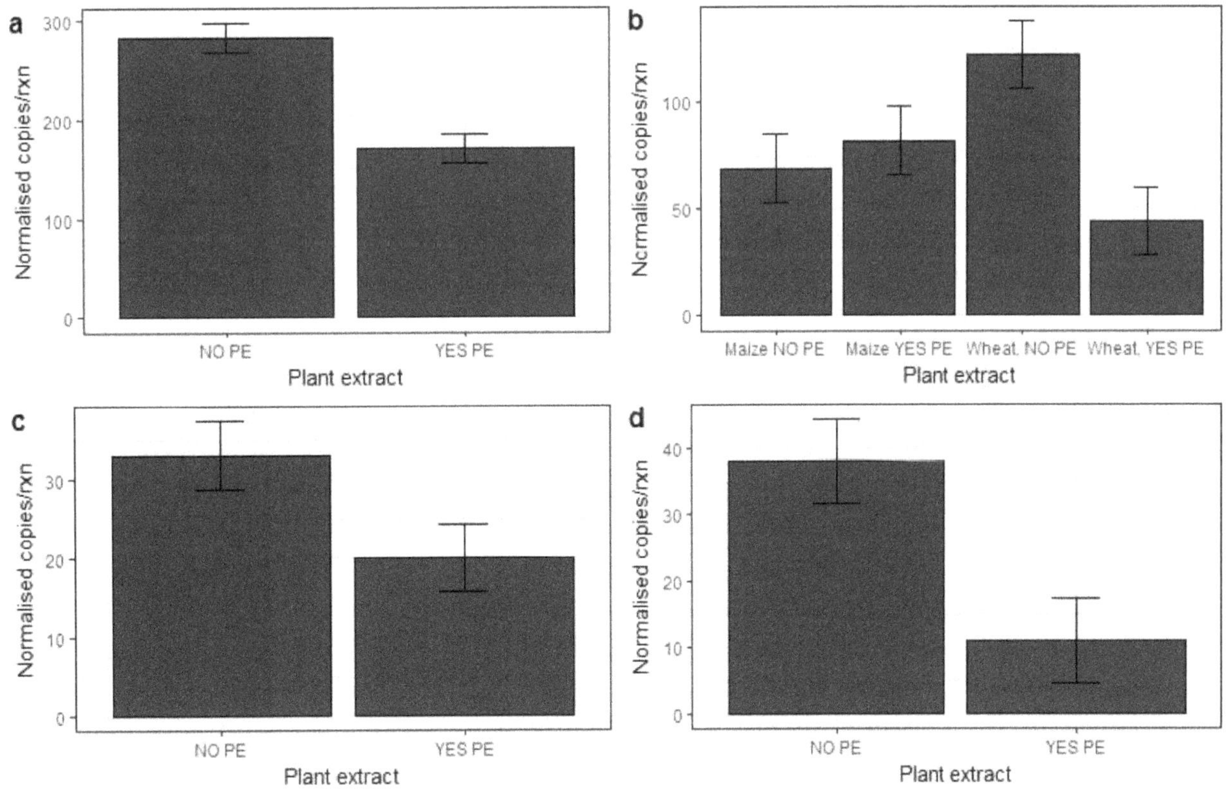

Figure 2. The effect of dietary plant extracts (PE) on the normalised mRNA copy number (per reaction) of (a) CD40 LG, (b) IL-12B, (c) INFG, (d) IL-6 in chicken caecal tonsils. Error bars represent ±1 pooled SEM.

for product specificity (single peak) and the presence of primer dimers. All primers were designed to be intron-spanning so that any residual gDNA present could not be detected and avoided known SNP and secondary structure. Assays were designed by qStandard (www.qstandard.co.uk) and were tested for specificity by electrophoresis, efficiency >95%, sensitivity to 10 copies/rxn, and linearity over 7 log by qPCR. Copy numbers/reaction were derived from the standard curves using the Rotor-Gene software. The four reference genes identified as the most stable using geNorm software were B2M, GAPDH, PPIA and YWHAZ. The normalisation factor for each sample was used to normalise GOI copy numbers per reaction.

3.6. Statistical analysis of data

Data were statistically analysed by two way analysis of variance (ANOVA) using a 2 × 2 factorial arrangement of treatments, blocked by experiment. The main effects were the cereals (maize and wheat) and additives (with and without PE). All data were processed using the procedure of Genstat (18th Edition) statistical software (IACR, Rothamstead, Hertfordshire, UK). In all instances, differences were reported as significant at $P < 0.05$. Graphics (**Figure 2**) were produced in "ggplot2" package version 2.2.1. [41] using R version 3.4.1. [42].

4. Effect of PE on bird growth performance and dietary available energy

Dietary PE supplementation significantly improved ($P < 0.05$) gain to feed (G:F) ratio by 2 points and dietary NE by 0.34 MJ (**Table 2**). No changes ($P > 0.05$) were observed in dietary ME due to PE supplementation. The increase in feed efficiency is in agreement with the ability of spices and mixtures of spices to increase bile secretion, activity of the pancreatic, and brush border enzymes [43, 44]. Maize based diets produced higher ($P < 0.05$) daily FI and ME, although wheat based diets had higher NE ($P < 0.001$). The values of ME and NE were in similar to previous reports [9, 45]. In agreement with [24], there were dietary type x PE interactions ($P < 0.05$) observed in bird growth, as birds fed wheat diets did not respond ($P > 0.05$) to PE supplementation. Similar tendency ($P = 0.074$) was observed for daily feed intake. Compared to maize, wheat contains more water-soluble non-starch polysaccharide (NSP), a carbohydrate complex possessing antinutrient activity, which may reduce dietary nutrient availability [46], thus explaining the reduced performance of birds fed wheat based diets. The observed interaction may also be due to the relatively high fat content of the wheat compared to maize based diets, and not to the cereals alone. Widening the dietary ME to protein ratio is likely to affect body fat retention more than bird growth performance, suggesting an explanation for the inconsistency between weight gain and NE of birds fed wheat based diets. However, the impact of dietary formulation (cereals, protein sources, fat content etc.) on the effectiveness of supplementary PE in poultry nutrition warrants further investigation.

Although there is a lack of consistency between growth performance and dietary ME, this is in agreement with many studies [8, 10, 11] but is in disagreement with others [9]. The

Items treatment factor	FI[1] (g DM/b/d)	WG[1] (g/b/d)	G:F[1] (g/g)	ME[1] (MJ/kg DM)	NE[1] (MJ/kg DM)	Vit E[2] (μg/g)	CoQ_{10}[2] (μg/g)
Cereals							
W	42.1	31.7	0.753	14.05	10.00	82.4	91.4
M	43.6	32.6	0.747	14.23	9.47	86.7	79.4
PE							
no	42.1	31.1	0.739	14.08	9.56	72.5	74.7
yes	43.6	33.2	0.762	14.05	9.90	96.7	96.1
SEM	0.496	0.460	0.0064	0.061	0.092	7.03	9.80
Cereals & PE							
W + 0	42.0	31.4	0.746	13.93	9.76	63.7	77.1
W + PE	42.2	32.0	0.760	14.16	10.23	101.2	105.8
M + 0	42.3	30.8	0.732	14.22	9.37	81.3	72.3
M + PE	45.0	34.4	0.763	14.24	9.57	92.2	86.4
SEM	0.702	0.651	0.0091	0.087	0.127	9.95	13.85
Probabilities of statistical differences							
Cereals	0.030	0.166	0.499	0.037	<0.001	0.542	0.221
PE	0.037	0.002	0.015	0.159	0.008	<0.001	0.032
Cereals x PE	0.074	0.030	0.347	0.211	0.309	0.062	0.458

Source: adapted from [47–51].
W, wheat-based diet; M, maize-based diet; PE, supplemental plant extracts (100 g PE/t).
[1]There were 38 observations per treatment (three experiments involving male Ross 308 broilers).
[2]There were 24 observations per treatment (two experiments involving male Ross 308 broilers).

Table 2. The effect of supplemental plant extracts in wheat and maize based diets on broilers daily feed intake (FI), daily weight gain (WG), gain to feed (G:F) ratio, dietary apparent metaboilisable energy (ME), dietary net energy (NE), concentration of hepatic vitamin E and coenzyme Q_{10}.

results show an improvement in feed efficiency in association with improved NE but not with ME. The beneficial effects of supplementary PE to poultry diets may therefore be mediated via a decrease in the energy required for maintenance, thereby providing more energy for growth. The improvement in feed efficiency is likely explained by increases in dietary NE, suggesting that PE may be improving the metabolic efficiency of the conversion of energy into tissue. Usually NE is described as the ME of the diet corrected for the energy losses that result from the heat released during absorption of the dietary nutrients and accretion of body mass [35]. Changes in maintenance energy are more likely to be detected by determination of NE but not ME. Thus confirming that dietary ME may not be the most sensitive method to evaluate the feeding quality of supplementary PE. This is in agreement with previous reports suggesting that NE is a more meaningful measure of energy utilisation with regard to prediction of the nutritive value of poultry diets [35].

5. Effect of PE on hepatic antioxidant content

Dietary PE supplementation significantly improved hepatic vitamin E ($P < 0.001$) by 33.4% and coenzyme Q_{10} ($P < 0.05$) by 28.6% (**Table 2**). No changes ($P > 0.05$) were observed in hepatic antioxidants content due to dietary type ($P > 0.05$), although the response of wheat based diets tended ($P = 0.062$) to be higher compared to maize based diets. More importantly, the increase in G:F and NE is coupled with the increase in the hepatic concentrations of vitamin E and coenzyme Q_{10} [48].

Infectious diseases have been demonstrated to reduce tissue antioxidants [52], suggesting that higher concentrations of vitamin E and coenzyme Q_{10} in liver may decrease the challenge provoked by infectious diseases. In addition, feeding a combination of PE in the current study resulted in not only improved feed efficiency, but also increased hepatic antioxidants retention compared with the non-supplemented diet. When birds are reared under commercial farm conditions, where the potential for challenge is greater, and fed diets supplemented with PE, then there may be improvements to their overall nutrition, antioxidant and health status, and resistance to diseases [48]. The improvements observed may indicate that vitamin E and coenzyme Q_{10} may be effective at reducing production and effects of free radicals [53]. Coenzyme Q_{10} is provided by the diet, however significant levels are also produced in the body. Increased concentration of coenzyme Q_{10} in the liver of the growing chickens is therefore likely the result of dietary PE supplementation and dietary sources should thus be considered beneficial at improving the antioxidant status. It has also been reported [13] that PE, increased the activity of the antioxidant enzymes of the mucosal cells of rats, thus reducing the intestinal cell damage and cell turnover and sustaining the integrity of the intestinal mucosal layer.

6. Effect of PE on the immune status of birds

As shown in **Figure 2** the expression of CD 40 LG, IFN-G, and IL-6 was reduced ($P < 0.001$ and $P < 0.05$, respectively) in birds fed PE compared to the control fed chickens in accordance with other reports [18, 19]. There was a cereal X PE interaction for IL12B, showing that dietary PE reduced IL-12B expression in a wheat but not in a maize based diet ($P < 0.05$). Both, IL-6 and IFN-G, are major pro-inflammatory cytokines, so if the levels of these cytokines are decreased this would indicate that there are lower levels of inflammation than in the other groups, presumably due to plant extracts. Birds fed with diets supplemented with the same PE mixture also reduced the expression of CD40LG and IL-12B genes. The IFN-G cytokine belongs to the T helper (Th) type 1 response and is driven by IL-12 production. Th1 type response drives the cell mediated inflammatory responses largely to intracellular pathogens [54] but chronically high levels of these cytokines in the intestine may have a damaging effect on the gut integrity, compromising nutrient absorption and overall gut health. The results of this study suggest that feeding PE may dampen chronic gut inflammation that may be partially attributed to the improved feed efficiency and dietary net energy.

7. Conclusions

Plant extracts can be used as growth promoters in poultry production independent of enzyme supplementation. Dietary PE may maximise the nutritional value of feed through improving gut health by reducing intestinal inflammation. Their mode of action may therefore be associated with improved immune status of the birds. This immune modulating effect of PE may explain improvements in growth performance and dietary NE seen in the present study. However, dietary supplementation with PE may improve bird growth performance without corresponding improvements in dietary ME. Studies that have focused solely on the effect of PE on ME alone, may not have detected their full benefit to improve the efficiency of broiler meat production. More research is needed to study the effect of supplementary PE on immune status of birds in relation to dietary available energy and growth performance of birds in commercial conditions using different practical feed formulations.

Acknowledgements

The authors acknowledge the support of Derek Brown, Richard James and Ros Crocker for their technical assistance.

Conflict of interest

No conflicts of interest.

Notes

Chemical structure (2-D) images (**Figure 1**) reproduced from PubChem (see [55 – 57]).

Author details

Vasil Pirgozliev[1]*, Stephen C. Mansbridge[1], Paul Rose[1] and David Bravo[2]

*Address all correspondence to: vpirgozliev@harper-adams.ac.uk

1 The National Institute of Poultry Husbandry, Harper Adams University, England

2 Pancosma S.A., Geneva, Switzerland

References

[1] Windisch W, Schedle K, Plitzner C, Kroismayr A. Use of phytogenic products as feed additives for swine and poultry. Journal of Animal Science. 2008;**86**(14_suppl):E140-E148. DOI: 10.2527/jas.2007-0459

[2] Murugesan GR, Syed B, Haldar S, Pender C. Phytogenic feed additives as an alternative to antibiotic growth promoters in broiler chickens. Frontiers in Veterinary Science. 2015;**2**:21. DOI: 10.3389/fvets.2015.00021

[3] Acamovic T, Brooker JD. Biochemistry of plant secondary metabolites and their effects in animals. Proceedings of the Nutrition Society. 2005;**64**(3):403-412. DOI: 10.1079/PNS2005449

[4] Dibner JJ, Richards JD. Antibiotic growth promoters in agriculture: History and mode of action. Poultry Science. 2005;**84**:634-643. DOI: 10.1093/ps/84.4.634

[5] Applegate TJ, Klose V, Steiner T, Ganner A, Schatzmayr G. Probiotics and phytogenics for poultry: Myth or reality? Journal of Applied Poultry Research. 2010;**19**:194-210. DOI: 10.3382/japr.2010-00168

[6] Wallace RJ, Oleszek W, Franz C, Hahn I, Baser KHC, Mathe A, Teichmann K. Dietary plant bioactives for poultry health and productivity. British Poultry Science. 2010;**51**: 461-487. DOI: 10.1080/00071668.2010.506908

[7] Harborne JB. Twenty-five years of chemical ecology. Natural Product Reports. 2001;**18**: 361-379. DOI: 10.1039/B005311M

[8] Mountzouris KC, Paraskevas V, Tsirtsikos P, Palamidi I, Steiner T, Schatzmayr G, Fegeros K. Assessment of phytogenic feed additive effect on broiler growth performance, nutrient digestibility and caecal microflora composition. Animal Feed Science and Technology. 2010;**168**:223-231. DOI: 10.1016/j.anifeedsci.2011.03.020

[9] Bravo D, Utterback P, Parsons CM. Evaluation of a mixture of carvacrol, cinnamaldehyde, and capsicum oleoresin for improving growth performance and metabolizable energy in broiler chicks fed corn and soybean meal. Journal of Applied Poultry Research. 2011;**20**:115-120. DOI: 10.3382/japr.2010-00163

[10] Juin H, Elgaard T, Chicoteau P. Effect of a citrus extract (NOR-SPICE AB) on broiler performances. British Poultry Science. 2003;**44**:810-811. DOI: 10.1080/00071668.2003.10871381

[11] Cross DE, McDevitt RM, Hillman K, Acamovic T. The effect of herbs and their associated essential oils on performance, dietary digestibility and gut microflora in chickens from 7 to 28 days of age. British Poultry Science. 2007;**48**:496-506. DOI: 10.1080/00071660701463221

[12] Brenes A, Roura E. Essential oils in poultry nutrition: Main effects and modes of action. Animal Feed Science and Technology. 2010;**158**(1-2):1-14. DOI: 10.1016/j.anifeedsci.2010.03.007

[13] Dhuley JN. Anti-oxidant effects of cinnamon (Cinnamomum verum) bark and greater cardamom (Amomum subulatum) seeds in rats fed high fat diet. Indian Journal of Experimental Biology. 1999;**37**:238-242

[14] Allen PC, Fetterer RH. Recent advances in biology and immunobiology of Eimeria species and in diagnosis and control of infection with these coccidian parasites of poultry. Clinical Microbiology Reviews. 2002;**15**(1):58-65. DOI: 10.1128/CMR.15.1.58-65.2002

[15] Bakuridze AD, Kurtsikidze S, Pisarev VM, Makharadze RV, Berashvili DT. Immunomodulators of plant origin. Pharmaceutical Chemistry Journal. 1993;**27**:589-595. DOI: 10.1007/BF00779922

[16] Lebish IJ, Moraski RM. Mechanisms of immunomodulation by drugs. Toxicologic Pathology. 1987;**15**(3):338-345. DOI: 10.1177/019262338701500312

[17] Jantan I, Ahmad W, Bukhari SNA. Plant-derived immunomodulators: An insight on their preclinical evaluation and clinical trials. Frontiers in Plant Science. 2015;**6**:655. DOI: 10.3389/fpls.2015.00655

[18] Chao LK, Hua K-F, Hsu H-Y, Cheng S-S, Lin F, Chen C-J, Chen S-T, Chang S-T. Cinnamaldehyde inhibits pro-inflammatory cytokines secretion from monocytes/macrophages through suppression of intracellular signalling. Food and Chemical Toxicology. 2008;**46**:220-231. DOI: 10.1016/j.fct.2007.07.016

[19] Lee SH, Lillehoj HS, Jang SI, Lillehoj EP, Min W, Bravo D. Dietary supplementation of young broiler chickens with Capsicum and turmeric oleoresins increases resistance to necrotic enteritis. British Journal of Nutrition. 2013;**110**:840-847. DOI: 10.1017/S0007114512006083

[20] Lee SH, Lillehoj HS, Lillehoj EP, Cho SM, Park DW, Hong YH, Chun HK, Park HJ. Immunomodulatory properties of dietary plum on coccidiosis. Comparative Immunology, Microbiology and Infectious Diseases. 2008;**31**(5):389-402. DOI: 10.1016/j.cimid.2007.06.005

[21] Guo FC, Williams BA, Kwakkel RP, Li HS, Li XP, Luo JY, Li WK, Verstegen MWA. Effects of mushroom and herb polysaccharides, as alternatives for an antibiotic, on the cecal microbial ecosystem in broiler chickens. Poultry Science. 2004;**83**:175-182. DOI: 10.1093/ps/83.2.175

[22] Burt S. Essential oils: Their antibacterial properties and potential applications in foods–a review. International Journal of Food Microbiology. 2004;**94**:223-253. DOI: 10.1016/j.ijfoodmicro.2004.03.022

[23] Jamroz D, Orda J, Kamel C, Wiliczkiewicz A, Wertelecki T, Skorupinska J. The influence of phytogenic extracts on performance, nutrient digestibility, carcass characteristics, and gut microbial status in broiler chickens. Journal of Animal and Feed Sciences. 2003;**12**:583-596. DOI: 10.22358/jafs/67752/2003

[24] Jamroz D, Wiliczkiewicz A, Wertelecki T, Orda J, Skorupinska J. Use of active substances of plant origin in chicken diets based on maize and locally grown cereals. British Poultry Science. 2005;**46**:485-493. DOI: 10.1080/00071660500191056

[25] Mitsch P, Zitterl-Eglseer K, Kohler B, Gabler C, Losa R, Zimpernik I. The effect of two

different blends of essential oil components on the proliferation of *Clostridium perfringens* in the intestines of broiler chickens. Poultry Science. 2004;**83**:669-675. DOI: 10.1093/ps/83.4.669

[26] Lillehoj HS, Kim DK, Bravo DM, Lee SH. Effects of dietary plant-derived phytonutrients on the genome-wide profiles and coccidiosis resistance in the broiler chickens. BMC Proceedings. 2011;**5**(Suppl. 4):S34. DOI: 10.1186/1753-6561-5-S4-S34

[27] Lambert RJW, Skandamis PN, Coote PJ, Nychas GJ. A study of the minimum inhibitory concentration and mode of action of oregano essential oil, thymol and carvacrol. Journal of Applied Microbiology. 2001;**91**(3):453-462. DOI: 10.1046/j.1365-2672.2001.01428.x

[28] Arunasree KM. Anti-proliferative effects of carvacrol on a human metastatic breast cancer cell line, MDA-MB 231. Phytomedicine. 2010;**17**(8-9):581-588. DOI: 10.1016/j.phymed.2009.12.008

[29] Friedman M, Kozukue N, Harden LA. Cinnamaldehyde content in foods determined by gas chromatography – mass spectrometry. Journal of Agricultural and Food Chemistry. 2000;**48**(11):5702-5709. DOI: 10.1021/jf000585g

[30] Prescott J, Swain-Campbell N. Responses to repeated oral irritation by capsaicin, cinnamaldehyde and ethanol in PROP tasters and non-tasters. Chemical Senses. 2000;**25**(3):246. DOI: 10.1093/chemse/25.3.239

[31] Jordt SE, Julius D. Molecular basis for species-specific sensitivity to "hot" chili peppers. Cell. 2002;**108**(3):421-430. DOI: 10.1016/S0092-8674(02)00637-2

[32] Maga JA, Todd PH. Capsicum. Critical Reviews in Food Science & Nutrition. 1975;**6**(2): 177-199. DOI: 10.1080/10408397509527189

[33] AOAC. Official Methods of Analysis. 17th ed. Gaithersburg: The Association of Official Analytical Chemists; 2000

[34] Hill FW, Anderson DL. Comparison of metabolizable energy and productive energy determinations with growing chicks. Journal of Nutrition. 1958;**64**:587-603

[35] Pirgozliev V, Bedford MR. Energy utilisation and growth performance of chicken fed diets containing graded levels of supplementary bacterial phytase. British Journal of Nutrition. 2013;**109**:248-253. DOI: 10.1017/S0007114512000943

[36] Noblet J, Dubois S, Labussiere E, Carré van Milgen J. Metabolic utilization of energy in monogastric animals and its implementation in net energy systems. In: Proceedings of the 3rd international symposium on energy and protein metabolism and nutrition; Parma Italy: European Federation of Animal Science. 2010. p. 573-582

[37] Karadas F, Surai P, Grammenidis E, Sparks NHC, Acamovic T. Supplementation of the maternal diet with tomato powder and marigold extract: Effects on the antioxidant system of the developing quail. British Poultry Science. 2006;**47**:200-208. DOI: 10.1080/00071660600611003

[38] Karadas F, Pirgozliev V, Pappas AC, Acamovic T, Bedford MR. Effects of different dietary phytase activities on the concentration of antioxidants in the liver of growing broilers. Journal of Animal Physiology and Animal Nutrition. 2010;**94**:519-526. DOI: 10.1111/j.1439-0396.2009.00938.x

[39] Surai PF, Speake BK. Distribution of carotenoids from the yolk to the tissues of the chick embryo. The Journal of Nutritional Biochemistry. 1998;**9**:645-651. DOI: 10.1016/S0955-2863(98)00068-0

[40] Mattila P, Kumpulainen J. Coenzymes Q9 and Q10: Contents in foods and dietary intake. Journal of Food Composition and Analysis. 2001;**14**:409-417. DOI: 10.1006/jfca.2000.0983

[41] Wickham H. ggplot2: Elegant Graphics for Data Analysis. New York: Springer-Verlag; 2009. DOI: 10.1007/978-0-387-98141-3

[42] R Development Core Team. R: A Language and Environment for Statistical Computing. Vienna, Austria: R Foundation for Statistical Computing; 2017. ISBN 3-900051-07-0, URL http://www.R-project.org

[43] Platel K, Srinivasan K. A study of the digestive stimulant action of select spices in experimental rats. Journal of Food Science and Technology. 2001;**38**:358-361

[44] Platel K, Rao A, Saraswathi G, Srinivasan K. Digestive stimulant action of three Indian spice mixes in experimental rats. Molecular Nutrition & Food Research. 2002;**46**:394-398. DOI: 10.1002/1521-3803(20021101)46:6<394::AID-FOOD394>3.0.CO;2-D

[45] Swick RA, Wu S-B, Zuo J, Rodgers N, Barekatain MR, Choct M. Implications and development of a net energy system for broilers. Animal Production Science. 2013;**53**:1231-1237. DOI: 10.1071/AN13204

[46] Annison G, Hughes RJ, Choct M. Effects of enzyme supplementation on the nutritive value of dehulled lupins. British Poultry Science. 1996;**37**:157-172. DOI: 10.1080/00071669608417845

[47] Bravo D, Pirgozliev V, Rose SP. A mixture of carvacrol, cinnamaldehyde and capsicum oleoresin improves energy utilization and growth performance of broiler chickens fed maize based diet. Journal of Animal Science. 2014;**92**:1531-1536. DOI: 10.2527/jas.2013-6244

[48] Karadas F, Pirgozliev V, Rose SP, Dimitrov D, Oduguwa O, Bravo D. Dietary essential oils improve the hepatic anti-oxidative status of broiler chickens. British Poultry Science. 2014;**55**(3):329-334. DOI: 10.1080/00071668.2014.891098

[49] Pirgozliev V, Bravo D, Rose SP. Rearing conditions influence nutrient availability of plant extracts supplemented diets when fed to broiler chickens. Journal of Animal Physiology and Animal Nutrition. 2014;**98**:667-671. DOI: 10.1111/jpn.12119

[50] Pirgozliev V, Beccaccia A, Rose SP, Bravo D. Partitioning of dietary energy of chickens fed maize or wheat based diets with and without a commercial blend of phytogenic feed additives. Journal of Animal Science. 2015;**93**(4):1695-1702. DOI: 10.2527/jas.2014-8175

[51] Pirgozliev V, Bravo D, Mirza MW, Rose SP. Growth performance and endogenous losses of broilers fed wheat based diets with and without essential oils and xylanase supplementation. Poultry Science. 2015;**94**:1227-1232. DOI: 10.3382/ps/peu017

[52] Koutsos E, Clifford A, Calvert C, Klasing C. Maternal carotenoid status modified the incorporation of dietary carotenoids into immune tissue of growing chickens (Gallus gallus domesticus). Journal of Nutrition. 2003;**133**:1132-1138. DOI: 10.1093/jn/133.4.1132

[53] Surai PF. Natural Antioxidants in Avian Nutrition and Reproduction. Nottingham: Nottingham University Press; 2002

[54] Kaiser P, Staheli P. Avian cytokines and chemokines. In: Schat K, Kaspers B, Kaiser P, editors. Avian Immunology. 2nd ed. London: Academic Press; 2014

[55] Carvacrol: National Center for Biotechnology Information. PubChem Compound Database; CID = 10,364, https://pubchem.ncbi.nlm.nih.gov/compound/10364 [Accessed: March 21, 2018]

[56] Cinnamaldehyde: National Center for Biotechnology Information. PubChem Compound Database; CID = 637,511, https://pubchem.ncbi.nlm.nih.gov/compound/637511 [Accessed: March 21, 2018]

[57] Capsaicin: National Center for Biotechnology Information. PubChem Compound Database; CID = 1,548,943, https://pubchem.ncbi.nlm.nih.gov/compound/1548943 [Accessed: March 21, 2018]

4

Phytochemicals—God's Endowment of Curative Power in Plants

Olayinka Temitayo Ogunmefun

Abstract

Phytochemicals—God's Endowment of Curative Power in Plants tried to review the link between the knowledge of God's pronouncement on plants as man's source of food and drugs in the Holy Bible to the scientific proofs of the availability of phytochemicals in different species of plants. The abundance of plants in the world as vegetables, spices, fruits, etc. of which more than 80% of their chemical compositions have not been discovered emphasizes the reasons for the search of these phytochemicals as alternative drug sources which are safer and relatively cheaper. Literature is reviewed on different phytochemicals such as alkaloids, saponins, tannins, anthraquinones, and glycosides in the form of cardiac and cyanogenetic glycosides, flavonoids, carotenoids, and phenols considering their chemical properties and their usefulness to man. This review confirmed the outburst that said "the world is too much with us; late and soon, getting and spending, we lay waste our powers: Little we see in nature that is ours." Therefore, there is an urgent need to search for these various phytochemicals in plants so that we can utilize the potentials in these free gifts from God and not lay waste the curative power endowed on them purposely for man's health benefits.

Keywords: alternative drug, curative power, endowment, God, phytochemicals, plants

1. Introduction

God created plants for the use of mankind and ordered man to make use of these herbs and trees for food and for medicine as reflected in His words recorded in the Holy Bible in the books of *Genesis* and *Revelation*. The book of *Genesis* Chapter 1 verse 29 reported and God said "Behold, I have given you every herb bearing seed, which is upon the face of all the earth, and every tree, in which is the fruit of a tree yielding seed; to you it shall be for meat." The book of *Revelation* Chapter 22 verse 1 also declared "And he showed me a pure river of water of life, clear as crystal, proceeding out of the throne of God and of the Lamb." Also, in *Revelation* Chapter 22 verse 2, it was written "In the midst of the street of it, and on either side of the river, was there the tree of life, which bare twelve manner of fruits, and yielded her fruit every month: and the leaves of the tree were for the healing of the nation" [1].

From the work of creation, God made light on the first day followed by water on the second day and afterward created plants on the third day in the categories of grass, herb yielding seed, and tree yielding fruit, whose seed was in itself, that is, seed enclosed in fruit. This order was a divine one which no one can fathom as God is all-knowing and His understanding is unsearchable. God knew what the requirements for the growth of all these plants would be, and He ordered their creation after those requirements were met so that they could survive.

He created man lastly on the sixth day after all other things (creatures) had been made so that man could have dominion over them. He ordered man to use the herbs and tree bearing fruits for meat, that is, food, and for treating their illnesses as He understood the frailty of man. He knew all the requirements that man needed to survive and made provisions for them.

God created plants to serve man and put into these plants certain powers that are capable of healing and which in the modern times are now known as "phytochemicals." These phytochemicals are of different types according to their specificity in curing various diseases. Many individual plants were endowed with varieties of these chemical constituents, and the synergistic effects of these constituents also termed secondary metabolites endow on them their curative abilities. The healing properties of most plants are becoming more recognizable and preferable as most are associated with little or no side effect which is a common problem with the administration of most synthetic drugs (orthodox medicines) and the realization of the fact that many natural remedies carry their cures along with them [2]. Never are we reminded of Wordsworth's outburst: "The world is too much with us; late and soon, getting and spending, we lay waste our powers. Little we see in nature that is ours" [2].

1.1. Objectives of the study

- To acknowledge the curative powers in plants as God's gift and perfect plan for man's well-being
- To review the study of plants in relation to their medicinal properties
- To review some plants used in the treatment of certain diseases

1.1.1. The history of botany in relation to medicine

Botanical science in a pure sense is the study of plants, and botany is the applied science which has in its interest the study of human use of plants. The studies that are mostly obvious in applied botany are agriculture, forestry, horticulture, pharmacognosy, weed science, economic botany, plant pathology, and ethnobotany that fall outside of modern botany courses [3].

The knowledge of plants especially in uses for food and medicine increased during the Neolithic Revolution. Protobotany which was the first prescientific written record of plants did not begin with food but was born out of the medicinal literature of China, Egypt, India, and Mesopotamia [4]. It was observed by botanical historian, Alan Morton, that agriculture was the occupation of the poor and uneducated, while medicine was the profession of the socially influential shamans, priests, magicians, physicians, and apothecians who were more likely to put their knowledge in record for posterity [3].

1.1.2. The relevance of botany in medicine

Lists of different plants and herb concoctions for pharmaceutical purposes were dated back to 481 BC–221 BC in ancient China. Over the centuries, the written knowledge of herbal pharmaceuticals was contributed to by many Chinese writers [5]. The study of medicinal plants was not being neglected, and a full synthesis of ancient Greek pharmacology was compiled in *De Materia Medica* c. 60 AD by Pedanius Dioscorides (c. 40–90 AD) who was a Greek physician with the Roman army [6]. The lives of the European middle ages were based on agriculture in the fifteenth and sixteenth centuries until when printing came into limelight which did not publish dissertations on agriculture but rather preferred the lists of medicinal plants with descriptions of their attributes and inherent power (efficacy). Records had it in most ancient history that *Herbal* which was the first series of books written on plants indicated botany to form a part of medicine [3]. People who contributed to *Herbal* were mostly university gardens' curators [7], and compilations of classic texts in *Herbal* were mostly derived from *De Materia Medica.*

1.2. Separation of botany from medicine

The need for accurate and detailed plant descriptions meant that some herbals were more botanical than medicinal. Herbals made contributions to botany by initiating the science of plant description, classification, and botanical illustrations. Botany and medicine were the same up to the seventeenth century, but those books that emphasized medicinal aspects omitted the plant lore and eventually became the modern pharmacopeias; those that omitted medicine became more botanical which evolved into the modern plant description compilations called *Floras* and are often backed by specimens deposited in a herbarium (a collection of dried plants that verified the plant descriptions given in the *Floras*). The transition from *Herbal* to *Floras* marked the final separation of botany from medicine [8].

1.2.1. Relevance of medicinal plants

Medicinal plants are gaining popularity in usage due to a large number of people in search of health remedies with little or no side effect which is the problem of most chemically synthesized drugs. Considerable attention is presently given to the use of eco-friendly and bio-friendly products from plant origin for the prevention and cure of human and animal health challenges (diseases) [9, 10]. This problem of side effects of most chemically based drugs has spurred the Western world to looking into natural products that are safe, effective, and affordable. It has been documented that 80% of the world's population has a strong belief in traditional medicine, especially drugs from plant origin for their primary health care [9, 10]. Medicinal plants, for example, neem leaves and stem bark (*Azadirachta indica*), pawpaw leaves (*Carica papaya*), mango leaves and stem bark (*Mangifera indica*), and Cinchona bark have been in use in one form or the other traditionally. No doubt, the plant kingdom is rich in diverse array of plants whose medicinal attributes (potencies) are yet to be unraveled [9, 10]. The various uses of some common medicinal plants from Nigeria used for treating various diseases highlighting the parts of the plants used are represented in **Table 1**.

1.3. Harvest of medicinal plants

Medicinal plants should be harvested at the appropriate seasons as their medicinal properties vary with respect to different seasons. The medicinal properties may be located and restricted to a particular part of the plant, and the medicinal attributes is also affected by the age of the plant. A medicinal plant of a particular age for drug processing should therefore be harvested at the correct season of the year to prevent loss or changes in its phytochemical constituents. The period of storage in shade or sun and the geographical locations of the medicinal plants also play important roles in the medicinal properties of the plant [11].

1.4. Identification and standardization of active principles in medicinal plants

Medicinal plants are very rich in chemical compounds which they produce for their own defense and are known as secondary metabolites (phytochemicals) and their medicinal potencies are attributed to these chemical compounds [11]. A medicinal plant may contain a mixture of different phytochemicals, for example, saponins, which have ability to lower cholesterol; alkaloids which are rich in nitrogenous compounds and are stimulants; tannins which are natural antibiotics; anthraquinones used as laxative and dye; cardiac glycosides which are good cardiovascular drugs; and phenols and flavonoids which are rich in antioxidants. The ability to identify these biologically active compounds in a medicinal plant serves as a guide in its quality control and dose determination. Most medicinal plants in Nigeria have not been screened for their complete phytochemical compositions, and this would help in their dose determination and standardization. The entire world has more than 250,000 species of higher plants gathered from conservative studies, and only an insignificant percentage has been exhaustively studied for their potentials as drug sources [11].

1.5. Plant-based drugs

In the ancient times, plants served humankind as the source of all drugs with most therapeutic agents provided by the higher plants. The World Health Organization estimated that about 3.5–4 billion people in the world depend on traditional medicine as sources of drugs for their primary health care (80% of people in the developing countries and 85% of traditional medicine rely on plant extracts) [12]. Plant-derived drugs represent 25% of the prescription of drugs in the market in the United States of America [13], and from 1983 to 1994, 39% of the new approved drugs were of natural origin; this included original natural products, semi-synthetically derived products from natural origin and synthetic products based on models from natural products [14]. From 87 approved anticancer drugs, a survey revealed that 62% were of natural origin or is derived from modeling of the natural product parents [14]. Paclitaxel, vincristine, podophyllotoxin (a natural product precursor), and camptothecin (a natural precursor for water-soluble derivatives) are among those clinically useful drugs.

	Botanical (species) name	Family name	Local name(s)	Common names	Parts used	Medicinal use(s)
1	*Abelmoschus esculentus*	Malvaceae	Ila, okweje, kubewa	Okra, lady's finger	Fruit, seeds	Fevers, dysentery, catarrhal, antispasmodic, tonic, gonorrhea
2	*Acalypha fimbriata*	Euphorbiaceae	Jinwinini, kandiri	Acalypha	Leaves	Syphilis, ulcers, asthma, anthelmintic, antimicrobial
3	*Adansonia digitata*	Bombacaceae	Igi-ose, kukaa, ose, kulambali	Baobab	Leaves, fruit, pulp, bark	Malaria, skin diseases, caries, asthma, diarrhea, bladder diseases, antimicrobial
4	*Aframomum melegueta*	Zingiberaceae	Atare, ata-ire, itaye, citta, ose oji, gyandamaryaji	Alligator pepper, grains of paradise	Leaves, seeds	Anemia, wounds, stimulant, coughs, malaria, rheumatism, anthelmintics, smallpox, chicken pox
5	*Alafia barteri*	Apocynaceae	Agbari etu	Alafia chewing stick, guinea fowl's crest	Roots, leaves	Eye infections, toothache, sickle cell anemia, rheumatic pains
6	*Allium cepa*	Liliaceae	Alubosa, albasa, yabase, albasa gudaji	Onion	Bulb, leaves	Skin diseases, throat infection, tumor, weak erection, cough, antidiuretic, anthelmintic, rubefacient
7	*Allium sativum*	Liliaceae	Aayu	Garlic	Bulb	Asthma, anthelmintic, antibiotic, blood tonic, malaria, ringworm, antimicrobials, emmenagogue, flatulence
8	*Aloe vera*	Liliaceae	Ahon erin	Barbados aloe	Leaves' juice	Purgative, guinea worms, hair care, skin diseases, amenorrhea, immune booster, diabetes, breast cancer
9	*Azadirachta indica*	Meliaceae	Dongo-yaro, eke-oyibo	Neem tree	Leaves, stem bark, seeds	Malaria, syphilis, jaundice, eczema, laxative, ringworm, skin disease, sore throat, anthelmintic
10	*Bambusa vulgaris*	Poaceae	Oparun, atosi	Bamboo	Leaves, young shoots	Gonorrhea, abortifacient, skin rashes of HIV/AIDS, emmenagogue, anthelmintic
11	*Buchholzia coriacea*	Sterculiaceae	Uworo, obi-ata	Wonderful kola	Fruit, bark	Antimicrobials, anthelminthic, ulcer, fibroid, dysmenorrhea, chest pains, respiratory disorders

	Botanical (species) name	Family name	Local name(s)	Common names	Parts used	Medicinal use(s)
12	*Butyrospermum paradoxum* (*Vitellaria paradoxa*)	Sapotaceae	Emi-emi, emi, osisi, ka'danya	Shea butter tree	Seeds	Nasal decongestion, anthelmintic, hypertension, diuretic
13	*Cannabis sativa*	Cannabaceae	Igbo	Indian hemp	Leaves, female inflorescence, seeds, stem, twigs	Diarrhea, sores, dandruff, sedative, gonorrhea, whooping cough, migraine, dyspepsia
14	*Carica papaya*	Caricaceae	Ibepe, ojo, gwanda	Pawpaw	Leaves, seeds, fruits	Amoebic dysentery, syphilis, gonorrhea, abortifacient, diabetes, roundworms, convulsion, malaria, mental disorder, papain enzyme as meat tenderizer
15	*Catharanthus roseus*	Apocynaceae	Apabida pupa	Rose periwinkle	Leaves, whole plant	Diabetes, antileukemic properties, dysentery, hypertension, menorrhagia, antitumor
16	*Ceiba pentandra*	Bombacaceae	Araba	White silk cotton tree	Flowers, leaves, bark, exudate	Fever, syphilis, gonorrhea, diabetes, emetic, astringent, asthma, menorrhagia, emollient, demulcent
17	*Citrus aurantifolia*	Rutaceae	Osan-wewe, dankabuya, afotanta, epe nkirisi	Lime, swing	Leaves, stem, root, fruit	Fever, hypertensive recipe, jaundice, gonorrhea, measles, abdominal ulcer, flavoring agent, cough, scurvy, toothache, anthelmintic
18	*Cocos nucifera*	Palmae	Agbon	Coconut palm	Bark, root, nuts	Bronchitis, migraine, dysentery, antiseptic, toothache, hair loss, uterine disease, emollient, diuretic, laxative, anthelmintic, liver ailment
19	*Daniellia oliveri*	Leguminosae	Iya	African copaiba, balsam tree	Gum, bark	Toothache, astringent, diarrhea, dysentery, urinary infection
20	*Datura metel*	Solanaceae	Ajegun-eegun	Devil's trumpet, hairy thorn apple	Leaves	Asthma, convulsion, venereal diseases
21	*Elaeis guineensis*	Palmae	Igi-ope, ope	Red oil palm	Root, bark, kernels, palm oil	Diarrhea, asthma, measles, mental disorders, malaria

	Botanical (species) name	Family name	Local name(s)	Common names	Parts used	Medicinal use(s)
22	*Entandrophragma cylindricum*	Meliaceae	Ijebo, jebo	Cedar mahogany	Stem bark	Stimulant, gastrointestinal disorders, cough, diabetes, fever, black tongue
23	*Euphorbia hirta*	Euphorbiaceae	Emi-ile, iroko-iju, oro-elewe	Asthma weed	Whole plant, exudate	Asthma, catarrh, cough, hay fever, conjunctivitis, anthelmintic, amoebic dysentery, increased lactation and breast shape, antispasmodic, hypertension
24	*Funtumia elastica*	Apocynaceae	Ire	Silk rubber tree, wild rubber	Stem, twigs, latex	Piles, jaundice, impotence, antipyretics
25	*Garcinia kola*	Guttiferae	Orogbo	Bitter kola	Seeds, roots, fruits, stem bark	Antimicrobial, bronchitis, cough, dysentery, toothache, fever, throat and respiratory ailments, liver disorders, evacuant, headache, anticancer
26	*Hibiscus rosa-sinensis*	Malvaceae	Kekeke	Garden hibiscus	Leaves, stem, flower buds	Influenza, appendicitis, hypertension, asthma, stomach upset, antipyretic, oligospermia
27	*Ipomoea batatas*	Convolvulaceae	Anamo, odukun, kunkundukun, dankali, ekomako, jioyibo	Sweet potato	Leaves, tuber	Boils, diabetes, wounds, bronchial asthma, antimicrobials, purgative, breast swelling
28	*Irvingia gabonensis*	Irvingiaceae	Oro (ogbono)	Wild mango, bread tree	Fruits, seeds (kernel), leaves	Weight loss, antiulcer, spleen infection
29	*Jatropha curcas*	Euphorbiaceae	Lapalapa, botuje, zugu, oluluidu	Physic nut	Seed, stem, leaves, roots, sap	Eczema, ringworm, scabies, whitlow, fever, guinea worm, herpes, irregular menstruation, smallpox, convulsion
30	*Khaya ivorensis*	Meliaceae	Oganwo, ono, madachi	African mahogany	Stem, root, barks	Malaria, anemia, skin diseases, jaundice, arthritis, anthelmintic, emmenagogue
31	*Kigelia africana*	Bignoniaceae	Pandoro, iyan, rawuya, uturubein	Sausage tree	Leaves, stem, root, bark, fruits,	Kidney disorders, rheumatism, cough, malaria, spleen infection, dysentery, gonorrhea, astringent, leucorrhoea
32	*Lagenaria breviflorus*	Cucurbitaceae	Tagiri, eso-itagiri, eso-ito	Pseudocolocynth	Root, fruit	Anthelmintic, diabetes, purgative, small pox, abortifacient, chicken pox, lumbago, cathartic

	Botanical (species) name	Family name	Local name(s)	Common names	Parts used	Medicinal use(s)
33	*Lawsonia inermis*	Lythraceae	Laali, lali	Henna plant	Leaves, bark, flowers	Spermatorrhea, malaria, astringent, gonorrhea, ulcers, jaundice, skin diseases, menorrhagia
34	*Mentha piperita*	Lamiaceae	Mintii	Peppermint	Whole plant	Mouth wash, stomach ache, respiratory infections, chest pains
35	*Morinda lucida*	Rubiaceae	Oruwo, eruwo, eze ogu, njisi	Brimstone tree	Leaves, stem bark, root bark	Anticancer, malaria, heart diseases, jaundice, flatulence, diuretic, emetic
36	*Newbouldia laevis*	Bignoniaceae	Akoko, ogirisi, aduruku	Tree of life, fertility tree	Leaves, bark, root	Infertility, hernia, elephantiasis, yellow fever, migraine, roundworms, cough, dysentery, earache, stomachache
37	*Ocimum gratissimum*	Lamiaceae	Efinrin-nla, efinrin-aja, oromoba, saidoya, nchanwu	Tea bush, balsam, basil	Leaves, whole plant	Antimicrobials, bronchitis, diarrhea, insect repellant, piles, cold, cough, diabetes, anthelmintic, hypertension, colic, fever, convulsions
38	*Parkia biglobosa*	Leguminosae	Igba, igi-iru, dadawa, ogirili, dorowa	West African locust bean, Dadawa tree	Leaves, bark, fruits, seeds, pulp	Antitumor, diabetes, high blood pressure, malaria, tonic, wounds, mental disorder, intestinal disorder, obesity, astringent
39	*Talinum triangulare*	Portulacaceae	Gbure, ofe bake, ntu oka	Water lettuce, Ceylon spinach, fame flower, Surinam purslane	Roots, leaves	Anemia, scabies, schistosomiasis, fresh cuts, high blood pressure
40	*Zingiber officinale*	Zingiberaceae	Atale, jinja	Ginger	Rhizome	Asthma, rheumatism, piles, hepatitis, diuretic, headache, cold, stimulant, cough, anthelmintic, typhoid fever, obesity, malaria

[40, 52, 53].

Table 1. Some common medicinal plants from Nigeria used for treating various diseases.

These substances contain properties which are essential as new chemotherapeutic agents useful for treatment in the hospitals. There are some new approaches to drug discovery, such as combinatorial chemistry and computer-based molecular modeling design, and none of them can replace the role of natural products in drug discovery and development. Examples of plant-based drugs are artemisinin, gingerosome, and quinine.

1.6. Synergy in relation to pharmacological action of phytomedicine

Most herbs exhibit their effects on a variety of constituents, and the idea of synergy within and between them is gaining acceptance [15]. Most herbal medicines are not well documented to prove whether they are acting truly in a synergistic way or by additive effects. It is usually difficult to clinically evaluate herbal preparations without the knowledge of their synergistic effects. Biological activity may be absent in the crude drugs but may contain some components that can enhance their active components' potency. One of such examples is St. John's wort (*Hypericum perforatum*, family Hypericaceae), a clinically proven herb which has efficacy as an antidepressant. Hypericins responsible for its activity was found to be very weak, and impurities in the fraction used gave the additional results which suggest multiple (polyvalent) and synergistic effects. St. John's wort thus represents a good example of an herb which may exhibit synergism and polyvalent action [16]. The use of combinations of herbs can also result in synergism or enhancement of activity of herbal drugs. In case of multiple herb extracts, some of the herbs enhance the potency of the real effective herb, and in some cases, their constituents could reduce the toxic effects of the main herb, resulting in a safe herbal combination tolerable for consumption by the human system [17].

1.7. Phytoconstituents in medicinal plants

Phytochemicals are chemicals found in plants that protect plants against bacteria, viruses, and fungi. Eating large amount of brightly colored fruits and vegetables, whole grains/cereals, and beans containing phytochemicals may decrease the risk of developing certain cancers as well as diabetes, hypertension, and heart disease. The actions of phytochemicals vary by the type of the food and the color. They may act as antioxidants or nutrient protectors or prevent carcinogens from forming. The term phytochemical refers to a wide variety of compounds made by plants but is mainly used to describe those compounds that may affect human health. Scientists have identified thousands of phytochemicals, although only a small fraction has been studied closely. Some common examples of phytochemicals include beta-carotene (with other carotenoids), vitamin C, vitamin E, and folic acid [18]. Phytochemicals have shown various physiological actions [19, 20]. Among the numerous phytochemicals in existence are the following with their usefulness:

1.8. Alkaloids

These are the largest group of secondary metabolites made of ammonia compounds comprising basically nitrogen bases synthesized from amino acid building blocks having various radicals substituting one or more of the hydrogen atoms in the peptide ring, containing mostly oxygen [21]. The compounds have basic properties and are alkaline in reaction, turning red litmus paper blue. In fact, one or more nitrogen atoms that are present in an alkaloid, typically as 1°, 2°, or 3° amines, contribute to the basicity of the alkaloid. The degree of basicity varies considerably, depending on the structure of the molecule, presence, and location of the functional groups [22]. They react with acids to form crystalline salts without the production of water [21]. Alkaloids exist majorly in solid states as atropine, liquids containing carbon, hydrogen, and nitrogen.

Alkaloids are mostly readily soluble in alcohol but are sparingly soluble in water though their salts are usually soluble in water. Their solutions are usually very bitter; alkaloids defend plants against herbivores and pathogens and are used widely as stimulants, narcotics, pharmaceuticals, and poisons because of their biological potencies [23]. Alkaloids, in nature, are found in large quantities in the seeds and roots of plants and mostly in combination with vegetable acids. Alkaloids are useful as central nervous system (CNS) stimulants and anesthetics in pharmacological applications [23].

Alkaloids also find its usefulness as pain relievers [24]. Atropine is an alkaloid used widely in medicine as an antidote to organophosphate poisoning, while caffeine stimulates CNS and respiratory systems. Caffeine also serves as an antidote to barbiturate and morphine poisoning, while emetine (from *Cephaelis ipecacuanha*) root is useful in the treatment of protozoal infections, for example, amoebic dysentery.

1.9. Tannins

The tannin compounds are found mainly in many plant species which help to confer on them protection from predators and probably pesticides; they also help in regulating plant growth [25]. The dry and puckery feeling in the mouth after eating unripe fruits or red wine is attributed to the astringency from the tannins [26]. The destruction or modification of tannins with time in like manner plays an important role in the ripening of fruit and the aging of wine. They are acidic in reaction, and this is attributed to the presence of phenolics or carboxylic group [27]. They form complexes with proteins, carbohydrates, gelatin, and alkaloids.

Tannins are divided into hydrolysable tannins and condensed tannins. Hydrolysable tannins, when hydrolyzed, produce gallic acid and ellagic acid, and depending on the type of acid produced, the hydrolysable tannins are called gallotannins or ellagitannins; when tannins are heated, they form pyrogallic acid [25]. The presence of phenolic group in tannins confers on them their usefulness as an antiseptic [27]. Common examples of hydrolysable tannins include the aflavins (from tea), daidzein, genistein, and glycitein.

Plants that contain tannins have been reported to be astringent in nature and are useful in treating intestinal disorders like diarrhea and dysentery. This means that tannins possess antimicrobial activity [28, 29]. The antimicrobial activities possessed by these plants could support their use in West Africa for treating gastrointestinal disorders [30]. Tannins are also potent antioxidants [31, 32].

1.10. Saponins

Saponins are a class of phytochemicals present in abundance in numerous species of plants. They are specifically amphipathic glycosides and are grouped phenomenologically by their production of soap-like foaming when shaken in aqueous solutions (phenomenology—study of structures of consciousness as experienced from the first-person point of view). They are grouped structurally by possession of one or more hydrophilic glycoside moieties combined with a lipophilic triterpene derivative [33].

Two major groups of saponins exist which are steroid and triterpene saponins. Saponins are insoluble in ether but soluble in water, and on hydrolysis, they give aglycones like glycosides. They cause hemolysis of blood and cattle poisoning as they are known to be extremely poisonous (27). Apart from causing irritation to mucous membranes, they have a bitter and acrid taste. They are soluble in alcohol and water but insoluble in solvents like benzene and n-hexane that are organic and nonpolar; therefore, they are mostly amorphous in nature. Saponins are therapeutically important because they lower bad fats in the body (hypolipidemic) and have anticancer potentials. Saponins work in synergy with the cardiac glycosides [22].

Saponins are known to produce inhibitory effect on inflammation [34]. Saponins help in lowering cholesterol which will subsequently reduce the risk of cardiovascular diseases such as hypertension which usually leads to stroke [35].

1.11. Anthraquinones

Anthraquinones are phenolic and glycosidic compound derivatives and are solely derived from anthracene leading to the production of variable oxidized derivatives like anthrones and anthranols [36, 21]. Industrially, anthraquinones are used for washing of bowels (laxatives) and in dye production [37].

1.12. Glycosides

Glycosides are the condensation products of sugars (polysaccharides inclusive) with different varieties of organic hydroxyl (occasionally thiol) compounds. Glycosides are colorless, crystalline water-soluble plant constituents found in the cell sap. Glycosides chemically contain a carbohydrate (glucose) and a noncarbohydrate part (aglycones or genin) [27, 21]. Glycosides can be readily hydrolyzed into its components with mineral acids as they are neutral in reaction and are purely bitter principles commonly found in plants of the family Genitiaceae. The action of the bitters on the gustatory nerves results in increased flow of saliva and gastric juices [27, 21]. Some of the bitter principles due to the presence of tannic acid are either used in restricting flow of blood (as astringents), function in the reduction of thyroxin, and thereby regulate cell metabolism and growth or as antiprotozoal. Examples of glycosides include cardiac glycosides which act on the heart and anthracene glycosides act as purgative and for treatment of skin diseases, while chalcone glycosides are used as anticancer agents [22]. The extracts of plants containing cyanogenetic glycosides have been reported to be useful as flavoring agents in many pharmaceutical formulations. Amygdalin has been used in the treatment of cancer [hydrogen cyanide (HCN) liberated in stomach kills malignant cells] and also as a cough suppressant in various preparations. Intake of cyanogenetic glycosides in excess quantities can be dangerous [22].

1.13. Cardiac glycosides

Plants long used as arrow poisons (e.g., *Strophanthus*) or as heart drugs, for example, *digitalis*, contain cardiac cardiotonic glycosides [38]. Cardiac glycosides help in the treatment of congestive heart (cardiac) failure; that is, they help a weakened heart to be strengthened and function more efficiently [39].

1.14. Cyanogenetic glycosides

Cyanogenetic glycosides are a group of materials derived majorly from plants which on hydrolysis liberate hydrocyanic acid (HCN). They therefore call for attention and an object of concern because of their ability in causing damage by poisoning that are natural toxicants. Cassava, an example of a food plant (*Manihot esculenta*), produces cyanogenetic glycosides which require prolonged hydrolysis and boiling in preparation of the starchy tuberous roots to release and evaporate off the HCN before consumption [40].

1.15. Flavonoids

Flavonoids belong to a group of important polyphenols which are widely distributed among plants. They have more than one benzene ring in its structure and are used as antioxidants or free radical scavengers [27]. Flavans are parent compounds from which they are derived. Out of over 4,000 flavonoids that exist, some are found as pigments in higher plants. About 70% of plants contain common flavonoids such as quercetin, kaempferol, and quercitrin. Among other groups of flavonoids in existence are flavones, flavans, anthocyanidins, dihydroflavons, flavonols, chalcones, and catechin [27]. Flavonoids function to reduce the risk of coronary heart diseases [41] and possess anticoagulant, anti-inflammatory, and aphrodisiac properties [42].

1.16. Phenols

Phenols contribute to the prevention of various degenerative diseases that act as an antioxidant [41]. Phenols, phenolics, or polyphenolics are chemical constituents that are commonly present as natural color pigments giving fruits of plants their colors. The action of phenylalanine ammonia lyses (PAL) on phenylalanine leads to the synthesis of phenolics in plants. Among the various functions of phenols is in plant defense against pathogens and predators of herbivores and therefore used in the control of human infections caused by pathogens [43]. The most common of phenolic compounds widespread in plants is caffeic acid which is followed by chlorogenic acid, the causal agent of excessively sensitive inflammation of the skin (dermatitis) among humans [27]. Phenolics are natural antioxidants functioning as nutraceuticals and available in red wine, apples, and green tea. They serve as anticancer and anti-inflammatory agents as well as prevent heart diseases.

1.17. Steroids

Plant steroids also known as cardiac or steroid glycosides are one of the most naturally occurring plant phytoconstituents that are applied therapeutically as cardiac drugs or arrow poisons [21]. The cardiac glycosides are majorly steroids having a natural ability to exert specific and powerful action on the cardiac muscle mainly when injected into animal or man. Steroids (anabolic steroids) have the ability to promote nitrogen retention in osteoporosis (a disease following menopause in women causing bones to be porous and subjected to fracture) and in animals with wasting illness [36, 23]. Steroids have the ability to exhibit activities such as antifungal, antiviral, antileukemic, hypnotic, antipyretic, and muscle-relaxant activities and are found in large quantities in many plants [44].

1.18. Carotenoids

Carotenoids are coloring pigments in plants especially fruits and vegetables; these act as antioxidants to protect the body against the activities of free radicals [45].

1.18.1. Mechanism of action of phytochemicals

Phytochemicals may inhibit microorganisms, may interfere with some metabolic processes, or may modulate gene expression and signal transduction pathways [46–48]. Among the many uses, phytochemicals may either be used as chemotherapeutic or chemopreventive agents. Chemoprevention refers to the use of agents to inhibit, reverse, or retard tumorigenesis. In this sense chemopreventive phytochemicals are applicable to cancer therapy, and molecular mechanisms may be common to both chemoprevention and cancer therapy [49, 50].

The mechanism of action of phytochemicals in general is attributed to proton-motive force disruption, active transport, cytoplasmic membrane disturbance, electron flow, and cell contents' coagulation [51]. There are different modes of action of phytoconstituents which could be anticancer, anti-inflammatory, antioxidant, anti-ulcer, antidiabetic and may be a multifunctional target.

2. Conclusion

God is the creator of all things that are in existence of which plants which are in abundance and of various diversities are among. He put plants in place to serve man especially for food and medicine to heal their diseases. It is therefore imperative to search more into medicinal plants for phytochemicals which can provide a clue in terms of lead (active) compound discovery for the cure of many so-called incurable diseases like cancer, diabetes, hypertension, ulcer, and other degenerative diseases that are just being managed by medical practitioners till the patient passes on. It is realized that many natural remedies carry their cures along with them; therefore, it could be concluded that botanists (plant scientists), pharmacists, pharmacognosists, pharmacologists, chemists, biochemists, and all other fields related to the science of drug discovery should rise up to these challenges of sourcing from plant alternative medicines which God had placed into our hands only left to be discovered.

Author details

Olayinka Temitayo Ogunmefun

Address all correspondence to: yinkatayo_08@yahoo.com

Department of Biological Sciences, Afe Babalola University, Ado-Ekiti, Nigeria

References

[1] Version KJ. Life Application Study Bible (the Holy Bible). Carol Stream: Illinois: Tyndale House Publishers, Inc.; 2004. 2143p

[2] Thomson WAR. Herbs that Heal. London: A and C Black; 1976. 184p

[3] Morton AG. History of Botanical Science: An Account of the Development of Botany from Ancient Times to the Present Day. London: Academic Press; 1981. 474p

[4] Reed HS. A Short History of the Plant Sciences. New York: Ronald Press Company; 1942. 330p

[5] Needham J, Lu G-d, Huang H-T. Science and Civilisation in China Vol. 6; Part 1 Botany. Cambridge: Cambridge University Press; 1986

[6] Singer C. Herbals. The Edinburgh Review. 1923;**237**:95-112

[7] Sachs J. History of Botany (1530-1860). Translated by Garnsey, H.E.F., revised by Balfour, I.B. Oxford University Press: London; 1890. Retrieved 13 December, 2015

[8] Oliver FW. Makers of British Botany. Cambridge: Cambridge University Press; 1913. pp. 146-246 Retrieved 2010-01-12

[9] Gijtenbeek JMM, Vanden Bent MJ, Vent CJ. Cyclosporine neurotoxicity. Journal of Neurology 1999;**246**:339-346

[10] Johnson WC, William OW. Warfarin toxicity. Journal of Vascular Surgery. 2002;**35**:413-421

[11] Dubey NK, Kumar R, Tripathi P. Global promotion of herbal medicine: India's opportunity. *Current Science*. 2004;**86**(1):37-41

[12] Farnsworth NR. In: Wilson EO, editor. Biodiversity. Washington DC: National Academy Press; 1988. 419p

[13] Pezzuto JM. Plant-derived anticancer agents. Biochemical Pharmacology. 1997;**53**(2):121-133

[14] Cragg GM, Newman DJ, Snader KM. Natural products in drug discovery and development. Journal of Natural Products. 1997;**60**:52-60

[15] Duke JA, Bogenschutz-Godwin MJ. Natural Products from Plants. Boca Raton, FI, USA: CRC Press; 1999. 632p

[16] Whitley D. In: Evans WC, editor. CNS Drugs in: Trease and Evans Pharmacognosy. Edinburgh, London: W.B. Saunders; 2002. p. 52

[17] Miaorong P, Jing L. Proceedings of the 40th Annual Conference on Chinese Medicine. Beijing University; 1996. pp. 28-30

[18] Glaser TS, Doss LE, Shih G, et al. The Association of Dietary Lutein plus Zeaxanthin and B vitamins with cataracts in the age-related eye disease study AREDS report no.37. Ophtalmology. 2015;**122**(7):1471-1479

[19] Edeoga HO, Okwu DE, Mbaebie BO. Phytochemical constituents of some Nigerian medicinal plants. African Journal of Biotechnology. 2005;**4**(7):685-688

[20] Peteros NP, Uy MM. Antioxidant and Cytotoxic activities and Phytochemical screening of four Philippine medicinal plants. Journal of Medicinal Plants Research. 2010;**4**:407-414

[21] Firn R. Nature's Chemicals. Oxford: Oxford University Press; 2010. pp. 74-75

[22] Sarker SD, Nahar L. Chemistry for Pharmacy Students General, Organic and Natural Product Chemistry. England: John Wiley and Sons; 2007. 396p

[23] Madziga HA, Sanni S, Sandabe UK. Phytochemical and elemental analysis of Acalypha wilkesiana leaf. Journal of American Science. 2010;**6**(11):510-514

[24] Kokate P, Purohit AP, Gokhale SB. Pharmacognosy. 20th ed. India: Nirali Publication; 2002. pp. 1-14

[25] Kathie E, Ferrelli T, Richard W. Squirrels; The Animal Answer Guide. Baltimore: Johns Hopkins University press; 2006. 91p

[26] McGee H. On Food and Cooking? The Science and Lore of the Kitchen. NewYork: Scribner; 2004. 714p

[27] Kar A. Pharmaocgnosy and Pharmacobiotechnology (Revised-Expanded Second Edition). New Delhi, India: New Age International Limted Publishers; 2007. 898p

[28] Scalbert A. Antimicrobial properties of tannin. Phytochemistry. 1991;**30**(12):3875-3883

[29] Dharmananda S. Gall nuts and the uses of tannins in Chinese medicine. In: Proceedings of Institute for Traditional Medicine. Portland, Oregon; 2003. p. 26

[30] Burkill HM. The Useful Plants of West Tropical Africa. 2nd ed. Royal Botanic Gardens: Kew, UK; 1985. 960p. http://plants.jstor.org/upwta/2_580

[31] Harborne JB. Phytochemical Methods – A Guide to Modern Techniques of Plant Analysis. London: Chapman and Hall; 1998. pp. 182-190

[32] Trease GE, Evans WC. A Text Book of Pharmacognosy. 16th ed. London: Saunders Ltd; 2009. 616p

[33] Hostettmann K, Marson A. Chemistry and Pharmacology of Natural Products: Saponins. Cambridge: Cambridge University press; 2008. 562p

[34] Just MJ, Recsio MG, Gner RM, Cuellar MJ, Marez S, Bilia AR, Rios J. Anti-inflammatory activity of unusual lupine saponins from Bupleurum fruiticescens. Planta Medica. 1998;**64**(5):404-407

[35] Francis G, Kerem Z, Makkar HP, Becker K. The biological action of saponins in animal systems: A review. British Journal of Nutrition. 2002;**88**(6):587-605. DOI: 10.1079/BJN2002725

[36] Maurya R, Singh G, Yadav PP. Antiosteoporotic agents from natural sources. In: Rahman A-u, editor. Studies in Natural Products Chemistry. Vol. 35. Elsevier Publication; 2008. pp. 517-545

[37] Bien HS, Stawitz J, Wunderlich K. Anthraquinone dyes and intermediates in: Ullmann's Encyclopedia of Industrial Chemistry. Weinheim: Wiley-VCH; 2005; 2745. DOI:10.1002/14356007.a02_355

[38] Dewick PM. Medicinal Natural Products: A Biosynthetic Approach. 2nd ed. England: John Willey & Sons Limited; 2002. 241-244, 455-456

[39] Colin B, Shelia J. Cardiac glycosides. The Oxford Companion to the Body. Encyclopedia.com. 2001. http://www.encyclopedia.com

[40] Odugbemi T. A Textbook of Medicinal Plants from Nigeria. Akoka, Yaba – Lagos, Nigeria: © Tolu Odugbemi University of Lagos Press; 2008. 628p

[41] Rice-Evans CA, Miller NJ, Paganga G. Structure–antioxidant activity relationships of flavonoids and phenolic acids. Free Radical Biology and Medicine. 1996;**20**(7):933-938

[42] Houghton PJ, Hylands PJ, Mensah AY, Hensel A, Deters AM. *In vitro* tests and ethnopharmacological investigations: Wound healing as an example. Journal of Ethnopharmacology. 2005;**100**:100-107

[43] Puupponen-Pimiä R, Nohynek L, Alakomi H, Oksman-Caldentey K. The action of berry Phenolics against human intestinal pathogens. BioFactors. 2008;**23**(4):243-251

[44] Kokpol U, Chittawong V, Mills HD. Chemical constituents of the roots of *Acanthus illicifolius*. Journal of Natural Product. 1984;**49**:355-356

[45] Sims J, Odle T. Carotenoids. Gale Encyclopedia of Alternative Medicine. Encyclopedia.com. 2005. http://www.encyclopedia.com

[46] Kris-Etherton PM, Hecker KD, Bonanome A, Coval SM, Binkoski AE, Hilpert KF, Griel AE, Etherton TD. Bioactive compounds in foods: Their role in the prevention of cardiovascular disease and Cancer. American Journal of Medicine. 2002;**113**:71S-88S

[47] Manson MM. Cancer prevention – The potential for diet to modulate molecular Signalling. Trends in Molecular Medicine. 2003;**9**:11-18

[48] Surh YJ. Cancer chemoprevention with dietary Phytochemicals. Natural Reviews in Cancer. 2003;**3**:768-780

[49] D'Incalci M, Steward WP, Gescher AJ. Use of Cancer Chemopreventive Phytochemicals as Antineoplastic agents. Lancet Oncology. 2005;**6**:899-904

[50] Sarkar FH, Liu Y. Using Chemopreventive agents to enhance the efficacy of Cancer therapy. Cancer Research. 2006;**66**:3347-3350

[51] Kotzekidou P, Giannakidis P, Boulamatsis A. Antimicrobial activity of some plant extracts and essential oils against food borne pathogens in vitro and on the fate of inoculated pathogens in chocolate. LWT Food Science and Technology Journal. 2008;**41**:119-127

[52] Ngondi JL, Oben JE, Minka SR. The effect of *Irvingia gabonensis* seeds on body weight and blood lipids of obese subjects in Cameroon. Lipids in Health and Disease. 2005;**4**:12

[53] Ngondi JL, Etoundi BC, Nyangono CB, Mbofung CM, Oben JE. IGOB 131, a novel seed extract of the west African plant *Irvingia gabonensis* significantly reduces body weight and improves metabolic parameters in overweight humans in a randomized double – Blind placebo controlled investigation. Lipids in Health and Disease. 2009;**8**:7

5

Phytochemical Profiling of Soybean (*Glycine max* (L.) Merr.) Genotypes using GC-MS Analysis

Salem Alghamdi, Hussein Migdadi, Muhammad Khan, Ehab H. El-Harty, Megahed Ammar, Muhammad Farooq and Muhammad Afzal

Abstract

Twenty-four soybean genotypes collected from different regions and origin were evaluated for their quality performance to explore their nutritional and medicinal values. The proximate compositions showed considerable variations among soybean genotypes. The USA genotypes recorded the highest values for protein (43.1 g/100 g), total fat (23.61 g/100 g), phenolic content and flavonoids (1.77 and 2.13 mg/g). Using GC-MS analyses of methanolic extracts, a total of 88 compounds were identified in the genotypes and were classified to: 19 heterocyclic compounds, 13 compounds for ketones and esters, 9 for phenolic compound, 7 compounds for carboxylic acids and sugar moiety, 5 compounds for aldehydes and alcohols, 4 ether compounds, 3 amide, 2 alkanes and one alkene and one fatty acid ester. Indonesian genotypes recorded the highest number of phenolic and the Australian genotype A-1 had the maximum number of esters. Genotypes showed high levels of proximate compositions and pharmaceutical components, offering potential candidates for improving those traits in adapted genotypes through breeding program, as well as serving as a good source of mass production of pharmaceutical and medicinal components either through classical or in vitro production. Furthermore, platform was set for isolating and understanding the characteristics of each compound for it pharmacological properties.

Keywords: soybean, phenolic compounds, GC-MS, flavonoids, nutritional value

1. Introduction

Soybean (*Glycine max* (L.) Merr) considered among ancient cultivated crops, it was domesticated in the 11th century BC around Northeast of China. It is one of the most widely grown leguminous crops in the world. Its cultivated area was recorded in 95 countries more than 121 million hectare that produced 335 million tons of dry seeds [1] (FAOSTAT, 2016). Soybean had a wide variability, the USDA alone maintains more than 15 thousand soybean accession grouped into 13 maturity classes including both determinate and indeterminate soybean. Early maturing groups are adapted to short summer growing seasons in North USA and Canada while late maturity groups are adapted to southern or coastal plain counties [2]. Soybean occupies an advanced position among agricultural crops, being the most important source of proteins and vegetable oils [3]. Its seeds provided abundant and high quality protein and oil for human diet and animal feed. Its seeds contain more than 36% protein, 30% carbohydrates in addition to fiber, vitamins, and minerals [3]. It also contains about 20% oil, which makes soybean one of the most important edible oil crops. Soy oil has used as binding additives in manufacturing of papers, inks, paints, varnishes, cosmetics, and plastics. It was used also in production of farming pesticides and pharmaceuticals products [4]. Nowadays, biodiesel utilizing soy oil become a new industrial renewable sources of energy. Additionally, soybean as a nitrogen-fixing legume crop helps in reducing the chemical source of nitrogen fertilizers production [4].

Furthermore, tofu, soy milk, soy sauce, miso, etc., have been developed for human consumption, while soya meal (oil extraction by-product) is used as a nutritious animal feed [5]. Moreover, soybean is now regarded as a model legume crop owing to the availability of genome sequence information [6]. Keeping in mind its vast uses, there is huge number of justifications for crop improvement programs throughout the world. Having 53% global production share of all oilseed crops, USA, China, Brazil, Argentina and India gave soybean much attention in the agricultural production systems. Yield and total production of soybean increased over the last two decades due to genetic improvement of this crop [7].

In comparison with conventional legume and animal feed sources, soybean is considered one of the cheapest food resources with medicinal properties due to their highest protein content and no cholesterol due to its contents of Genistein, photochemical and isoflavones [8]. It can help in disease fighting due to its pharmacological properties and its phytochemicals constitutes, including antioxidant, estrogenic, antidiabetic, anti-hypercholesterolemic, anti-hyperlipidemic, anti-obesity, antihypertensive, anticancer, anti-mutagenic, hepatoprotective, anti-osteoporotic, antiviral, bifidogenic, anti-inflammatory, immunomodulatory, neuroprotective, wound healing, antimicrobial, goitrogenic anti-skin aging, anti-photoaging activity and the effects of anti-nutritional factors [3]. A 111 volatile compounds in fermented soybean curds were reported by Chung [9] and an 83 in commercial plain sufu [10]. Messina [11] reported that the presence of isoflavones in soybean is behind the pharmacological attributes of this crop. Chemical composition included Phenolic acids, flavonoids, isoflavones, saponins, phytosterols and sphingolipids were recorded in soybean [12–14]. Due to importance of this crop and its products, this study was amid at estimating the most active constitutes of 24 soybean genotypes including total phenolic, flavonoid and protein content and phytochemicals using GC-MS.

2. Materials and methods

2.1. Plant materials

Twenty-four soybean genotypes were grown in Dirab Agriculture Research Station, King Saud University, Riyadh, Kingdom of Saudi Arabia (24_25049.200 N 46_22012.500E) on August, 2014 and were collected from nine countries (Argentina, Australia, China, Egypt, India, Indonesia, USA, and Pakistan). The name and geographical origin of these genotypes are presented in the **Table 1**.

2.2. Chemical analysis

2.2.1. Proximate composition

Triplicate sample is used to determine the proximate analysis of soybean genotypes for crude proteins, moisture, total ash, fat and carbohydrate by using the methods described in AOAC, [15]. Protein content was estimated using Kjeldahl method with titration and percent nitrogen was determined using [16] equation.

Entry no.	Genotype name	Source/origin	Entry no.	Genotype name	Source/origin
1	Admaril	Pakistan	13	Giza 111	Egypt
2	Romal-1	Pakistan	14	Clark	USA
3	NARC-2	Pakistan	15	3803	Syria
4	Williams 82	USA	15	A-1	Australia
5	X 32	Egypt	17	Ijen	Indonesia
6	Giza 22	Egypt	18	Indo-black	Indonesia
7	Giza 21	Egypt	29	Indo-I	Indonesia
8	X2 L 12	Egypt	20	Indo-II	Indonesia
9	Giza 83	Egypt	21	USA-1	USA
10	Crawford	USA	22	Indian	India
11	Giza 35	Egypt	23	Chinese	China
12	X 30	Egypt	24	Argentinian	Argentina

Table 1. Name and source of the 24 soybean genotypes invistigated in the study.

2.2.2. Antioxidants determination

Soybean samples approximately (1 g) were powdered and homogenized in 10 ml 80% methanol. The mixture was shaken at 300 rpm at room temperature for 3 h. Then the extract was centrifuged for 10 min at 3000 rpm and upper aqueous phase were transferred to new Eppndorf tubes. Moreover, the residues were again extracted with 5 ml 80% methanol overnight. The extraction was performed in three replicates, later on extracts combined and stored in dark at 4°C. The Folin-Ciocalteu reagent was used to determine the total phenolic compounds from the extracts using gallic acid calibration curve as standard. The total phenolics were expressed as mg/g gallic acid equivalents (GAE). An extract was aliquot (50 μl) and mixed with Folin-Ciocalteu reagent of 250 μl and 7.5% sodium carbonate of 750 μl. The volume was increased to 5 ml with water and sample was incubated for 2 h. The absorbance was measured at 765 nm against distilled water as blank. The flavonoid determination was measure by aluminum chloride method with the help of Quercetin equivalent as standard. An aliquot of extract (250 μl) was mixed with ddH2O and 5% $NaNO_2$ (15:1, v/v). After 6 min, 150 μl of 10% $AlCl_3$ was added to the mixture. A 500 μl of 1 M NaOH was added to the mixture at the 5th min, and volume made up to 2.5 ml with distills water and the absorbance was measured spectrophotometrically at 410 nm.

2.2.3. Gas chromatography-mass spectroscopy

The GC-MS analysis of fractions were performed using a TSQ™ 8000 Evo Triple Quadrupole GC-MS/MS (Thermo Fisher Scientific) equipped with an Elite-5 capillary column (length 30 nm and inner diameter 0.25 mm and film thickness 0.25 μm) and mass detector was operated in electron impact (EI) mode with full scan (50–550 amu). Helium was used as the carrier gas at constant flow rate 1 mL/min and an injection volume of 1 μL. The oven injector temperature was programmed from 50°C with an increase of 8°C/min to 200°C, then 7°C/min to 290°C/min. The results were compared using the database of National Institute Standard and Technology (NIST).

2.3. Data analysis

The data were subjected to descriptive statistics (mean, standard deviation, coefficient of variability, minimum and maximum values) and principal component analysis (PCA) using statistical software Past3 program [17].

3. Results and discussion

3.1. Proximate analysis

The proximate analysis values of 24 soybean genotypes (crude protein, ash fat, carbohydrate, and moisture contents) values and total phenolic and flavonoid contents are shown in **Table 2**, and the detailed proximate analysis estimates are presented in **Table S1**. The minimum crude protein value was recorded for Argentinian (35.63%), while maximum recorded for Clark genotypes (43.13%). The genotypes, i.e., Clark, Indo-1, Indo-black, Ijen, Romal-1, X 30 and 3803 recorded higher than 40% crude protein. The significant variations for crude proteins among genotypes were recorded and that might observed due to differences in genetic background and/or origin. The higher protein content in the genotypes is also reported previously which ranged from 43 to 45% [18]. These results are also in line with Zarkadas et al. [19, 20] who reported crude protein contents in soybean ranging from 33.67 to 42.11%. The minimum moisture contents were recorded in Giza 83 (3.08%) while maximum was recorded for Indo-1 (5.88%) with an average (4.90%) mean value showing non-significant difference. Ash contents ranged from 4.55 to 6.28% with an average of 5.44%. The maximum was recorded for Giza 111 (6.28%) genotype while Romal-1 genotype had the lowest (4.55%) of ash contents. The moisture and ash contents values were recorded lower than that reported by [21]. Total fat ranged from 16.92 to 22.94% with a mean value of 21.16%. The genotype Indo-black contained the lowest while the genotype 3803 recorded the highest content. Soybean is considered about 47% of its energy value in fat content [22, 23] which is compared to other legumes. Our results regarding total fat were in line with that of [24] who reported that that total fat value ranged 18 and 22 g/100 g in soybean genotypes. The minimum carbohydrate content in Clark (26.11%) while maximum in Argentinian (33.18%), with an average (29.48%) was recorded among soybean genotypes.

3.2. Flavonoid and phenolic contents

Flavonoid and phenolic compounds are the important phytochemicals and natural antioxidants founds in fruits, vegetable and cereals grains. It serves as multiple biological functions, i.e., defense against cardiovascular disease, cancer and aging [25]. The results regarding total phenolic and flavonoids contents for 24 soybean genotypes are presented in **Table S1**, and significant differences were recorded for all soybean genotypes. The seed extracted results indicated that the maximum phenolic contents was recorded in Romal-1 (1.7 mg/g) while minimum in Giza 111 (1.15 mg/g) with an average 1.45 GAE/g mg/g (**Table 2**). However, total flavonoid content ranged 0.68 to 2.13 mg QE/g (**Table 2**). Phenolic content is strongly linked with antioxidant capacity [26, 27] and can contribute towards antioxidants activities [28]. The use and demands of phenolic are increasing rapidly in food industry to enhance nutritional value and quality of food [29].

	Crude protein (g/100 g)	Moisture (g/100 g)	Ash (g/100 g)	Total fat (g/100 g)	Carbohydrate (g/100 g)	Total phenolic content (TPC)	Total flavonoid content (TFC)
N	24	24	24	24	24	24	24
Min	35.63	3.08	4.55	16.92	26.11	1.15	0.68
Max	43.13	5.88	6.28	23.61	33.18	1.77	2.13
Mean	39.02	4.90	5.44	21.16	29.48	1.45	1.24
Stand. dev.	2.09	0.65	0.33	1.41	1.86	0.16	0.36
Coeff. Var.	5.35	13.26	6.11	6.68	6.30	11.58	29.32

Table 2. Descriptive statistics of chemical composition in 24 soybean genotypes.

3.3. GC-MS analysis

Methanolic extracts of 24 soybean genotypes using GC-MS analysis were used to identify a large number of phytochemical. Based on peak area, retention time and molecular formula, about 88 compounds were recognized. A large number of bioactive phytochemicals including flavonoids, phenolic acids, saponins, isoflavones, sphingolipids and phytosterols were also reported previously for soybean [12–14]. The carbamide was the first compound that identified at 3.67 min retention time, whereas, last compound identified at 48.53 min retention time was methyl 10 Trans, 12-cisoctadecadienoate recognized at 48.53 min retention time (**Table S2**). A wide difference was recorded for composition of phytochemical in 24 soybean genotypes. The phytocompounds and their biological activities in soybean genotypes were presented in **Table 3**. The phytocompounds of the studied soybean genotypes divided into different groups (**Figure 1**). The resulted 88 compounds were categorized into heterocyclic compounds (19), aldehydes (5), alcohols (5), esters (13), amide (3), sugar moiety (7), ether (4),

	Compound	Other names	Nature	Activity	RT	MW
22	2H-1-Benzopyran,3,5,6,8a-tetrahydro-2,5,5,8a-tetramethyl-,(2S-cis)-	Edulan II	Heterocyclic compound		7.58	192
27	1,2-Cyclopentanedione		Ketone	Antioxidant	7.98	98
28	Pyran-4-Carboxylic acid, 4-(4-methoxyphenyl)-tetrahydro-		Heterocyclic compound		8.02	236
34	2,4-Dihydroxy-2,5-dimethyl-3(2H)-furan-3-one		Ketone		9.74	144
36	2H-Pyran-2,6(3H)-dione	Glutaconic anhydride	Heterocyclic compound		10.75	112
39	2-Pyrrolidinone, 1-methyl	M-Pyrol	Ketone		11.86	99
42	2,5-Dimethyl-4-hydroxy-3(2H)-furanone		Ketone		12.28	128
44	Phenol, 2-methoxy-		Phenolic compound	Antimicrobial, antioxidant, anti-inflammatory, analgesic	13.83	124
49	4H-Pyran-4-one,3-hydroxy-2-methyl-	Maltol	Heterocyclic compound	Flavor enhancer	14.78	126
50	5-Hepten-3-one, 5-methyl-		Ketone compound		15.09	126
52	3,5-Dihydroxy-6-methyl-2,3-dihydro-4H-pyran-4-one		Heterocyclic compound	Antimicrobial, anti-inflammatory	16.61	144
57	Phenol, 4-ethenyl-, acetate	4-Vinylphenyl acetate	Phenolic compound	Antimicrobial, antioxidant, anti-inflammatory	19.29	162
60	Benzofuran, 2,3-dihydro	Coumaran	Heterocyclic compound	Antihelminthic, anti-inflammatory, antidiarrheal	20.16	120
62	Benzeneacetaldehyde, 3-methyl	m-Tolualdehyde	Aldehyde	Antimicrobial	20.34	120

	Compound	Other names	Nature	Activity	RT	MW
61	1,2-Benzenediol,3-methoxy-	Pyrocatechol, 3-methoxy	Phenolic compound	Antioxidant	21.01	140
64	2-Methoxy-4-vinylphenol	Phenol, 4-ethenyl-2-methoxy-	Phenolic compound	Antimicrobial, antioxidant, anti-inflammatory	23.35	150
68	Phenol, 2,6-dimethoxy-	Pyrogallol 1,3-dimethyl ether	Phenolic compound	Antimicrobial, antioxidant, anti-inflammatory	24.99	154
70	Phenol,2,6-bis(1,1-dimethylethyl)-4-methyl-	Butylated hydroxytoluene	Phenolic compound	Antimicrobial, antioxidant, anti-inflammatory, analgesic	30.99	220
71	Phenol, 2,4-bis(1,1-dimethylethyl)-	Phenol, 2,4-di-tert-butyl-	Phenolic compound	Antimicrobial, antioxidant, anti-inflammatory	31.19	206
72	5-tert-Butyl-1,2,3-benzenetriol	5-Tert-butylpyrogallol	Phenolic compound	Antioxidant, antiseptic, antibacterial, anti-dermatitic fungicide, pesticide	31.91	182
76	3,5-Dimethoxyacetophenone		Ketone	Antioxidant	33.65	180
85	Hexadecanoic acid, methyl ester	Palmitic acid, methyl ester	Ester	Antioxidant, flavor, hypocholesterolemic, nematicide	46.13	270

Table 3. List of important phytocompounds identified in the methanolic seed extract of soybean genotypes by GC-MS.

phenolic compound (9), carboxylic acids (7), ketones (13), alkanes (2), one fatty acid ester and one Alkene. A typical chromatogram of one soybean genotype was shown in **Figure 2**. The GC-MS analyses showed that the methanolic extract is largely composed of heterocyclic compound, ester and phenolic compound. Hexadecanoic acid, methyl ester, 2,6-dimethoxy, 3,5-dimethoxyacetophenone, 2-methoxy-4-vinylphenol, phenol and 1,2-cyclopentanedione were noticed in most of the genotypes. These phytochemicals are involved in various pharmacological actions, i.e., antioxidants and antimicrobial activities [30]. These chemicals are also active in many biological activities that were listed (**Table S2**). Phytochemicals also possess antioxidant activities, anti-cancer, anticarcinogenic, antibacterial, antiviral, or anti-inflammatory activities and play an important role for plant metabolism [30, 31]. The five compounds belong to aldehyde group (benzeneacetaldehyde, 3,4-dimethylbenzaldehyde, methoxy-propanal, p-hydroxyphenyl, glyoxal and propanal, 2-(benzoyloxy)-, benzeneacetaldehyde), were detected in 10 genotypes (**Table S2**). Admiral and Williams 82 contains 3-methoxy-propanal while indo-black, Indo-1 and Indo-II contains 3,4-dimethylbenzaldehyde, whereas Giza 35 and X30 contains p-hydroxyphenyl) glyoxal and propanal, 2-benzoyloxy, respectively. The highest number of aldehyde compounds is present in William 82 genotype (2). It is also reported that; aldehyde possess powerful antimicrobial activity due to their highly electronegative arrangement of conjugated group C=C double bond [32], as the electronegativity increase, antimicrobial activity also increases in those genotypes [33, 34]. These compounds react with vital nitrogen components such as protein and nucleic acid, consequently inhibit microorganism. Thirteen ketone related compounds were identified, i.e., 1-(dimethylamino)-,

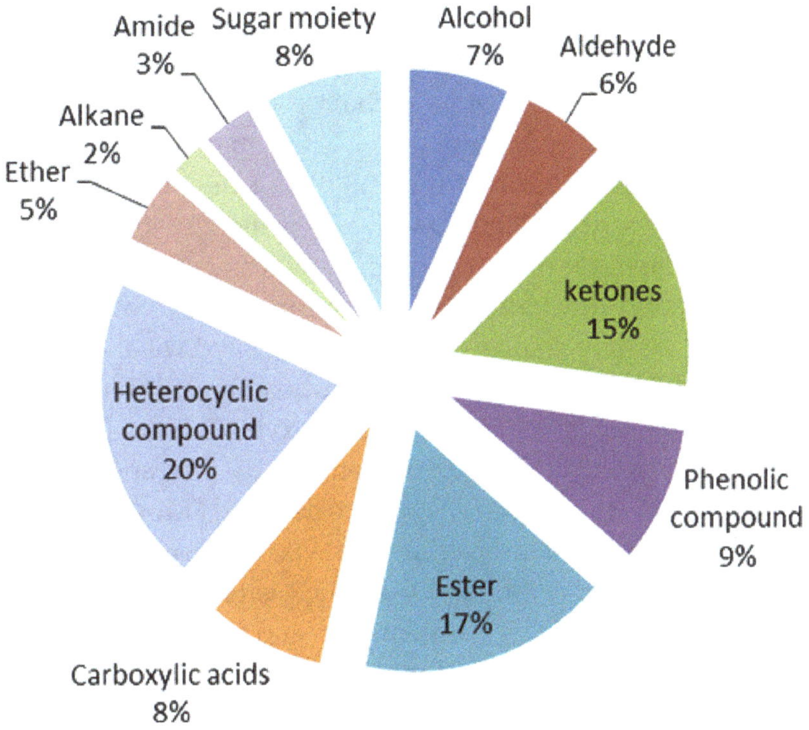

Figure 1. Pie diagram showing the percentage of phytochemical groups identified in 24 soybean genotypes.

1,2-propanone, 1,2-cyclopentanedione and 6-Oxa-bicyclo [3.1.0] hexan-3-one, 2,4-dihydroxy-2,5-dimethyl-3(2H)-furan-3-one,2-acetyl-2,3,5,6-tetrahydro-1,4-thiazine,butyrolactone, 2,5-Dimethyl-4-hydroxy-3(2H)-furanone, 5-hepten-3-one, 5-methyl-, dihydroxyacetone, 2-pyrrolidinone, 1-methyl, 2,4,6,-cycloheptatrien-1-one,4-methyl-, 3,5-dimethoxyacetophenone. The indo-11 and 3803 genotypes recorded highest ketonic compounds (8) followed by present in Giza 35 and USA-1 genotypes that contained 6ketonic group each. Ketones might be formed by beta-oxidation of fatty acid and have some important flavor compounds [35]. During fatty

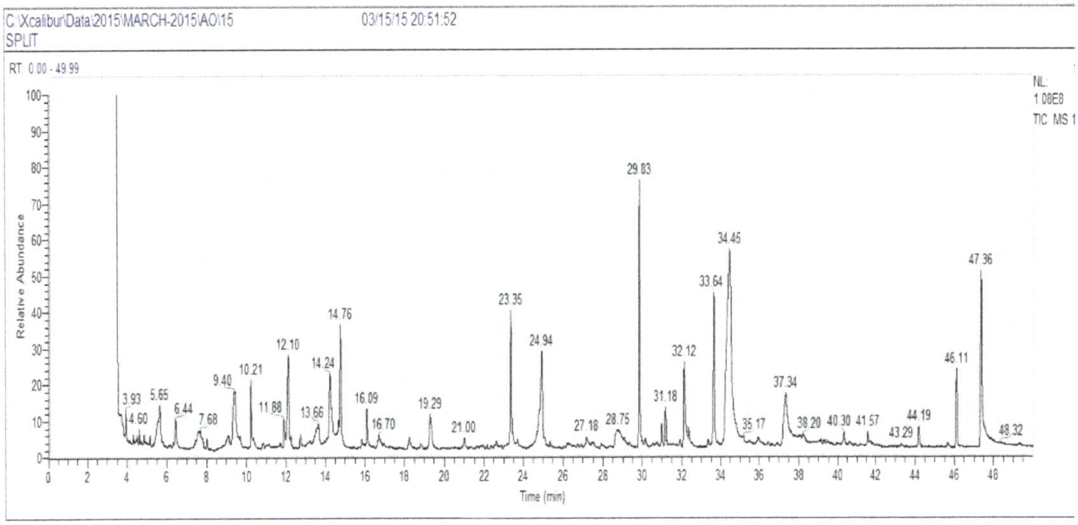

Figure 2. A typical GC-MS profile of seeds of soybean genotype.

acid metabolism, many volatile compounds are also formed, producing alcohols, acids and esters. Many alcoholic compounds are derived from bioremediation of unsaturated fatty acids and are prerequisite for the formation of long chain esters. These identified compounds in soybean genotypes are 4-methyl-2-haptanol, 1,2,3-propanetriol, isosorbide (D-glucitol, 1,4,3,6-dianhydro), 1-undecanol alcohol, and 1,3-dioxolane-4-methanol (glycerol formal). 4-Methyl-2-haptanol was present in Genotype Giza 35 while 1,2,3-propanetriol was present in nine genotypes and isosorbide was detected in three soybean genotypes. The highest alcoholic compounds (3) were detected in Clark genotype as compared to other genotypes. Alcohols also possess antibacterial activity against vegetative cell. Glycerol and derivatives also show bacterial inhibiting effect [36]. The following seven carboxylic acids namely acetic acid, 2-pyridinecarboxylic acid (also called picolinic acid), 2,2-[oxybis(2,1-ethanediyloxy)]bis, butanoic acid, 4-hydroxy-, propyl-(also called 2-propylmalonic acid), propanedioic acid, benzoic acid, butanoic acid, 4,4-dithiobis[2-amino-,[S-(R/,R/)] were detected (**Table S2**). Five genotypes were having acetic acid and 2-pyridinecarboxylic acid was present in five genotypes. Three genotypes have butanoic acid and 4-hydroxy-was appeared in three genotypes while one genotype has benzoic acid. Giza 35, X30, Argentinian and Chinese compassed the maximum numbers of carboxylic acids compounds. Thirteen esters were identified. The butyrolactone, acetic acid, 2-(dimethylamino)ethyl ester, formic acid, 3-methylbut-2-yl ester, pentanoic acid, 2-isopropoxyphenyl ester, phthalic acid, hex-3-yl-isobutyl ester, hexadecanoic acid, methyl ester, phthalic acid, butyl undecyl ester, 5,8,11-heptadecatriynoic acid methyl ester, methyl 10-trans, 12-cis-octadecadienoate, 9,12-octadecadienoic acid(Z,Z)-methyl ester, benzoic acid, 4-ethoxy-, ethyl ester, 1,2-benzenedicarboxylic acid, dibutyl ester, and pentanoic acid, 2,2-4-trimethyl-3-carboxyisopropyl, isobutyl, ester were identified. The genotype A-1 had maximum six esters compounds followed by others genotypes (Giza 83, Romal-1, Clark, Argentinian and 3803) having five (5) esters compounds. Hexadecanoic acid ethyl ester shows antioxidant, nematicidal activities and hypocholesterolemic [37]. Regarding phenolic compound, a total of nine compounds were identified. 1,2-benzenediol,3-methoxy-, 5-tert-butyl-1,2,3-benzenetriol, phenol, 4-ethenyl-, acetate, phenol, 2,6-dimethoxy-, 2-methoxy-4-vinylphenol, phenol,2,6-bis(1,1-dimethylethyl)-4-methy l-, phenol, 2,4-bis(1,1-dimethylethyl)-, and phenol, 2-methoxy. The genotypes Indo-1 and Ijen and recorded the highest number of phenolic compounds which is five while the genotypes Clark, NARC-2, Giza 35, USA-1 and Indo-11 contained the four (4) phenolic compounds each. The plant phenolics compounds are of great interest to human due to their anti-oxidative and possible anticarcinogenic activities. The dietary phenolics are considered anti-carcinogens because of antioxidants, but there is no clear proof supporting this supposition [38]. Phenolic may inhibit carcinogenesis by interfering the molecular events in initiation, promotion, and progression stages. Isoflavones and lignans from soybean may distract tumor formation by mediating estrogen-related activities and also modulate the growth of benign and malignant prostatic epithelial cells in vitro [39]. The following sugar moiety, L-galactose, 6-deoxy-, 3,4-0-isopropylidene-d-galactose, a-methyl-D-m annopyranoside, 3-O-methyl-d-glucose a-D-galactopyranoside, methyl were appeared among soybean studied genotypes. The relatively notable amounts of heterocyclic compounds were identified including 3,5-dihydroxy-6-methyl-2, 2,6-diisoprpylnapthalene, 4H-pyran-4-one, 3-dihydro-4Hpyran-4-one, 3-hydroxy-2-methyl-, pyrazine, ethyl-, oxirane, 2-ethyl-2-methyl, 1H-indazole, 4,5,6,7-tetrahydro, N-aminomorpholine, and benzofuran, 2,3-dihydro. The genotype X30 had four sugars compounds while genotypes USA-1, Indo-1, and Indo-11 had three sugars compounds each. Benzofurans are considered to possess anti-oxidant, antimicrobial effect and anti-inflammatory [40]. The compounds detected in this study have reported to have potentials as therapeutic agents, antioxidant, antimicrobial, and anti-inflammatory compounds and demonstrating that different compounds can exhibit similar activity and this might be due to presence of similar functional groups (**Table S2**). Antioxidant properties of soybean extract could be the basis for the presence of various antioxidant and anti-inflammatory compounds.

3.4. Principal component analysis (PCA)

The first three principal components explained 78.64% of total variations among genotypes (**Table 4** and **Figure 3**). The first component described 59.65% of total variation, and positively correlated with phytochemical classes of ether, alcohol, sugar moiety ketone and phenolic compounds. Genotypes Ijen, Clark, A-1, USA-1, Indo-II, 3803, X 30, Giza 35, Indo-black and Indo-I showed the most variability according to these components and can be selected for these classes. PC2 illustrated 10.63% of the total variance, and the amide, sugar moiety, ether, alkane, ketone and carboxylic acid positively correlated with this component. The genotypes showed most variability were Giza 111, Giza 35, X 30, X 32, Indo-II and 3803. Alkane, Aldehyde, Carboxylic acid and Phenolic compound were positively correlated with the third component. The genotypes Giza 35, X 32 showed most variability based on this component. In this study, genotypes Giza 35, X 30, Indo-II and genotype 3803 showed positive loading in at least two out of the three PCs, which can be utilized in breeding for ceratin class of phytochemical. Utilizing PCA effectively reduces the number of variables needed to classify cultivars

	PC 1	PC 2	PC 3
Eigen values	0.17	0.03	0.02
Percent of variance	59.65	10.63	8.36
Cumulative percentage	59.65	70.28	78.64
Alcohol	0.42	0.11	−0.12
Aldehyde	−0.14	0.00	0.24
Alkane	−0.01	0.29	0.75
Amide	−0.59	0.67	−0.28
Sugar moiety	0.39	0.44	−0.06
Carboxylic acid	0.03	0.06	0.31
Ester	0.12	−0.25	−0.26
Ether	0.45	0.34	0.02
Heterocyclic compound	0.05	0.14	−0.16
Ketone	0.27	0.21	−0.18
Phenolic compound	0.11	−0.09	0.24

Table 4. Eigen values and proportion of the variance explained for the three principal components of the 24 soybean genotypes based on phytochemical components.

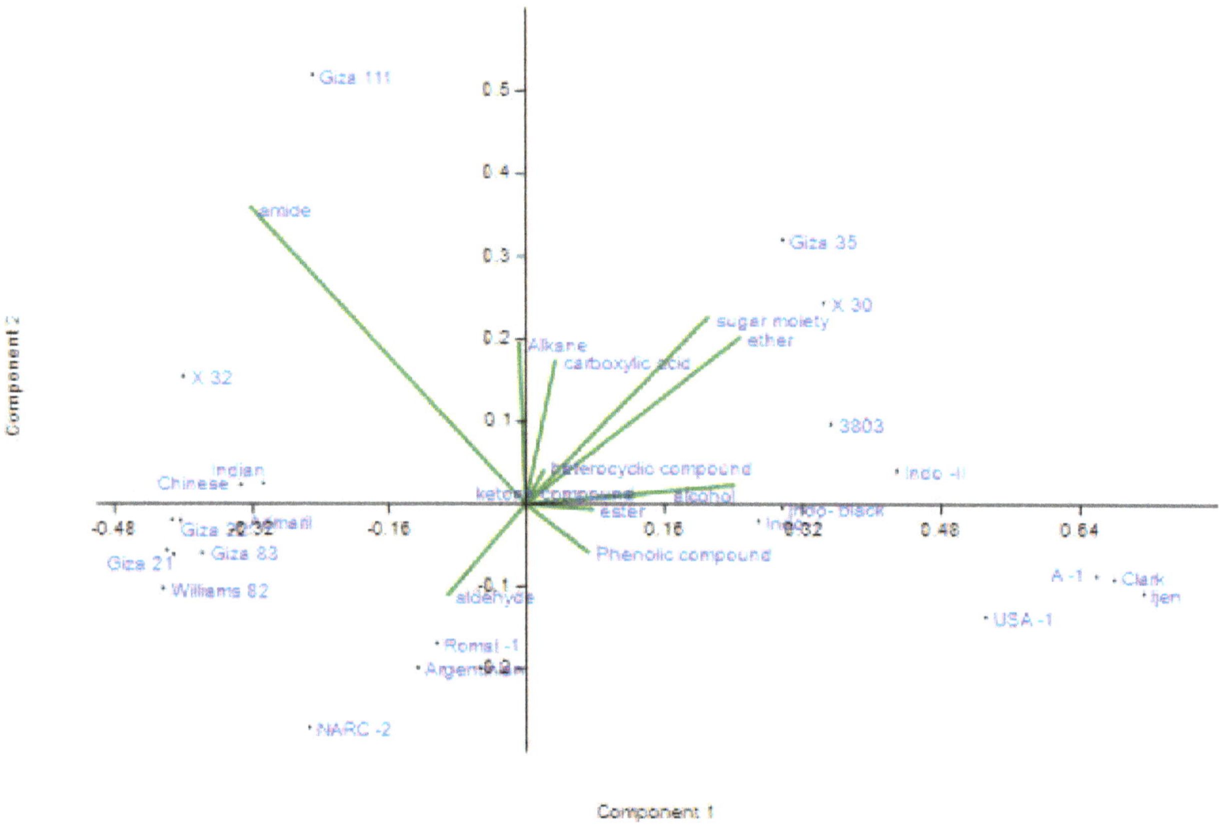

Figure 3. Two-dimensional biplot ordination of 24 soybean genotypes on principal component axes according to 11 phytochemical classes.

and permitted soybean researchers to more easily develop significant relationships between important soybean characteristics. Soybean cultivars have been classified using (PCA) of the fatty acid data [41]. The first four principal components generated in total 81.49% of the variance, where PC1 positively correlated with oleic, linoleic, and gondoic acids, PC2 with stearic, linolenic and arachidic acids, PC3 behenic and lignoceric acids, and PC4 by palmitic acid. Moreover, due to the ability of PCA to manage and interpret large data sets, it has been used in studying relationships that exist in fatty acid characterization [42]. Although soybean oil has been included in some chemometric studies comparing vegetable oils, soybean cultivars have yet to be extensively classified using multivariate techniques [43, 44].

4. Conclusion

The results revealed that soybean genotypes cover variable patterns of total proteins flavonoids, phenolic and various bioactive volatile compounds. The mass spectrometry analysis results demonstrated that, majority of soybean genotypes are a source bioactive compounds with antioxidant, anti-inflammatory, antimicrobial and other functions. 2-Methoxy-4-vinylphenol, phenol, 2,6-dimethoxy-, 3,5-dimethoxyacetophenone, hexadecanoic acid methyl ester, 1,2-cyclopentanedione, and 3,5-dihydroxy-6-methyl-2,3-dihydro-4H-pyran-4-one were present in majority of genotypes. However, the genotypes Ijen and Indo-1 contributed more phenolic compound than others genotype. Genotype A-1 has the maximum compound in esters compounds. The genotypes Indo-11 and 3803 contribute maximum ketone compounds while Giza 111 contributes more in heterocyclic compounds. Some genotypes may have good therapeutic potential and could be served as a potential source in drug wdevelopment as a health supplement. This study also provides a platform for isolating and understanding the properties of each compound for it pharmacological properties.

A. Appendix (supplementary materials)

Genotype name	Crude protein (g/100 g)	Moisture (g/100 g)	Ash (g/100 g)	Total fat (g/100 g)	Carbohydrate (g/100 g)	Total phenolic content mg/g	Total flavonoid content mg/g
Admaril	37.84	4.56	5.27	21.65	30.68	1.30	0.975
Romal-1	40.93	4.79	4.55	20.35	29.38	1.75	1
NARC-2	38.01	4.84	5.79	21.16	30.2	1.50	1.25
Williams 82	38.23	4.97	5.65	22.79	28.36	1.42	1.05
X 32	39.8	4.31	5.54	21.04	29.31	1.25	0.875
Holladay	37.04	4.35	5.55	23.61	29.45	1.35	0.75
Giza 22	39.82	4.45	5.55	21.91	28.27	1.37	0.675
Giza 21	39.84	4.4	5.56	21.72	28.48	1.40	0.8
X2 L 12	38.26	4.26	5.29	21.96	30.23	1.42	1.2
Giza 83	38.29	3.08	5.39	21.42	31.82	1.38	0.925
Crawford	39.43	4.84	5.58	22.38	27.77	1.30	1.125
Giza 35	38.8	3.77	5.49	21.78	30.16	1.32	1.025
X 30	40.05	4.99	5.64	21.78	27.54	1.70	1.0375
Giza 111	36.89	5.34	6.28	22.07	29.42	1.15	1.75
Clark	43.13	5.41	5.77	19.58	26.11	1.35	1.375
3803	40	5.12	5.45	22.94	26.49	1.33	1.625
A - 1	39.01	5.19	4.8	20.69	30.31	1.37	1.45
Ijen	41.7	5.54	5.54	18.66	28.56	1.65	1.25
Indo-black	42.71	5.88	5.36	16.92	29.13	1.65	1.025
Indo-I	42.74	5.88	5.7	19.33	26.35	1.62	1.775
Indo-II	37.87	5.51	5.14	21.17	30.31	1.32	1.375
USA-1	36.89	5.34	5.24	21.34	31.19	1.77	2.125
Indian	36.59	5.43	5.25	20.88	31.85	1.65	1.7625
Chinese	35.98	5.19	5.26	21.06	32.51	1.50	1.35
Argentinian	35.63	5.12	5.3	20.77	33.18	1.37	1.325

Table S1. Proximate analysis, total phenolic and flavonoid in the seeds of 24 soybean genotypes seeds (on a dry weight basis).

Sr. no	Compound	Other name	Nature	Activity	RT	MW
1	Carbamide	Urea	Amide		3.67	60
2	Propanal, 3-methoxy	3-Methoxy-propanal	Aldehyde	Antibacterial	3.75	88
3	n-Hexane		Alkane	Antibacterial	3.8	86
4	Acetamide, oxime		Amide	Antimicribial	3.86	74
5	1,2-Naphthalenedione, 4 chloro		Heterocyclic compound		3.92	192
6	1,3-Dioxolane-4-methanol	Glycerol formal	Alcohol		3.93	104
7	1-Monolinoleoyglycerol trimethylsilyl ether		Ether		4.02	498
8	Acetic acid		Carboxylic acid		4.17	60
9	Acetic acid, 2,2-[oxybis(2,1-ethanediyloxy)]bis	(2-[2-(Carboxymethoxy)ethoxy] ethoxy)acetic acid	Carboxylic acid		4.24	222
10	Ethyl(dimethyl)isopropoxysilane	Ethyl(dimethyl)silyl isopropyl ether	Ether		4.54	146
11	Silane, triethylmethoxy-	Methyl trethylsilyl ether	Ether		4.6	146
12	Butanoic acid, 4,4-dithiobis[2-amino-,[S-(R*,R*)]		Carboxylic acid		4.73	268
13	2-Pyridinecarboxylic acid	Picolinic acid	Carboxylic acid	Natural chelator	4.73	123
14	2-Propanone, 1-(dimethylamino)-	(Dimethylamino)acetone	Ketone compound		4.89	101
15	2,2-Bioxirane	Butane1,2:3,4-diepoxy-	Heterocyclic compound		4.92	86
16	Cyclotrisiloxane, hexamethyl	Dimethylsiloxane cyclic trimer	Heterocyclic compound		5.3	222
17	Pyrimidine, 2-methyl-	2-Methylpyrimidine	Heterocyclic compound		5.61	94
18	L-Galactose, 6-deoxy-	6-Deoxyhexose	Sugar moiety	Preservative	6.39	164
19	2-Propenamide	Acrylamide	Amide		6.43	71
20	1,2,4-Triazole, 4-(4-methoxybenzylidenamino)-5-methyl-3-(3,5-dimethylpyrazol-1-yl		Heterocyclic compound		7.54	310

Sr. no	Compound	Other name	Nature	Activity	RT	MW
21	Acetic acid, 2-(dimethylamino)ethyl ester	Dimethylaminoethanol acetate	Ester		7.57	131
22	2H-1-Benzopyran, 3,5,6,8a-tetrahydro-2,5,5,8a-tetramethyl-,(2S-cis)-	Edulan II	Heterocyclic compound		7.58	192
23	Pyrazine, ethyl-	Ethylpyrazine	Heterocyclic compound		7.67	108
24	Oxirane, 2-ethyl-2-methyl	Butane, 1,2-epoxy-2-methyl	Heterocyclic compound		7.77	86
25	Butyrolactone		Ketone compound		7.88	86
26	4-Methyl-2-haptanol		Alcohol		7.96	130
27	1,2-Cyclopentanedione		Ketone compound	Antioxidant	7.98	98
28	Pyran-4-carboxylic acid, 4-(4-methoxyphenyl)-tetrahydro-		Heterocyclic compound		8.02	236
29	6-Oxa-bicyclo[3.1.0]hexan-3-one		Ketone compound		8.09	98
30	Dihydroxyacetone	2-Propanone, 1,3-dihydroxy-	Ketone compound		8.18	90
31	Butanoic acid, 4-hydroxy-		Carboxylic acid		8.54	104
32	Propanedioic acid, Propyl-	2-Propylmalonic acid	Carboxylic acid		9.1	146
33	1,2,3-Propanetriol	Glycerin	Alcohol		9.33	92
34	2,4-Dihydroxy-2,5-dimethyl-3(2H)-furan-3-one		Ketone compound		9.74	144
35	Oxirane, [(2-propenyloxy)methyl}-	Propane, 1-(allyloxy)2,3-epoxy-	Heterocyclic compound		10.26	114
37	HEPES[4-(2-Hydroxyethyl)-1-piperazineethanesuffonic acis)]		Heterocyclic compound		10.26	238

Sr. no	Compound	Other name	Nature	Activity	RT	MW
37	2H-Pyran-2,6(3H)-dione	Glutaconic anhydride	Heterocyclic compound		10.75	112
38	1H-Indazole, 4,5, 6, 7-tetrahydro		Heterocyclic compound		11.54	122
39	2-Pyrrolidinone, 1-methyl	M-Pyrol	Ketone compound		11.86	99
40	Benzeneacetaldehyde		Aldehyde	Antibacterial	12	120
41	2,4,6,-Cycloheptatrien-1-one,4-methyl-		Ketone compound		12.06	120
42	2,5-Dimethyl-4-hydroxy-3(2H)-furanone		Ketone compound		12.28	128
43	a-D-Glucopyranoside, O-a-D-glucopyranosyl-(1. fwdarw.3)-a-D-fructofuranosyl		Sugar moiety		12.81	504
44	Phenol, 2-methoxy-		Phenolic compound	Antimicrobial, antioxidant, anti-inflammatory, analgesic	13.83	124
46	Formic acid, 3-methylbut-2-yl ester		Ester		14.24	116
45	1-Butanol,3-methyl-, formate (isopentyl alcohol, formate)	Isopentyl alcohol, formate	Fatty acid ester	Antimicrobial activity	14.24	116
47	1,5-Hexadien-3-ol		Alkene		14.36	98
48	Cyclopentane, (1,1-dimethylethyl)-{Tert-Butylcyclopentane}	Tert-Butylcyclopentane	Alkane	Antibacterial	14.68	126
49	4H-Pyran-4-one,3-hydroxy-2-methyl-	Maltol	Heterocyclic compound	Flavor enhancer	14.78	126
50	5-Hepten-3-one, 5-methyl-		Ketone compound		15.09	126
51	2-Acetyl-2,3,5,6-tetrahydro-1,4-thiazine	1-(3-Thiomorpholinylethanone	Ketone compound		15.85	145
52	3,5-Dihydroxy-6-methyl-2,3-dihydro-4H-pyran-4-one		Heterocyclic compound	Antimicrobial, anti-inflammatory, anti-proliferative	16.61	144

Sr. no	Compound	Other name	Nature	Activity	RT	MW
53	Propanal, 2-(benzoyloxy)-,®	1-Methyl-2-oxoethyl benzoate	Aldehyde		16.69	178
54	Benzoic Acid		Carboxylic acid		16.76	122
55	N-aminomorpholine	4-Aminomorpholine	Heterocyclic compound		16.95	102
56	Pentanoic acid, 2-isopropoxyphenyl ester	2-Isopropoxyphenyl pentanoate	Ester		18.26	236
57	Phenol, 4-ethenyl-, acetate	4-Vinylphenyl acetate	Phenolic compound	Antimicrobial, antioxidant, anti-inflammatory, analgesic	19.29	162
58	Benzaldehyde, 3,4-dimethyl-	3,4-dimethylbenzaldehyde	Aldehyde	Antibacterial	19.3	134
59	Benzene, (ethenyloxy)-	Ether, phenyl vinyl	Ether		19.31	120
60	Benzofuran, 2,3-dihydro	Coumaran	Heterocyclic compound	Antihelminthic, anti-inflammatory, anti-diarrhoeal	20.16	120
61	Benzeneacetaldehyde, 3-methyl	m-Tolualdehyde	Aldehyde	Antimicrobial	20.34	120
62	1,2-Benzenediol,3-methoxy	Pyrocatechol, 3-methoxy	Phenolic compound	Antioxidant	21.01	140
63	Isosorbide	D-Glucitol, 1,4,3,6-dianhydro	Alcohol		22.61	146
64	2-Methoxy-4-vinylphenol	phenol, 4-ethenyl-2-methoxy-	Phenolic compound	Antimicrobial, antioxidant, anti-inflammatory, analgesic	23.35	150
65	(p-Hydroxyphenyl)glyoxal	Benzeneacetaldehyde, 4-hydroxy-a-0x0	Aldehyde	Antibacterial	23.71	150
66	2-Acetamido-2-deoxy-d-mannolactone		Sugar moiety	Anti-bacterial	24.8	217
67	Phenol, 2,6-dimethoxy-	Pyrogallol 1,3-dimethyl ether	Phenolic compound	Antimicrobial, antioxidant, anti-inflammatory, analgesic	24.99	154
68	1-Undecanol alcohol	Undecyl alcohol	Alcohol		29.83	172
69	Phenol,2,6-bis(1,1-dimethylethyl)-4-methyl-	Butylated hydroxytoluene	Phenolic compound	Antimicrobial, antioxidant, anti-inflammatory, analgesic	30.99	220
70	Phenol, 2,4-bis(1,1-dimethylethyl)-	Phenol, 2,4-di-tert-butyl-	Phenolic compound	Antimicrobial, antioxidant, anti-inflammatory, analgesic	31.19	206

Sr. no	Compound	Other name	Nature	Activity	RT	MW
71	5-Tert-butyl-1,2,3-benzenetriol	5-Tert-butylpyrogallol	Phenolic compound	Antioxidant, antiseptic antibacterial, anti-dermatitic fungicide, pesticide	31.91	182
72	Benzoic acid, 4-ethoxy-, ethyl ester		Ester		32.12	194
73	3,4-0-Isopropylidene-d-galactose	3,4,0-(1-Methylethylidene) hexopyranose	Sugar moiety	Preservative	32.35	220
74	Pentanoic acid, 2,2-4-trimethyl-3-carboxyisopropyl,isobutyl ester		Ester		32.97	286
75	3,5-Dimethoxyacetophenone		Ketone compound	antioxidant	33.65	180
76	a-Methyl-D-mannopyranoside		Sugar moiety	Preservative	34.35	194
77	a-D-Galactopyranoside, methyl	Galactopyranoside, methyl, a-D-	Sugar moiety	Preservative	34.61	194
78	3-O-methyl-d-glucose	3-O-methylhexose	Sugar moiety	Preservative	37.68	194
79	2,6-Diisopropylnapthalene		Hetercyclic compound		37.71	212
80	Dodecyl acrylate	n-Lauryl acrylate	Ester		38.17	240
81	Cyclopenta [1,3][cyclopropa [1,2]cyclohepten-3(3ah)one, 1,2,3b,6,7,8-hexahydro-6,6-dimethyl-		Ketone compound		40.31	190
82	5-Tert.butyloxy carboxamido-2,3,3-trimethyl-3H-indole	Tert-butyl 2, 3,3-trimethyl-3H-indole-5-ylcarbamate	Heterocyclic compound		41.6	274
83	Phthalic acid, hex-3-yl-isobutyl ester		Ester		42.4	306
84	Hexadecanoic acid, methyl ester	Palmitic acid, methyl ester	Ester	Antioxidant, flavor, hypocholesterolemic, nematicide	46.13	270
85	5,8, 11-Heptadecatriynoic acid methyl ester		Ester		46.2	272
86	Phthalic acid, butyl undecyl ester		Ester		47.36	376
87	1,2-Benzenedicarboxylic acid, dibutyl ester	Dibutyl phthalate	Ester	Plasticizer, antimicrobial, antifouling	47.37	278
88	Methyl 10 trans, 12-cis-octadecadienoate		Ester		48.53	294

Table S2. List and basic features of identified phytocomponents in the methanolic extract of soybean genotypes by GCMS analysis.

Acknowledgements

The authors of this project in number AT-34-58 are highly appreciated the encouragement and the assistances provided by the King Abdulaziz City for Science and Technology.

Conflict of interest

The authors have declared that no conflict of interest exists.

Author details

Salem Alghamdi[1], Hussein Migdadi[1*], Muhammad Khan[1], Ehab H. El-Harty[1], Megahed Ammar[2], Muhammad Farooq[1,3,4] and Muhammad Afzal[1]

*Address all correspondence to: h.migdadi@gmail.com

1 Legume Research Group, Plant Production Department, Faculty of Food and Agricultural Sciences, King Saud University, Riyadh, Saudi Arabia

2 Rice Research and Training Center, Kafr El Sheikh, Egypt

3 Department of Agronomy, University of Agriculture, Faisalabad, Pakistan

4 Department of Crop Sciences, College of Agricultural and Marine Sciences, Sultan Qaboos University, Al-Khoud, Oman

References

[1] FAOSTAT. Food and Agriculture Organization of the United Nations. 2016. Available from http://www.fao.org/statistics/en [Accessed: March, 2018]

[2] Acquaah G. Breeding soybean. In: Acqaah G, editor. Principles of Plant Genetics and Breeding Book. Malden, MA, USA: Blackwell Publishing Ltd; 2007. p. 519

[3] Lim TK. Edible Medicinal and Non-Medicinal Plants. Vol. 2, Fruits. New York: Springer Science, Business Media B.V; 2012

[4] Gupta SK. Technological Innovations in Major World Oil Crops. New York, USA: Springer; 2012

[5] Probst H, Judd RW. Origin, US history and development, and world distribution. In: Caldwell BE, editor. Soybean, Improvement, Production, and Uses. Madison, USA: American Soci ety of Agronomy; 1973. pp. 1-15

[6] Schmutz J, Cannon S, Schlueter J, Ma J, Mitros T, Nelson W, Hyten DL, Song Q, Thelen J, Cheng A, et al. Genome sequence of the paleopolyploid soybean. Nature. 2010;**463**:178-183

[7] Pratap A, Gupta SK, Kumar J, Solanki RK, Soybean. In: Gupta SK, editor. Technological Innovations in Major World Oil Crops, Vol. 1: Breeding. New York: Springer Science Business Media; 2012. pp. 293-321. DOI: 10.1007/978-1-4614-0356-2_12

[8] El-Shemy H, Soybean. Nutrition and health. In: El-Shemy, editor. Soybean-BioActive Compounds. Rijeka: InTech; 2013. pp. 453-473

[9] Chung HY. Volatile components in fermented soybean (*Glycine max*) curds. Journal of Agricultural and Food Chemistry. 1999;**47**(7):2690-2696

[10] Chung HY, Fung PK, Kim JS. Aroma impact components in commercial plain sufu. Journal of Agricultural and Food Chemistry. 2005;**53**(5):1684-1691

[11] Messina M. Soybean isoflavone exposure does not have feminizing effects on men, a critical examination of the clinical evidence. Fertility and Sterility. 2010;**93**:2095-2104

[12] Luthria DL, Biswas R, Natarajan S. Comparison of extraction solvents and techniques used for the assay of isoflavones from soybean. Food Chemistry. 2007;**105**:325-333

[13] Lee SJ, Kim JJ, Moon HI, Ahn JK, Chun SC, Jung WS, Lee OK, Chung IM. Analysis of isoflavones and phenolic compounds in Korean soybean *Glycine max* (L.) seeds of different seed weights. Journal of Agricultural and Food Chemistry. 2008;**56**:2751-2758

[14] Gutierrez E, Wang T, Fehr WR. Quantification of sphingolipids in soybeans. Journal of the American Oil Chemists' Society. 2004;**81**:737-742

[15] AOAC, editor. Official Methods of Analysis of the AOAC. 15th ed. Washington DC, USA: AOAC International; 1990

[16] Markham R. Distillation apparatus suitable for micro-Kjeldahl analysis. The Biochemical Journal. 1942;**36**:970-791

[17] Hammer O, Harper DA, Ryan PD. PAST, paleontological statistics software package for education and data analysis. Palaeontologia Electronica. 2001;**4**:1-9

[18] Machado FP, Queróz JH, Oliveira MG, Piovesan ND, Peluzio MC, Costa NMB, et al. Effects of heating on protein quality of soybean flour devoid of Kunitz inhibitor and lectin. Food Chemistry. 2008;**107**:649-655

[19] Zarkadas CG, Yu ZR, Voldeng HD, Minero-Amador A. Assessment of the protein quality of a new high-protein soybean cultivar by amino acid analysis. Journal of Agricultural and Food Chemistry. 1993;**41**:616-623

[20] Zarkadas CG, Voldeng HD, Yu ZR, Choi V. Assessment of the protein quality of nine northern adapted yellow and brown seed coated soybean cultivars by amino acid analysis. Journal of Agricultural and Food Chemistry. 1999;**47**:5009-5018

[21] Monteiro MR, Costa NM, Oliveira MG, Pires CV, Moreira MA. Qualidade proteica de linhagens de soja com ausência do inibidor de tripsina kunitz e das isoenzimas lipoxigenases. Revista de Nutrição. 2004;**17**:195-205

[22] Liu K. Chemistry and nutritional value of soybean components. In: Liu K, editor. Soybeans, Chemistry, Technology and Utilization. New York, USA: Chapman & Hall; 1997. pp. 25-113

[23] Messina M. Legumes and soybeans, overview of their nutritional profiles and health effects. The American Journal of Clinical Nutrition. 1999;**70**:439-450

[24] Guillon F, Champ MM. Carbohydrate fractions of legumes, uses in human nutrition and potential for health. The British Journal of Nutrition. 2002;**8**:293-306

[25] Karimi E, Oskoueian E, Hendra R, Jaafar HZ. Evaluation of *Crocus sativus* L. stigma phenolic and flavonoid compounds and its antioxidant activity. Molecules. 2010;**15**:6244-6256

[26] Zheng W, Wang SY. Antioxidant activity and phenolic compounds in selected herbs. Journal of Agricultural and Food Chemistry. 2001;**49**:5165-5170

[27] Skerget M, Kotnik P, Hadolin M, Hras AR, Simonic M, Knez Z. Phenols, proanthocyanidins, flavones and flavonols in some plant materials and their antioxidant activities. Food Chemistry. 2005;**89**:191-198

[28] Duh PD, Tu YY, Yen GC. Antioxidative activity of water extracts of Harng Jyur (*Chrysanthemum morifolium*). Journal of Food Science and Technology. 1999;**32**:269-277

[29] Aneta W, Jan O, Renate C. Antioxidant activity and phenolic compounds in 32 selected herbs. Food Chemistry. 2007;**105**:940-949

[30] Tapiero H, Tew KD, Nguyen BG, Mathe G. Polyphenols, do they play a role in the prevention of human pathologies? Biomedicine & Pharmacotherapy. 2002;**56**:200-207

[31] Wei Y, Liu ZQ, Liu ZL. Antioxidant effect of coumarin derivatives on free radical initiated and photosensitized peroxidation of linoleic acid in micelles. Journal of the Chemical Society, Perkin Transactions. 1999;**2**:969-974

[32] Moleyar V, Narasimham P. Antifungal activity of some essential oil components. Food Microbiology. 1986;**3**:331-336

[33] Kurita N, Miyaji M, Kurane R. Antifungal activity and molecular orbital energies of aldehyde compounds from oils of higher plants. Agricultural and Biological Chemistry. 1979;**43**:2365-2371

[34] Kurita N, Miyaji M, Kurane R, Takahara Y. Antifungal activity of components of essential oils. Agricultural and Biological Chemistry. 1981;**45**:945-952

[35] Yu AN, Sun BG, Tian DT, Qu WY. Analysis of volatile compounds in traditional smoke-cured bacon (CSCB) with different fibber coatings using SPME. Food Chemistry. 2008;**110**:233-238

[36] Saegeman VS, Ectors NL, Lismont D, Verduykt B, Verhaegen J. Short and long term bacterial inhibiting effect of high concentration of glycerol used in preservation of skin allografts. Burns. 2008;**34**:205-211

[37] Priya K, Vijaylakshmi VK. Determination of bioactive components of *Cynodon dactylon* by GC-MS analysis. New York Science Journal. 2011;**4**:16-20

[38] Yang CS, Landau JM, Huang MT, Newmark HL. Inhibition of carcinogenesis by dietary polyphenolic compounds. Annual Review of Nutrition. 2001;**21**:381-406

[39] Hedlund TE, Johannes WU, Miller GJ. Soy isoflavonoid equol modulates the growth of benign and malignant prostatic epithelial cells in vitro. The Prostate. 2003;**54**:68-78

[40] Kamal M, Shakya AK, Jawid T. Benzofurans: A new profile of biological activities. International Journal of Medicine and Pharmaceutical Sciences. 2011;**1**:1-15

[41] Shin E, Hwang CE, Lee BW, Kim HT, Ko JM, Baek IY, Lee Y, Choi J, Cho EJ, Seo WT, Cho KM. Chemometric approach to fatty acid profiles in soybean cultivars by principal component analysis (PCA). Preventive Nutrition and Food Science. 2012;**17**:184-191

[42] Brodnjak-Voncina D, Kodba ZC, Novic M. Multivariate data analysis in classification of vegetable oils characterized by the content of fatty acids. Chemometrics and Intelligent Laboratory Systems. 2005;**75**:31-43

[43] Zagonel GF, Peralta-Zamora P, Ramos LP. Multivariate monitoring of soybean oil ethanolysis by FTIR. Talanta. 2004;**63**:1021-1025

[44] Brandao LF, Braga JW, Suarez PA. Determination of vegetable oils and fats adulterants in diesel oil by high performance liquid chromatography and multivariate methods. Journal of Chromatography. 2012;**1225**:150-157

6

Phytochemicals and Disease Prevention

Md Asaduzzaman and Toshiki Asao

1. Introduction

Phytochemicals, the nonnutritive chemical compounds derived from plants, play a significant role in human disease prevention. Phytochemicals such as secondary metabolites and antioxidants have important medicinal properties. This chapter will briefly outline the source of phytochemicals, their role in disease prevention, phytochemicals produced due to stress conditions, and accumulation of bioactive compounds in fruits and vegetables. It will also discuss the role of allelochemicals as phytochemicals that produced under stressed environment in the plant rhizosphere and neighboring plants leaving significant ecological role. The purpose of this chapter is to provide a general description of phytochemicals and their roles in major diseases prevention.

2. Role of phytochemicals in disease prevention in human

Phytochemicals present in medicinal plants, such as alkaloids, tannins, saponins, flavonoids, phenols, steroids, carotenoids, etc., have several disease prevention activity [1]. These plant-derived chemical compounds play important preventive activities mainly anti-inflammatory, antidiabetic, antiaging, antimicrobial, antiparasitic, antidepressant, anticancer, antioxidant, and wound healing [2]. They also have great role in stress tolerance of plants and accumulation of many important bioactive compounds in fruits and vegetables.

Flavonoids are the most common bioactive compounds found in medicinal plants [3]. They have several preventive activities in human disease such as antimicrobial, antioxidant, anticancer, anti-inflammatory, and wound-healing capacity [4–6]. Anticarcinogenic flavonoids have been reported to be found in a number of fruits and vegetables [7, 8]. Apple and berries found to have cardioprotective properties and showed positive impact on blood pressure [9].

Anthocyanins are the flavonoid constituents abundant in cell vacuole responsible for pigmentation in flowers, fruits, and vegetables and produced generally during plant under environmental stress [10, 11]. *In vitro* studies showed antioxidative activities of anthocyanins in cell culture systems such as colon, liver, breast, leukemic cell, and keratinocytes [12–15].

Carotenoids are considered as the potential natural antioxidant found in fruits and vegetables. They include xanthophyll and carotenes having scavenging of peroxyl radical [16]. Lycopene is common in tomato and berries, while β-carotenes are orange-colored carotenoids abundant in yellow-orange and dark-green leafy vegetables [17].

3. Allelochemicals as phytochemicals in the plant rhizosphere and its ecological role

Plant releases a numerous phytochemicals in order to protect it from environmental stresses such as drought, submergence, chemical pollution, UV exposure, pest and disease infection, and several other unfavorable conditions [18, 19]. Through this process, plant produces secondary metabolites and bioactive compounds having potential antioxidative roles [20]. In general, under natural ecosystem, plant releases numerous chemical compounds to the environment from its body and maintains its normal growth and development. However, plant produces several other chemicals/allelochemicals under environmental stress conditions [21–23]. The released allelochemicals create both heterotoxic and autotoxic conditions for the plant and its neighboring species [24]. Under replanting conditions and recycled hydroponics, plant found to produce a number of allelochemicals that inhibit its own growth and development, and this phenomenon has been reported in beans, taro, strawberry, lettuce, several other leafy vegetables, and ornamentals [25–29]. On the other hand, these allelochemicals may play a significant ecological role in controlling weeds, pests, and plant diseases [30, 31].

4. Conclusion

Fruits and vegetables are the great source of phytochemicals that play protective role in many age-related diseases. Phytochemical supplementation can benefit human health through supplying specific antioxidative/bioactive compounds which have preventive role in several diseases. Flavonoids are the most common phytochemicals that provide antimicrobial, antioxidant, anticancer, anti-inflammatory, and wound-healing activities. Plant under stress also produces allelochemicals that can inhibit either its own growth or neighboring plant species. Under stress condition, plant-produced allelochemicals may also play significant ecological roles through controlling weeds, plant disease, and insect pests.

Author details

Md Asaduzzaman[1,2]* and Toshiki Asao[1]

*Address all correspondence to: asadcbt@bari.gov.bd

1 Department of Agriculture, Faculty of Life and Environmental Science, Shimane University, Matsue, Shimane, Japan

2 Olericulture Division, Horticulture Research Center, Bangladesh Agricultural Research Institute, Gazipur, Bangladesh

References

[1] Barbosa A, Silveira GD, de Menezes I, Neto J, Bitencurt J, Estavam CD, et al. Antidiabetic effect of the *Chrysobalanus icaco* L. aqueous extract in rats. Journal of Medicinal Food. 2013;**16**:538-543. DOI: 10.1089/jmf.2012.0084

[2] Bahramsoltani R, Farzaei MH, Rahimi R. Medicinal plants and their natural components as future drugs for the treatment of burn wounds: An integrative review. Archives of Dermatological Research. 2014;**306**:601-617. DOI: 10.1007/s00403-014-1474-6

[3] Pietta PG. Flavonoids as antioxidants. Journal of Natural Products. 2000;**63**:1035-1042. DOI: 10.1021/np9904509

[4] Cushnie TPT, Lamb AJ. Antimicrobial activity of flavonoids. International Journal of Antimicrobial Agents. 2005;**26**:343-356. DOI: 10.1016/j.ijantimicag.2005.09.002

[5] Procházková D, Boušová I, Wilhelmová N. Antioxidant and prooxidant properties of flavonoids. Fitoterapia. 2011;**82**:513-523. DOI: 10.1016/j.fitote.2011.01.018

[6] Chirumbolo S. Flavonoids in propolis acting on mast cell-mediated wound healing. Inflammopharmacology. 2012;**20**:99-102. DOI: 10.1007/s10787-012-0125-9

[7] Barrientos S, Brem H, Stojadinovic O, Tomic-Canic M. Clinical application of growth factors and cytokines in wound healing. Wound Repair and Regeneration. 2014;**22**:569-578. DOI: 10.1111/wrr.12205

[8] Ahmed SA, Nazim S, Siraj S, Siddik PM, Wahid CA. *Euphorbia neriifolia* Linn: A phytopharmacological review. International Research Journal of Pharmacy. 2011;**2**:41-48

[9] Toh JY, Tan VMH, Lim PCY, Lim ST, Chong MFF. Flavonoids from fruit and vegetables: A focus on cardiovascular risk factors. Current Atherosclerosis Reports. 2013;**15**:368. DOI: 10.1007/s11883-013-0368-y

[10] Chalker-Scott L. Environmental significance of anthocyanins in plant stress responses. Photochemistry and Photobiology. 1999;**70**:1-9. DOI: 10.1111/j.1751-1097.1999.tb01944.x

[11] Heerboth S, Housman G, Leary M, Longacre M, Byler S, Lapinska K, et al. EMT and tumor metastasis. Clinical and Translational Medicine. 2015;**4**:6. DOI: 10.1186/s40169-015-0048-3

[12] Parry J, Su L, Moore J, Cheng Z, Luther M, Rao JN, et al. Chemical compositions, antioxidant capacities, and antiproliferative activities of selected fruit seed flours. Journal of Agricultural and Food Chemistry. 2006;**54**:3773-3778. DOI: 10.1021/jf060325k

[13] Shin DY, Lee WS, Kim SH, Kim MJ, Yun JW, Lu JN, et al. Anti-invasive activity of anthocyanins isolated from *Vitis coignetiae* in human hepatocarcinoma cells. Journal of Medicinal Food. 2009;**12**:967-972. DOI: 10.1089/jmf.2008.1338

[14] Takikawa M, Inoue S, Horio F, Tsuda T. Dietary anthocyanin-rich bilberry extract ameliorates hyperglycemia and insulin sensitivity via activation of amp-activated protein kinase in diabetic mice. The Journal of Nutrition. 2010;**140**:527-533. DOI: 10.3945/jn.109.118216

[15] Olsson ME, Gustavsson KE, Andersson S, Nilsson A, Duan RD. Inhibition of cancer cell proliferation *in vitro* by fruit and berry extracts and correlations with antioxidant levels. Journal of Agricultural and Food Chemistry. 2004;**52**:7264-7271. DOI: 10.1021/jf030479p

[16] Stahl W, Sies H. Antioxidant activity of carotenoids. Molecular Aspects of Medicine. 2003;**24**:345-351. DOI: 10.1016/S0098-2997(03)00030-X

[17] Rao AV, Rao LG. Carotenoids and human health. Pharmacological Research. 2007;**55**:207-216. DOI: 10.1016/j.phrs.2007.01.012

[18] Gibson EL, Wardel J, Watts CJ. Fruit and vegetable consumption, nutritional knowledge and beliefs in mothers and children. Appetite. 1998;**31**:205-228. DOI: 10.1006/appe.1998.0180

[19] Mathai K. Nutrition in the adult years. In: Mahan LK, Escott-Stump S, editors. Krause's Food, Nutrition, and Diet Therapy. 10th ed. Philadelphia, Pa: W.B. Saunders; 2000. pp. 274-275. https://trove.nla.gov.au/version/44576287

[20] Rao N. Bioactive phytochemicals in Indian foods and their potential in health promotion and disease prevention. Asia Pacific Journal of Clinical Nutrition. 2003;**12**:9-22

[21] Putnam AR. Allelopathic research in agriculture: Past highlights and potential. In: Thompson AC, editor. The Chemistry of Allelopathy: Biochemical Interactions among Plants. Washington DC: American Chemical Society; 1985. pp. 1-8. DOI: 10.1021/bk-1985-0268.ch001

[22] Miller DA. Allelopathy in forage crop systems. Agronomy Journal. 1996;**88**:854-859. DOI: 10.2134/agronj1996.00021962003600060003x

[23] Singh HP, Batish DR, Kohli RK. Autotoxicity: Concept, organisms and ecological significance. Critical Reviews in Plant Sciences. 1999;**18**:757-772. DOI: 10.1080/07352689991309478

[24] Asaduzzaman M, Fuad Mondal M, Ban T, Asao T. Selection of ideal succeeding crops after asparagus, taro and beans replanting field in seedling growth bioassay. Allelopathy Journal. 2013;**32**:1-22

[25] Asaduzzaman M, Asao T. Autotoxicity in beans and their allelochemicals. Scientia Horticulturae. 2012;**134**:26-31. DOI: 10.1016/j.scienta.2011.11.035

[26] Asao T, Hasegawa K, Sueda Y, Tomita K, Taniguchi K, Hosoki T, et al. Autotoxicity of root exudates from taro. Scientia Horticulturae. 2003;**97**:389-396. DOI: 10.1016/S0304-4238(02)00197-8

[27] Kitazawa H, Asao T, Ban T, Pramanik MHR, Hosoki T. Autotoxicity of root exudates from strawberry. The Journal of Horticultural Science and Biotechnology. 2005;**80**:677-680. DOI: 10.1080/14620316.2005.11511997

[28] Lee JG, Lee BY, Lee HJ. Accumulation of phytotoxic organic acids in reused nutrient solution during hydroponic cultivation of lettuce (*Lactuca sativa* L.). Scientia Horticulturae. 2006;**110**:119-128. DOI: 10.1016/j.scienta.2006.06.013

[29] Asao T, Kitazawa H, Ushio K, Sueda Y, Ban T, Pramanik MHR. Autotoxicity in some ornamentals with the means to overcome it. Hortscience. 2007;**42**:1346-1350

[30] Rizvi SJH, Rizvi V. Exploitation of allelochemicals in improving crop productivity. In: Rizvi SJH, Rizvi V, editors. Allelopathy: Basic and Applied Aspects. London: Chapman and Hall; 1992. pp. 443-472. DOI: 10.1007/978-94-011-2376-1

[31] Kohli RK, Batish D, Singh HP. Allelopathy and its implications in agroecosystems. Journal of Crop Production. 1998;**1**:169-202. DOI: 10.1300/J144v01n01_08

7

An Evaluation of the Impact of Novel Processing Technologies on the Phytochemical Composition of Fruits and Vegetables

Vishal Ganessingh, Raeesah Sahibdeen and Rohanie Maharaj

Abstract

Phytochemicals are highly beneficial in lowering the risk of several noncommunicable diseases. There is a need to provide novel technologies that can ensure the maintenance of desired phytochemicals in fruits and vegetables when compared to the traditional chemical or thermal treatments for the preservation of such crops. The development of physical nonthermal treatments such as pulsed electric field (PEF), pulsed light (PL), ultra sound (US), high pressure processing (HPP) and cold plasma (CP) techniques have been promising in maintaining the integrity of phytochemicals and the nutritional quality of fruits and vegetables. This chapter will focus on the effects such novel technologies can have on food quality and stability on phytochemicals in fruit and vegetable products.

Keywords: phytochemicals, novel processing technologies, nonthermal treatments, fruits and vegetables

1. Introduction

According to the Centers for Disease Prevention and Control (CDC), presently the most preventable and chronic health conditions are cardiovascular diseases, cancer, type 2 diabetes and obesity [1]. These diet related diseases account for an estimated number of 678,000 deaths annually [2]. Consumer demand for high quality, fresh and nutritious foods has increased over the years due to the need for a healthy diet and the associated consumption of fruits and vegetables, which is required for improved health. Organizations such as the World Health Organization (WHO), the Food and Agriculture Organization (FAO), the United States Department of Agriculture (USDA) and the European Food Safety Authority (EFSA) have recommended the consumption of fruits and vegetables to lower the risk of cardiovascular diseases and cancer due to their high content of micronutrients and fibers [3]. Thus, the main contributor to the protective effect of fruits and vegetables against chronic diseases are largely due to their phytochemical content.

Phytochemicals are nonnutrient, biologically active compounds and are commonly found in vegetables, fruits, grains and other crop plants. The major groups of phytochemicals based on their chemical structure are polyphenols, terpenoids, sulfur compounds, and alkaloids [4]. In the fight against diseases, phytochemicals act as antioxidant, antibacterial, antifungals, antivirals, anti-inflammatory and cholesterol reducing agents [5]. Studies have shown that polyphenols found in potatoes have the ability to inhibit the enzymes responsible for Alzheimer's disease [6]. Consumption of blueberries containing high levels of phenolic acids, flavonols, anthocyanins and proanthocyanidins were associated with the prevention of degenerative and chronic diseases [7].

In developed countries, approximately 75% of all deaths are due to non–communicable diseases (NCDs) related to an unbalanced diet [8]. Developing countries are also overburdened due to over and under nutrition [8]. Associated with an increasing demand for fresh cut fruits and vegetables in developed countries, developing countries are now following suit due to an increased level of education and awareness for healthy food amongst consumers [3, 7]. The need for nutritious, ready to eat convenience foods has thus given rise to minimally processed fruits and vegetables (MPVFs) [7, 9], which are mildly processed such that they possess "fresh-like" attributes [9]. Some key attributes that ensure the marketability of MPVFs are the maintenance of nutritional value especially phytochemical content, flavor, color, texture, appearance and shelf life.

Some methods used to minimally process fruits and vegetables, negatively affect its phytochemical content and thus, the consumer does not benefit from the desired health benefits. Thermal processing allows for a longer shelf life by reducing microbial load and inhibiting enzymes that leads to deterioration, but it also decreases the level of phytochemicals in the fruits and vegetables [7, 10, 11]. Thus, this has prompted food scientists and researchers to find new ways to process fruits and vegetables without compromising the nutritional content and quality. Novel, nonthermal processing such as pulsed electric field (PEF), pulsed light (PL), ultra sound (US), high pressure processing (HPP) and cold plasma (CP) techniques have been promising in maintaining the integrity of phytochemicals and the nutritional quality of fruits and vegetables, inclusive of minimally processed ones [10]. Such technologies have the potential to be adapted in developing countries. This chapter will explore the use of nonthermal processing technologies and their effects on key phytochemicals such as carotenoids, flavonoids and phenolic acids in several fruits and vegetables with a focus on health benefits.

2. Sources of phytochemicals and functions

Scientific evidence has shown that phytochemicals are highly beneficial in lowering the risk of several noncommunicable diseases [10]. They are known to have the ability to treat diseases such as stroke, cancer and metabolic syndromes. Phytochemicals are grouped based on their chemical structure and function. To date thousands of phytochemicals have been identified in fruits, vegetables and grains and the most important groups are phenolic compounds, nitrogen-containing compounds, alkaloids, organosulfur compounds, phytosterols, and carotenoids [11]. The most studied groups of dietary phytochemicals related to human health are carotenoids and phenolic acids [11].

2.1. Carotenoids

Carotenoids are the red, yellow and orange color plant pigments of fruits and vegetables. To date approximately 600 types of carotenoids have been identified. They are mostly present as fat soluble, colored pigments in plants [12]. They can be separated into two groups; carotenes and xanthophylls. The two primary forms of carotenoids are β-carotene and α-carotene [12]. Other essential carotenoids include zeaxanthin, lutein and lycopene. The health benefits of carotenoids are due mainly to their antioxidant effects and physiological functions as provitamins. However, post-harvest technologies and processing greatly affect the composition and bioavailability of carotenoids in fruits and vegetables. Fruits and vegetables such as papaya, mangoes, carrots, sweet potatoes, pumpkin and cantaloupes are rich in β-carotene, whilst tomatoes, pink grapefruits, and watermelons contains high levels of lycopene [10]. In a study by Leoung and Oey, it was found that the highest content of carotenoids was found in red peppers followed by carrots, apricots, plums and peaches, whilst cherries contained the lowest amount of carotenoids [13].

Since carotenoids are a precursor of vitamin A, they have been found to decrease the incidence of diseases such as cancer of the lungs, pancreas and gastrointestinal tracts, cardiovascular diseases and eye-related diseases [14]. According to Toniolo et al., a case-control study conducted in New York between the years 1985–1994, showed that the carotenoids lutein, zeaxanthin, lycopene, α carotene and β carotene were responsible for decreasing the risk of breast cancer [15]. In another study by Giovannucci, it was observed that a decrease in prostate cancer was associated with a consumption of tomatoes due to their high lycopene content [16]. With respect to cardiovascular diseases, studies showed that the blood plasma of patients suffering with coronary artery disease, contained lower levels of zeaxanthin, lycopene, β carotene and α carotene [17]. This is in agreement with a study conducted by Knekt et al. who showed that a higher intake of β carotene and several carotenoids, led to a lower risk of major coronary heart diseases [18].

2.2. Phenolic compounds

Phenolic compounds most commonly occur as antioxidants in fruits, and vegetables. Amongst the major classes of phenolic compounds with health benefits are flavonoids such as anthocyanins and non-flavonoids such as phenolic acids [19]. The many benefits of phenolic compounds include; antioxidant, anti-carcinogenic, antimutagenic and anti-inflammatory effects [20]. Amongst the most common phenolics are flavonoids. These are found in plant tissues and are often responsible along with carotenoids and chlorophylls for the blue, purple, yellow, orange and red colors in fruits and vegetables [20]. Within the group of flavonoids, are anthocyanins, which is responsible for reducing cardiovascular diseases. Anthocyanins are mainly found in red fruits like berries and grapes [21]. Non-flavonoid phenolic compounds, such as phenolic acids can be grouped into two major constituents; hydroxybenzoic acids

(HBAs) and hydroxycinnamic acids (HCAs). Phenolic acids are seldom found in mangoes, berries, citrus fruits, red wine and plums. Their main benefits to human health are the prevention of stroke, cancer and coronary heart diseases [22].

2.2.1. *Anthocyanins*

Anthocyanins belong to the widespread group of plant constituents called flavonoids. In fruits and vegetables, they are responsible for the orange, red, purple and blue colors. Such dietary antioxidants aid in preventing neuronal diseases, heart diseases, cancer, diabetes and inflammation [23]. According to a study by Zhao et al. various commercial extracts of anthocyanin rich grapes, bilberry and chokeberry were prepared. When investigated for their chemopreventitive effects against colon cancer, it was found that all of the extracts inhibited the growth of HT-29 colon cancer cells [24]. In another study conducted by Wang and Mazza [25], the inhibitory effects of anthocyanins found in selected berries against nitric oxide (NO) were investigated. Since NO is associated with many chronic inflammatory diseases, the strong inhibition of anthocyanins on NO production indicated that anthocyanins can aid in the prevention of chronic inflammatory diseases [25].

2.2.2. *Phenolic acids*

Phenolic acids are a major source of dietary phenolics belonging to the non-flavonoid group of phytochemicals. Two major groups are HBAs and HCAs as noted above [25]. HCAs are found in many conjugated forms, with p-coumaric, caffeic, ferulic and sinapic acids being the most common and in HBAs; p-hydroxybenzoic, vanillic, syringic and protocatechuic are the most common. Phenolic acids are often found in berries such as strawberries, raspberries and blackberries [26]. Studies conducted on caffeic acid have shown that phenolic acids possess the ability to inhibit antitumor activity against colon carcinogenesis [27].

3. Advanced nonthermal technologies

Conventional thermal processing such as blanching and pasteurization can result in oxidation and other deleterious reactions that lower the levels of phytonutrients in processed foods [28–30]. For example, canned fruits and vegetables undergo retort processing temperatures in excess of 100°C to obtain commercial sterility. This can lead to significant losses in anthocyanin content, up to 70%, observed in the processing of strawberries into jam. Advanced nonthermal technologies are able to achieve preserving effects at sub-lethal temperatures (up to 40°C). These methods retain higher phytochemical content whilst minimally changing the sensorial properties of the food [29]. The stability of phytochemicals in thermally processed fruits and vegetables decreases exponentially with a linear increase in both the magnitude and duration of the heating process [30]. The use of nonthermal treatments at successfully lower temperatures and times provide real alternatives from traditional thermal processing through the production of additional health promoting-benefits and maintaining the desired *"fresh-like"* quality of foods for consumers [28, 29]. The present review will focus on the effects of the following novel technologies: pulsed electric field (PEF), high pressure processing (HPP), pulsed light (PL), cold plasma (CP) and ultrasound (US) on food quality and stability of phytochemicals particularly in fruit and vegetable products. These findings are reported below and summarized in **Table 1**.

Technology and process conditions	Food matrix	Results	Source
Pulsed electric field (PEF)			
38 kV/cm, 15–24 μs, 70–120 Hz	Mango nectar	High retention of carotene (94.2%), monoterpene (Z)-Ocimene; reduction in HMF; minimal changes in TSS, pH, acidity, color	Kumar et al. [33, 44]
35 kV/cm, 59 μs, ≈ 60°C	Orange juice	Less degradation of vitamin C, carotenoid, polyphenol, volatile aroma compounds	Cited in Buckow et al. [35]
5 kV/cm; 1.8 kJ/kg and 10 kV/cm; 6.7 kJ/kg	Grape skin	Total polyphenols index in PEF-treated wines was 13.7% higher (5 kV/cm treatment) and 29.0% higher (10 kV/cm treatment) with improved color	Cited in Ricci et al. [31]
1–3 kV/cm, 20 μs, 20 Hz; mechanical pressing (1.32 bar/6 min)	Red raspberries	Increase bioaccessibility of total phenolics (up to 22%) and total anthocyanins (up to 26%); increased juice recovery (9–25%)	Lamanauskas et al. [36]
0.3–2.5 kV/cm, 20 μs, 100 Hz	Sweet cherry	Enhanced production of desirable C6 aldehyde and alcohol volatiles	Sotelo et al. [37]
High pressure processing (HPP)			
Mild-temperature (300, 600 MPa/15 min)	Strawberry puree	Reduction in vitamin C, anthocyanin content of 20% and 5% higher at 600 MPa than at 300 MPa	Marszałek et al. [40]
Combination (300, 600, 900 MPa/60, 70, 80°C)	Pumpkin puree	Higher pressures effective in maintaining and/or increasing lutein, α-carotene, β-carotene)	Garcia-Parra et al. [42]
Thermal-assisted (250 MPa/60°C/3 min)	Grapefruit juice	Reduction in PME, PPO activity; improvement in total carotenoid, anthocyanin, flavanol, flavonoid and antioxidant capacity	Aadil et al. [43]
Ultrasound (US)			
Combination (blanching 100°C/4 min + sonication 20 kHz/70%/2 min)	Carrot juice	Significant increase in total carotenoid, lycopene, lutein; improvement in retention of sucrose, fructose, glucose, chlorogenic acid, Na, K	Jabbar et al. [45]
25 kHz, 70%, 20°C, 30/60/90 min	Apple juice	Improved ascorbic acid, phenols, antioxidant capacity; no significant changes in TSS, pH, TA	Abid et al. [46]

Technology and process conditions	Food matrix	Results	Source
40 kHz, $0.5Wcm^{-1}$, 20/40/60 min	Blueberry juice	Enhancement of viscosity, color; improvement in TSS, polyphenol, anthocyanin; increase in antioxidant scavenging activity	Zou, Hou [47]
19 kHz, 20–100%, 2–10 min	Soursop juice	Increasing sonication intensity resulted in lower phenolic content, ascorbic acid; minimal impact on overall color	Dias et al. [48]
200–500 W, 15–90 min	Blueberry extract	Degradation of cyanidin-3-glucoside and antioxidant activity with increasing sonication power and prolonged treatment time	Yao et al. [49]
Pulsed light (PL)			
17.5 J/cm, 0.5 μs, 0.5 Hz	Fresh-cut apple	Reduction in browning and slight retention in firmness during storage of irradiated samples	Manzocco et al. [54]
0.7 J/cm, 250 μs, 4 pulses per day	Fresh-cut mango	Reduced color and fresh mass loss; increase in total carotenoid and antioxidant activity.	Lopes et al. [55]
2.7, 7.8, 11.7, 15.6 J/cm at 9, 26, 39 and 52 pulses respectively	Fresh-cut cantaloupe	Retention in firmness, pH, TSS, TA, color; no significant effect on phenols; ascorbic acid content decreased significantly on stored samples subjected to higher-fluence	Koh et al. [56]
2-4 J/cm, 360 μs, 3 pulses	Uncut tomato and Annurca apple	Significant increase in total carotenoid, lycopene, phenolics and antioxidant activity noted in both fruits	Pataro et al. [57]
Cold plasma (CP)			
60 kV, 50 Hz, RH 42%	Strawberry	Minimal impact on color and firmness; significant reduction in microbial flora	Misra et al. [63]
30 kV, 50 Hz, RH 45% 7.5–15 kV, 30 s, RH 42%	Uncut cherry; uncut tomato	Insignificant changes on pH, color, firmness, weight loss in both varieties	Misra et al. [61] Vukic et al. [64]
15 kV, RH 60%, 10/20/30 min for apple; 30/60 min for melon	Fresh-cut apple; and fresh-cut melon	Significant loss in *"crunchiness"* in apple texture, melons exhibited no significant texture impact; linear reduction in PPO and POD activity	Tappi et al. [65, 66]
15 kV, RH 60%, 1/5/10 min treatment	Fresh-cut kiwifruit	Slight initial reduction in chlorophyll and carotenoid but improved color retention during storage; slight reduction in phenols but no significant impact on antioxidant activity	Ramazinna et al. [67]

Table 1. Impact of nonthermal processes on food quality and phytochemical compounds.

3.1. Pulsed electric field (PEF)

Pulsed electric field (PEF) involves the direct application of short, high current voltage pulses that create an intense electric field, applied to a food matrix placed between two electrodes [31]. PEF has been used as an alternative nonthermal treatment in the pasteurization of liquid or pumpable foods. Fruit juices, milk, smoothies, yogurt, sauces, wine, and soup-based products contain large amounts of water and dipolar molecules making them more conductive for passage of electrical currents compared to solid type foods. The PEF system discharges a high voltage pulse uniformly throughout the food in a treatment chamber (see **Figure 1a**) [29, 32]. Typical field strengths varies from 0.1 to 80 kV/cm with the time duration of the pulse cycles ranging from *μs* to *ms* depending on the application of PEF. The mechanism of PEF is best explained using the *"electroporation"* model in which the strong electric fields generated induce either reversible or irreversible (depending on electric field intensity) perforation of the cytoplasmic membrane promoting cell leakage (see **Figure 1b**) [31]. This effect has shown inactivation of microorganisms and food spoilage enzymes, thereby enhancing food safety, quality and phytochemical yield and extraction.

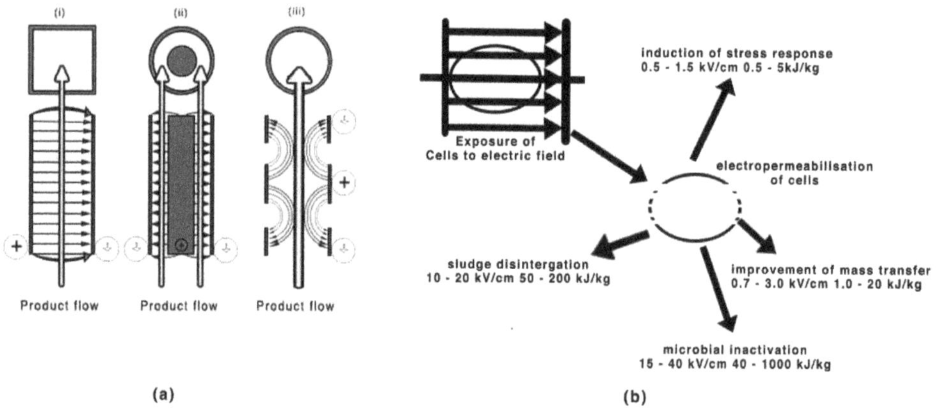

Figure 1. (a) Configuration of treatment chambers for continuous PEF processing: (i) parallel plate, (ii) coaxial, and (iii) co-linear; and (b) effects of exposure of biological cells at different electric field strengths and applications in food. Adapted from Toepfl et al. [32].

Kumar et al. on investigating the effect of PEF on carotenoids, microbial stability and different physicochemical changes on ready-to-drink (RTD) mango nectar, noted a high retention of carotene content (94.2%) and minimal changes in total soluble solids (TSS), pH acidity and color [33]. In a separate study [34], a higher retention of volatile monoterpene compounds, in particular (Z)-Ocimene, in mango nectar pasteurized at 96°C for 300 and 600 s was observed. Sensory scores conducted also found PEF samples to be insignificantly different from control samples owing to retention in volatile components and reduction in nonenzymatic 5-hydroxy methyl furfural (HMF) brown compounds. As cited in Buckow et al. several studies surveyed the effects of PEF on orange juice treated at ≤68°C, resulted in maintenance of vitamin C, carotenoid, polyphenol, and volatile aroma compounds compared to thermal pasteurization (95°C for 30 s) both after processing and refrigerated storage [35].

PEF is capable of extracting compounds such as pigments, antioxidants and flavors through the ability of the electric fields to induce cell membrane breakdown in plant tissue, increasing the bioaccessibility of phytochemicals [29, 31]. As cited in Ricci et al. investigations using PEF assisted maceration on Tempranillo grape skin with treatments of 5 and 10 kV/cm increased the polyphenol and anthocyanin extraction in wine processing [31]. Results showed total polyphenols index in PEF treated wines was 13.7% higher (5 kV/cm treatment) and 29.0% higher (10 kV/cm treatment) with respect to the control after 96 h maceration; and at the end of fermentation color intensity also improved of 23.93 (control), 27.04 (5 kV/cm treatment), and 29.33 (10 kV/cm treatment). Increased juice recovery (9–25%) and higher amounts of total phenolics (up to 22%) and total anthocyanins (up to 26%) in PEF treated raspberries and press cakes extracts were reported [36]. With sweet cherries, PEF applied at low field strengths, increased production of volatiles, (aldehydes and alcohols) known to have desirable odors was reported by Sotelo et al. [37].

3.2. High pressure processing (HPP)

High pressure processing (HPP), also known as high-hydrostatic pressure (HHP) or ultra-high pressure (UHP), is capable of inactivating both pathogenic and vegetative spoilage microorganisms by using pressure rather than heat [38]. HPP mainly uses water as a medium to transmit pressure ranging from 100 to 800 MPa to foods [29]. The basic components of an HPP system include a pressurization vessel, a pressure transmitting fluid, a material handling unit, and supporting heating and cooling system components (see **Figure 2**) [39]. During HPP, food in flexible packages/containers is placed in a holding basket and lowered into the reaction chamber. High hydrostatic pressure is generated through the action of a piston or pump, which compresses the pressure-transmitting fluid allowing for uniform distribution throughout the product matrix [29]. Vitamins, flavor compounds and pigments survive the process while denaturation of proteins, gelation, hydrophobic reactions, lipid phase changes and ionization of molecules is able to modify the integrity of cell walls and membranes [38]. By optimizing HPP parameters of pressure (P), temperature (T) and duration time (t); important foodborne pathogens can be inactivated whilst preserving and/or enhancing the nutritional and organoleptic properties of food and vegetables [29].

On investigating the effects of mild temperature (50°C) and HPP (300 and 600 MPa) on the shelf life of strawberry purée, Marszałek et al. showed that higher pressure values resulted in prolonging shelf life from 4 to 28 weeks [40]. However, HPP was unable to preserve vitamin C and anthocyanin content in the treated purée, resulting in significant degradation of 20 and 5% higher at 600 than at 300 MPa respectively. The inactivation of endogenous enzymes such as β-glucosidase, polyphenol oxidase (PPO) and peroxidase (POD) are mainly responsible for anthocyanin degradation during storage. However, other factors such as temperature, light, pH, sugars, presence of oxygen, sulfites, ascorbic acid, metal ions and co-pigments may also destabilize anthocyanin compounds and accelerate its decomposition [41].

Garcia-Parra et al. investigated the effect of thermal assisted HPP to preserve pumpkin puree under varying combinations of pressure and temperature (300, 600, 900 MPa/60, 70, 80°C < 71 min) and found that treatments at higher pressures were effective in maintaining and/or increasing the individual carotenoids (lutein, α-carotene and β-carotene) [42]. Similar studies on orange, carrot and tomato juices/purees also showed significant increases in carotenoid content and antioxidant activity [28]. It is believed that the mechanism of pressure-induced disruption of cell

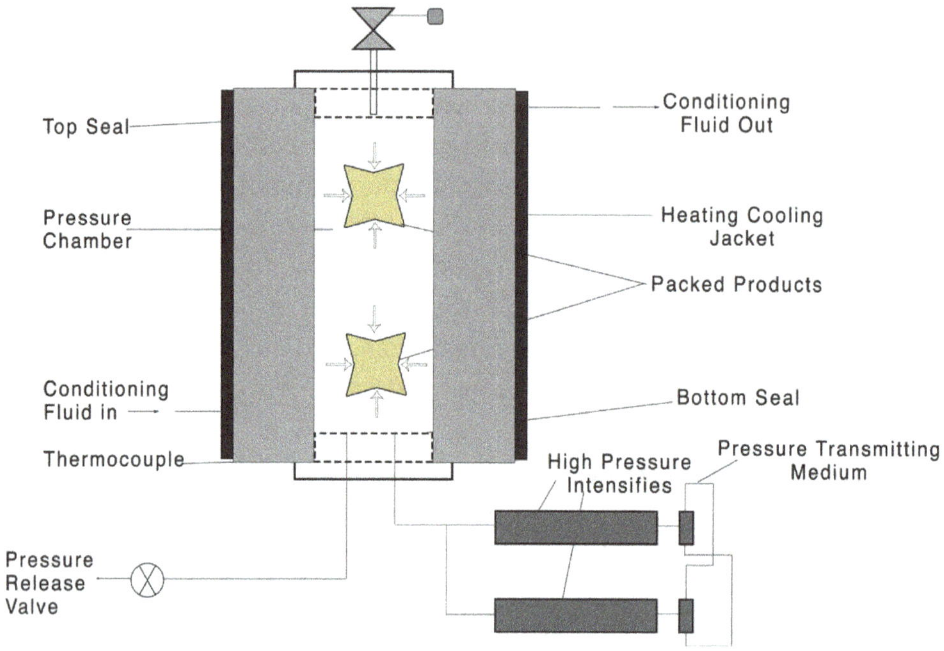

Figure 2. Schematic of a batch high pressure processing setup. Adapted from Chakraborty et al. [39].

walls and membranes, proteins and enzymes also facilitate the release and extraction of bound carotenoid from the cellular matrix, increasing its bioaccessibility [29]. Aadil et al. studied the effects of thermal-assisted HPP versus thermal processing of grapefruit juice and observed that processed juice at 250 MPa/60°C/3 min had an improvement in total carotenoid and anthocyanin content compared to control and thermally treated samples [43]. In the same study, ascorbic acid contents were reduced from 25.58 to 19.32 (mg/100 ml) in HPP and 17.28 (mg/100 ml) in thermal processed samples. While retention of vitamin C was higher under HPP compared to thermal processing, the elevated temperatures are most likely responsible for its depletion in both cases.

3.3. Ultrasound (US)

Ultrasound (US) employs mechanical sound waves at frequencies between 20 kHz and 500 MHz, and has emerged as an alternative technique, capable of inactivating microorganisms for food preservation [29, 44]. US systems are either batch or continuous type, that include sonication baths, ultrasonic probes and vibrating systems, and can be applied to liquid foods or solid type matrices embedded in a transmitting liquid medium (typically water) (see **Figure 3**) [45]. US mode of action is attributed to the *"cavitation"* phenomenon in which micro-bubbles generated in the transmitting medium by the sonication device, oscillate, grow in size and eventually collapse producing shock waves that induce a number of thermal, mechanical and chemical effects. As stated by Majid et al. the high temperatures, pressures, shear forces and free radicals generated in the cavitation zone affects cell walls and membranes for microbial inactivation, whilst retaining sensory, nutritional and functional characteristics of the food [44].

Jabbar et al. in evaluating the combined effects of blanching and sonication (frequency 20 kHz, amplitude level 70%) on carrot juice, reported improvements in the retention of chlorogenic acid, total carotenoids, lycopene and lutein content [45]. The increase in the bioavailability of these

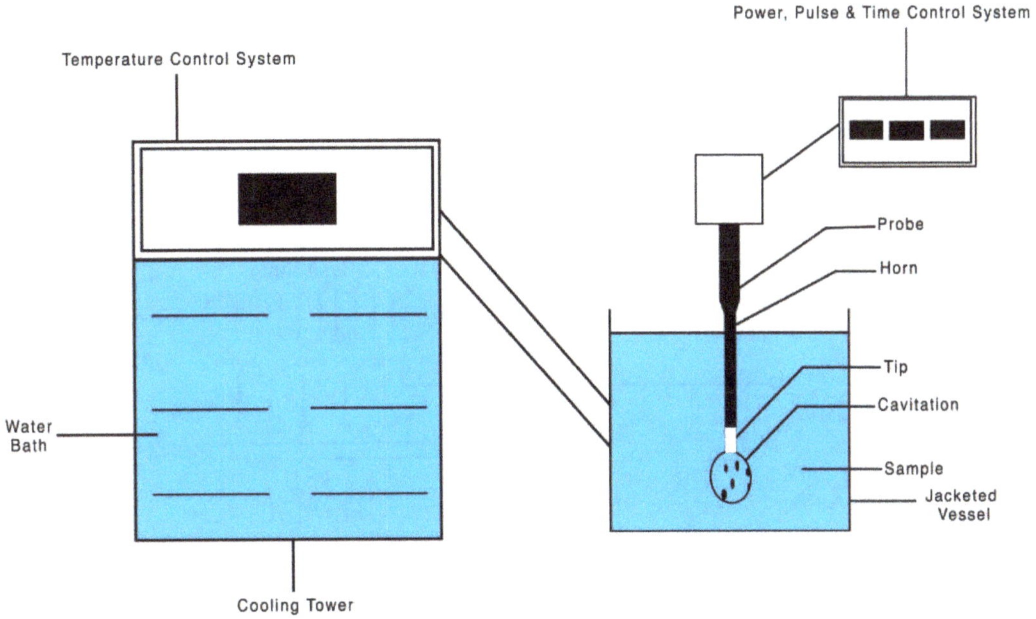

Figure 3. Schematic of a probe-type sonication system. Adapted from Jabbar et al. [45].

compounds might be attributed to the breakdown of cell walls and disruption of chromoplasts created by cavitation pressures allowing for release of membrane bound carotenoids. These results were similar to Abid et al. and Zou and Hou, when investigating US on different quality parameters of apple and blue berry juice respectively [46, 47]. Sonication showed increased levels of ascorbic acid, total phenolics, flavanols and flavonoids, and increased antioxidant activity due to the extraction and availability of these compounds. In a contrasting study by Dias et al. soursop juice subjected to varying levels of sonication energy, showed that increasing US intensity resulted in lower levels of phenols, ascorbic acid and higher levels of total color difference between sonicated and untreated samples [48]. The apparent decreases in overall phytonutrient content was attributed to increasing temperature and free radical formation that produced strong oxidizing effects during cavitation. Yao et al. investigating the effects of US on cyanidin-3-glucoside in blueberries, demonstrated that the pathway for degradation was the pyrolysis of water molecules creating –OH radicals involved in the opening of anthocyanin ring formation [49]. US-assisted extraction of various phytochemicals has grown in interest because of the potential industrial application to provide an efficient and energy saving extractive method.

3.4. Pulsed light (PL)

Pulsed light (PL) involves the use of intense, short duration pulses of light over a broad spectrum of wavelengths ranging from UV (180–380 nm), visible light (380–700 nm) to near-infrared (700–1100 nm); mainly used for decontamination of surface microorganisms on food and packaging [50, 51]. The basic components of a PL system incorporates three main parts: a lamp (xenon gas lamp), a power supply and a pulse configuration device (controller); configured in either batch or continuous flow design depending on the food material to process (see **Figure 4**) [52]. The mechanism of PL on microbial inactivation is attributed to both photochemical and photothermal effects. UV radiation is absorbed by carbon–carbon double bonds in

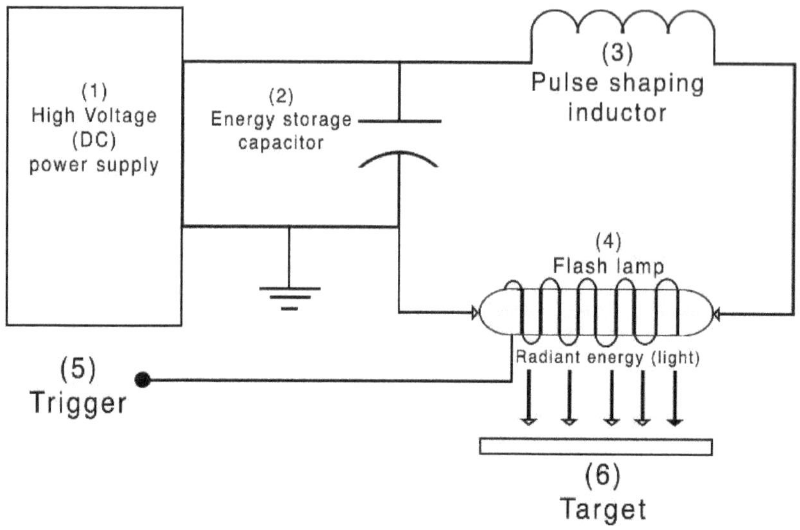

Figure 4. Schematic diagram of a high intensity pulsed-light system. Adapted from Abida et al. [52].

nucleic acids and proteins disrupting DNA and RNA structures, as well as rupturing bacterial cells due to localized overheating from absorption [50–52]. Similarly, the nonionizing effects of UV-C radiation at low doses has been the subject of numerous studies and documented by Maharaj et al. as having positive impacts on phytochemicals and sensory properties, either by preserving its content in fruits and vegetables or increasing it following treatment [53].

Manzocco et al. on studying the effect of PL on fresh-cut apple of increasing fluence ranges of 0, 8.8 and 17.5 J/cm^2 showed a significant decrease in browning of PL treated samples attributed to the modification of metabolic respiration and controlling the formation of brown polyphenols [54]. Similar studies on the effects of PL support this theory as observed by Lopes et al. On the effects of the exposure mode of light treatment on fresh-cut mangoes. PL treatments of 1 pulse (0.7 J/cm^2), 4 pulses (2.8 J/cm^2) and 1 pulse for 4 days (2.8 J/cm^2) reduced the respiration rate with positive impacts on maintenance of yellow color and lower mass loss during storage [55]. Significant improvements in firmness were most likely associated with higher levels of UV-C, which either directly suppress cell wall hydrolase activity or indirectly via increase polyamine content that inhibit the enzyme. In the same study, there were marked increases in carotenoid and ascorbic acid content at the higher fluence intensity treatments. The authors noted the increase in the biosynthesis of these compounds with antioxidant activity could be an adapted photo-protective response to increasing oxidative stresses caused by UV-radiation. Koh et al. demonstrated that PL treatment on fresh-cut cantaloupe, a nonacidic fruit, resulted in the retention of phenolic and ascorbic acid content, albeit at much lower levels when compared to other studies on acidic types [56]. The study also highlighted that at much higher fluence treatments of 11.7 and 15.6 J/cm^2 there was a significant reduction in ascorbic acid content attributed to photothermal degradation of heat labile ascorbic acid at the higher intensities. At low PL dosage rates of 2 and 4 J/cm^2, Pataro et al. recorded significant increases in total carotenoids, lycopene and phenolics in whole, uncut tomatoes and Annurca apples [57]. Investigations on raspberries known to be high in antioxidant compounds showed that PL in combination with sanitizer washing was able to significantly increase the total phenolic and anthocyanin content both directly after treatment, and retain higher levels after 3 months of frozen storage compared to untreated samples [58]. Both UV light and thermal stress created by PL induce the production of phenolic compounds through increased activity of phenylalanine ammonia lyase (PAL). However, increasing the duration of treatment (20–30 s) leads to over dosage of thermal stress producing severe damages to plant tissue, discoloration of the fruit skin and loss in bioactive content.

3.5. Cold plasma (CP)

Plasma is a quasi-neutral gas state, considered the *"fourth"* state of matter, and composed of a mixture of partially ionized gas molecules, ions, atoms and free electrons in their fundamental or excited state with an overall net neutral charge [59]. Plasma can be generated by using several types of energies to excite molecules. In the food industry, the general approach of producing plasma is to subject atmospheric air to an electric or electromagnetic field of constant or alternating amplitude, to induce electron collisions and generation of the ionized species [60]. The dielectric barrier discharge (DBD) and the plasma jet (see **Figure 5**) [59] are two common design types used to breakdown gas in a stationary electric field between electrodes to create the ionizing effect. The term cold plasma (CP) is considered a nonthermal technique from the fact that the temperature of electrons (T_e) is much higher than the temperature of the ions, neutrals and global gas (T_g) in the plasma ($T_e >> T_g$) [61]. Thus the overall temperature of CP is at ambient temperature without raising the temperature of the surrounding medium. Under Atmospheric cold plasma (ACP), several reactive oxygen species (ROS); as well as reactive nitrogen species (RNS) are formed with high lethal effects, capable of inactivating a wide range of microorganisms [62]. The nonthermal nature of CP technology, coupled with its high antimicrobial effects, has provided an alternative treatment for the decontamination of fruits and vegetables whilst minimizing deleterious quality impacts.

Misra et al. studied the effects of ACP on fresh strawberries and demonstrated significant reductions of 2.4 and 3.3 log cycles for mesophiles and surface yeast and mold respectively, with minimal impact to color and firmness between treated and control samples [63]. This is in agreement with other studies conducted on whole cherry tomatoes where CP did not induce metabolic changes that adversely affect critical quality parameters of color, firmness, pH and weight loss [61, 64]. Studies conducted by Tappi et al. on the effect of CP on fresh-cut apples and melon had variable changes on texture. Whilst apples showed a significant loss in *"crunchiness"* in texture, melons exhibited no significant differences in the cut fruit [65, 66]. However,

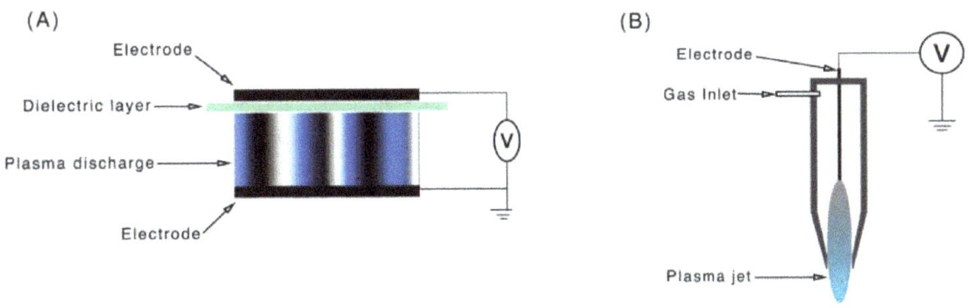

Figure 5. Schematic diagram of (A) dielectric barrier discharge; and (B) plasma jet system. Adapted from Pankaj et al. [59].

common to both cut apples and melons, was significant improvement in a reduction in brown color formed from enzymatic degradation products. By increasing CP treatment time, an observed linear reduction was noted for PPO and POD activity. The inhibitory effect of CP on enzyme activity was attributed to chemically reactive oxygen and nitrogen species modifying amino acids within the 3-D structure of proteins resulting in loss in enzyme function.

While the effects of CP on phytochemical composition is in its infant stage, Ramazzina et al. attempted to evaluate the effects of CP on bioactive compounds in minimally processed kiwifruit [67]. In the study, a significant reduction in chlorophyll and carotenoid content was observed in CP treated samples followed by better retention in these pigments during storage. This was attributed to the breakdown and oxidation of chlorophyll and carotenoids mediated by reactive species during the initial stage of treatment, followed by a slower rate of deterioration during storage due to partial protein denaturation and reduction in enzyme activity as previously described [65]. Analysis of health promoting ascorbic acid and phenolic compounds in the same study showed no significant changes in their content in the kiwifruit. While the investigators did note a slight initial decrease in total phenolic content, it did not significantly affect the overall antioxidant activity between CP and control treatments. It was noted that plasma induced oxidation of phenols at the initial stage of treatment, could be counteracted by tissue response/defense mechanisms that synthesize new phenolic compounds through increased activity of the enzyme (PAL) [67].

4. Conclusion

The recent global rise in consumer health awareness has prompted some food producers to utilize nonchemical preservation treatments to maintain and enhance the integrity of food products. Enhancing the competitiveness of the food industry requires technological innovation for improving quality, nutritious and safe ready to eat foods. Some studies have shown that unlike traditional thermal processing, nonthermal alternatives such as pulsed electric field (PEF), pulsed light (PL), ultra sound (US), high pressure processing (HPP) and cold plasma (CP) techniques have the ability to preserve and in some cases elicit increased phytochemical content of some fruits and vegetables. Such novel food preservation technologies have shown promising evidence in producing foods capable of reducing noncommunicable diseases with benefits to both domestic and export markets. In summary, the review has focused on both the application and impact of nonthermal technologies on the bioavailability of phytochemicals in fruits and vegetables which can positively impact the Food and Beverage industry.

Author details

Vishal Ganessingh, Raeesah Sahibdeen and Rohanie Maharaj*

*Address all correspondence to: rohanie.maharaj@utt.edu.tt

Biosciences, Agriculture and Food Technologies (BAFT), ECIAF Campus, The University of Trinidad and Tobago, Trinidad & Tobago

References

[1] Chronic Disease Overview. Publications Chronic Disease Prevention and Health Promotion. CDC [Internet]. [cited 2018 Mar 28]. Available from: https://www.cdc.gov/chronicdisease/overview/index.htm

[2] Why Good Nutrition is Important. Center for Science in the Public Interest [Internet]. [cited 2018 Mar 28]. Available from: https://cspinet.org/eating-healthy/why-good-nutrition-important

[3] Ramos B, Miller FA, Brandão TRS, Teixeira P, Silva CLM. Fresh fruits and vegetables—An overview on applied methodologies to improve its quality and safety. Innovative Food Science and Emerging Technologies [Internet]. 2013 [cited 2018 Mar 28];**20**:1-15. Available from: http://eduteka.icesi.edu.co/gp/upload/5b815520c1a83b3fccc89c6590ed229b.pdf

[4] Desjardins Y. Horticulture: Plants for People and Places. In: Dixon RG, Aldous ED, editors. 1st ed. Vol. 3. Netherlands: Springer; 2014. pp. 965-975

[5] Oz AT, Kafkas E. Phytochemicals in fruits and vegetables. In: Superfood and Functional Food–An Overview of their Processing and Utilization [Internet]. Rijeka, Crotia: InTech; 2017 [cited 2018 Mar 28]. Available from: http://www.intechopen.com/books/superfood-and-functional-food-an-overview-of-their-processing-and-utilization/phytochemicals-in-fruits-and-vegetables

[6] Laib I, Barkat M. Optimization of conditions for extraction of polyphenols and the determination of the impact of cooking on total polyphenolic, antioxidant, and anticholinesterase activities of potato. Foods [Internet]. 2018 Mar 9 [cited 2018 Apr 3];**7**(3):36. Available from: http://www.mdpi.com/2304-8158/7/3/36

[7] Zambiazi RC, Jansen C, Bueno-Costa FM, Silva SSS, Hartwig N. Bioactive compounds and antioxidant activity of blueberry toppings with honey. International Food Research Journal. 2016;**23**(6):2375-2383

[8] Mastorci F, Vassalle C, Chatzianagnostou K, Marabotti C, Siddiqui K, Eba A, et al. Undernutrition and overnutrition burden for diseases in developing countries: The role of oxidative stress biomarkers to assess disease risk and interventional strategies. Antioxidants. 2017 Jun 8;**6**(2):41 Available from: http://www.mdpi.com/2076-3921/6/2/41

[9] Rodgers S. Minimally Processed Functional Foods: Technological and Operational Pathways. [cited 2018 Apr 3]; Available from: https://onlinelibrary.wiley.com/doi/pdf/10.1111/1750-3841.13422

[10] Liu RH. Potential synergy of phytochemicals in cancer prevention: Mechanism of action. In: International Research Conference on Food, Nutrition and Cancer. 2004

[11] Liu RH. Health-promoting components of fruits and vegetables in the diet. Advances in Nutrition. 2013;**4**(3):384S-392S. Available from: http://www.ncbi.nlm.nih.gov/pubmed/23674808

[12] Khoo HE, Prasad KN, Kong KW, Jiang Y, Ismail A. Carotenoids and their isomers: Color pigments in fruits and vegetables. Molecules. 2011;**16**(2):1710-1738

[13] Leong SY, Oey I. Effects of Processing on Anthocyanins, Carotenoids and Vitamin C in Summer Fruits and Vegetables. 2012. Available from: http://ucce.ucdavis.edu/files/datastore/608-90.pdf

[14] Rao V. In: Rao V, editor. Phytochemicals–A Global Perspective of their Role in Nutrition and Health. Janeza Trdine Rijeka, Crotia: Intech; 2012. p. 548

[15] Toniolo P, Van Kappel AL, Akhmedkhanov A, Ferrari P, Kato I, Shore RE, et al. Serum carotenoids and breast cancer. American Journal of Epidemiology. 2001 Jun 15;**153**(12):1142-1147. Available from: https://academic.oup.com/aje/article-lookup/doi/10.1093/aje/153.12.1142

[16] Giovannucci E. A review of epidemiologic studies of tomatoes, lycopene, and prostate cancer. Experimental Biology and Medicine. 2002;**227**(10):852-859. Available from: http://journals.sagepub.com/doi/10.1177/153537020222701003

[17] Sesso HD, Buring JE, Norkus EP, Gaziano JM. Plasma lycopene, other carotenoids, and retinol and the risk of cardiovascular disease in women. The American Journal of Clinical Nutrition. 2004;**79**(1):47-53. Available from: https://academic.oup.com/ajcn/article/79/1/47/4690068

[18] Knekt P, Ritz J, Pereira MA, O'Reilly EJ, Augustsson K, Fraser GE, et al. Antioxidant vitamins and coronary heart disease risk: A pooled analysis of 9 cohorts. The American Journal of Clinical Nutrition. 2004;**80**(6):1508-1520. Available from: https://academic.oup.com/ajcn/article/80/6/1508/4690474

[19] Garcia-Salas P, Morales-Soto A, Segura-Carretero A, Fernández-Gutiérrez A. Phenolic-compound-extraction systems for fruit and vegetable samples. Molecules. 2010;**15**(12):8813-8826

[20] Huang W-Y, Cai Y-Z, Zhang Y. Natural phenolic compounds from medicinal herbs and dietary plants: Potential use for cancer prevention. Nutrition and Cancer. 2009;**62**(1):1-20. Available from: http://www.tandfonline.com/doi/abs/10.1080/01635580903191585

[21] De Pascual-Teresa S, Moreno DA, García-Viguera C. Flavanols and anthocyanins in cardiovascular health: A review of current evidence. International Journal of Molecular Sciences. 2010;**11**(4):1679-1703. Available from: http://www.mdpi.com/1422-0067/11/4/1679

[22] Goleniowski M, Bonfill M, Cusido R, Palazon J. Phenolic Acids. In Natural Products: Phytochemistry, Botany and Metabolism of Alkaloids, Phenolics and Terpenes. Berlin, Heidelberg: Springer Berlin Heidelberg. https://doi.org/10.1007/978-3-642-22144-6_64 2013. pp. 1951-1973

[23] Yousuf B, Gul K, Wani AA, Singh P. Health benefits of anthocyanins and their encapsulation for potential use in food systems: A review. Critical *Reviews in* Food Science *and* Nutrition. 2016;**56**(13):2223-2230. Available from: http://www.tandfonline.com/doi/full/10.1080/10408398.2013.805316

[24] Zhao Cuiwei, Monica Giusti M, Malik Minnie, Moyer MP, Magnuson BA. Effects of Commercial Anthocyanin-Rich Extracts on Colonic Cancer and Nontumorigenic Colonic Cell Growth. Journal of Agricultural and Food Chemistry. 2004;**52**(20):6122-6128. Available from: https://pubs.acs.org/doi/abs/10.1021/jf049517a

[25] Wang J, Mazza G. Inhibitory Effects of Anthocyanins and Other Phenolic Compounds on Nitric Oxide Production in LPS/IFN-γ-Activated RAW 264.7 Macrophages. Journal of Agricultural and Food Chemistry. 2002;**50**(4):850-857. Available from: https://pubs.acs.org/doi/abs/10.1021/jf010976a

[26] Basli A, Belkacem N, Amrani I. Health benefits of phenolic compounds against cancers. Phenolic Compd - Biol Act. 2017;March:193-210 Rijeka, Crotia: Intech; Available from: http://www.intechopen.com/books/phenolic-compounds-biological-activity/health-benefits-of-phenolic-compounds-against-cancers

[27] Olthof MR, PCH H, Katan MB. Chlorogenic acid and caffeic acid are absorbed in humans. Journal of Nutrition. 2001;**131**(1):66-71. Available from: https://academic.oup.com/jn/article/131/1/66/4686566

[28] Barrett DM, Lloyd B. Advanced preservation methods and nutrient retention in fruits and vegetables. Journal of the Science of Food and Agriculture. 2011 November;**92**(1): 7-22. DOI: 10.1002/jsfa.4718

[29] Barba FJ, Mariutti LRB, Braganolo N, Mercadante AZ, Barbosa-Canovas GV, Orlien V. Bioaccessibility of bioactive compounds from fruits and vegetables after thermal and non-thermal processing. Trends in Food Science and Technology. 2017 September;**67**. DOI: 10.1016/j.tifs.2017.07.006

[30] Tiwari U, Cummins E. Factors influencing levels of phytochemicals in selected fruit and vegetables during pre- and post-harvest food processing operations. Food Research International. 2013 March;**50**(2):497-506

[31] Ricci A, Parpinello GP, Versari A. Recent advances and applications of pulsed electric fields (PEF) to improve polyphenol extraction and colour release during red winemaking. Beverages. 2018 January;**4**(1):8

[32] Toepfl S, Heinz V. New Food Magazine - Pulsed Electric Field Processing of Foods. [Online]. 2007. Available from: https://www.newfoodmagazine.com/article/1594/pulsed-electric-field-processing-of-foods/

[33] Kumar R, Bawa AS, Kathiravan T, Nadanasabapathi S. Optimization of pulsed electric field parameters for mango nectar processing using response surface methodology. International Food Research Journal. 2015 December;**22**(1):1353-1360

[34] Kumar R, Bawa AS, RRK KT. Pulsed electric field and combination processing of mango nectar: Effect on volatile compounds and HMF formation. Croatian Journal of Food Science and Technology. 2015;**7**(2):58-67. DOI: 10.17508/CJFST.2015.7.2.02

[35] Buckow R, Ng S, Toepfl S. Pulsed electric field processing of orange juice: A review on micro-

bial, enzymatic, nutritional, and sensory quality and stability. Comprehensive Reviews in Food Science and Food Safety. 2013;**12**(5):455-467. DOI: 10.1111/1541-4337.12026

[36] Lamanauskas N, Pataro G, Bobinas Č, Šatkauskas S, Viškelis P, Bobinaitė R, et al. Impact of pulsed electric field treatment on juice yield and recovery of bioactive compounds from raspberries and their by-products. Zemdirbyste-Agriculture. 2016;**103**(1):83-90. DOI: 10.13080/z-a.2016.103.011

[37] Sotelo KAG, Hamid N, Oey I, Gutierrez-Maddox N, Ma Q, Leong SY. Effect of pulsed electric fields on the flavour profile of red-fleshed sweet cherries (Prunus avium var. Stella). Molecules. 2015 March;**20**(3):5223-5238. DOI: 10.3390/molecules20035223

[38] Muntean M, Marian O, Barbieru V, Catunescu G, Ranta O, Drocas I, et al. High pressure processing in the food industry–Characteristics and applications. In 5th International Conference "Agriculture for Life, Life for Agriculture"; 2016; Bucharest. pp. 377-383

[39] Chakraborty S, Rao PS. Food and Beverage News–Impact of HPP on Antioxidant Capacity of Fruit Beverages. [Online]. 2015. Available from: http://www.fnbnews.com/Beverage/impact-of-hpp-on-antioxidant-capacity-of-fruit-beverages-37935

[40] Marszałek K, Woźniak Ł, Skąpska S. The application of high pressure–mild temperature processing for prolonging the shelf life of strawberry purée. High Pressure Research. 2016;**36**(2):220-234. DOI: 10.1080/08957959.2016.1172072

[41] Marszałek K, Woźniak Ł, Kruszewski B, Skąpska S. The effect of high pressure techniques on the stability of anthocyanins in fruit and vegetables. International Journal of Molecular Sciences. 2017 January;**18**:277. DOI: 10.3390/ijms18020277

[42] Garcia-Parra J, Gonzdlez-Cebrino F, Delgado J, Cava R, Ramirez R. High pressure assisted thermal processing of pumpkin puree: Effect on microbial counts, color, bioactive compounds and polyphenoloxidase enzyme. Food and Bioproducts Processing. 2016;**98**: 124-132

[43] Aadil RM, Zeng XA, Jabbar S, Nazir A, Mann AA, Khan MKI, et al. Quality evaluation of grapefruit juice by thermal and high pressure processing treatment. Pakistan Journal of Agricultural Research. 2017 September;**30**(3):249-257

[44] Majid I, Nayik GA, Nanda V. Ultrasonication and food technology: A review. Cogent Food & Agriculture. 2015;**1**:1071022. DOI: 10.1080/23311932.2015.1071022

[45] Jabbar S, Abid M, Hu B, Wu T, Hashim MM, Lei S, et al. Quality of carrot juice as influenced by blanching and sonication treatments. LWT - Food Science and Technology. 2014 January;**55**(1):16-21

[46] Abid M, Jabbar S, Wu T, Hashim MM, Hu B, Lei S, et al. Effect of ultrasound on different quality parameters of apple juice. Ultrasonics Sonochemistry. 2013 September; **20**(5):1182-1187

[47] Zou Y, Hou X. Sonication enhances quality and antioxidant activity of blueberry juice. The Food Science and Technology Journal (Campinas). 2017 Dec;**37**(4):599-603

[48] Dias DRC, Barros ZMP, Oliveira de Carvalho CB, Honorato FA, Guerra NB, Azoubel PM. Effect of sonication on soursop juice quality. LWT - Food Science and Technology. 2015 June;**62**(1):883-889

[49] Yao GL, Ma XH, Cao XY, Chen J. Effects of power ultrasound on stability of cyanidin-3-glucoside obtained from blueberry. Molecules. 2016 November;**21**:11. DOI: 10.3390/molecules21111564

[50] Bhavya ML, Umesh Hebbar H. Pulsed light processing of foods for microbial safety. Food Quality and Safety. 2017 August;**1**(3):187-201. DOI: 10.1093/fqsafe/fyx017

[51] Elmnasser N, Guillo S, Leroi F, Orange N, Bakhrouf A, Federighi M. Pulsed-light system as a novel decontamination technology: A review. Canada Journal of Microbiology. 2007;**53**:813-821. DOI: 10.1139/W07-042

[52] Abida J, Rbmfa. Pulsed light technology: A novel method for food preservation. International Food Research Journal. 2014 January;**21**(3):839-848

[53] Maharaj R, Mohammed A. Significance of UV-C hormesis and its relation to some phytochemicals in ripening and senescence process. In Montanaro G, editor. Advances in Selected Plant Physiology Aspects. InTech. 2012. pp. 251-268. DOI: 10.5772/26694. Available from: https://www.intechopen.com/books/advances-in-selected-plant-physiology-aspects/significance-of-uv-c-hormesis-and-its-relation-to-some-phytochemicals-in-ripening-and-senescence-pro

[54] Manzocco L, Comuzzo P, Scampicchio M, Nicoli MC. Effect of pulsed light on selected properties of cut apple. Italian Journal of Food Science. 2017;**29**:317-328

[55] Lopes MMA, Silva EO, Laurent S, Charles F, Urban L, Miranda MRA. The influence of pulsed light exposure mode on quality and bioactive compounds of fresh-cut mangoes. Journal of Food Science and Technology. 2017 June;**54**:2332. DOI: 10.1007/s13197-017-2673-x

[56] Koh PC, Noranizan MA, Karim R, Hanani ZAN. Microbiological stability and quality of pulsed light treated cantaloupe (Cucumis melo L. reticulatus cv. Glamour) based on cut type and light fluence. Journal of Food Science and Technology. 2016 April;**53**(4):1798-1810. DOI: 10.1007/s13197-015-2139-y

[57] Pataro G, Donsi G, Ferrari G. Post-harvest UV-C and PL irradiation of fruits and vegetables. Chemical Engineering Transactions. 2015;**44**:31-36. DOI: 10.3303/CET1544006

[58] Xu W, Chen H, Wu C. Salmonella and Escherichia coli 0 1 57:H7 inactivation, color, and bioactive compounds enhancement on raspberries during frozen storage after decontamination using new formula sanitizer washing or pulsed light. Journal o f Food Protection. 2016;**79**(7):1107-1114. DOI: 10.4315/0362-028X.JFP-15-379

[59] Pankaj SK, Wan Z, Keener KM. Effects of cold plasma on food quality: A review. Food. 2018 January;**7**:4. DOI: 10.3390/foods7010004

[60] Thirumdas R, Sarangapani C, Annapure US. Cold plasma: A novel non-thermal tech-

nology for food processing. Food Biophysics. 2014 November;**1**:10. DOI: 10.1007/s11483-014-9382-z

[61] Misra NN, Keener KM, Bourke P, Mosnier JP, Cullen PJ. In-package atmospheric pressure cold plasma treatment of cherry tomatoes. Journal of Bioscience and Bioengineering. 2014;**118**(2):177-182. DOI: 10.1016/j.jbiosc.2014.02.005

[62] Stoica M, Alexe P, Mihalcea L. Atmospheric cold plasma as new strategy for food processing–An overview. Innovative Romanian Food Biotechnology. 2014 November;**15**:1-8

[63] Misra NN, Patil S, Moiseev T, Bourke P, Mosnier JP, Keener KM, et al. In-package atmospheric pressure cold plasma treatment of strawberries. Journal of Food Engineering. 2014 March;**125**:131-138. DOI: 10.1016/j.jfoodeng.2013.10.023

[64] Vukić M, Vujadinović D, Gojković V, Grujić R. Influence of cold plasma treatment on textural and color characteristics of two tomato varieties. Quality of Life. 2016;**7**(1-2):12-16. DOI: 10.7251/QOL16012V

[65] Tappi S, Berardinelli A, Ragni L, Rosa MD, Guarnieri A, Rocculi P. Atmospheric gas plasma treatment of fresh-cut apples. Innovative Food Science and Emerging Technologies. 2014 October;**24**:114-122. DOI: 10.1016/j.ifset.2013.09.012

[66] Tappi S, Gozzi G, Vannini L, Berardinelli A, Romani S, Ragni L, et al. Cold plasma treatment for fresh-cut melon stabilization. Innovative Food Science and Emerging Technologies. 2016 December;**33**:225-233. DOI: 10.1016/j.ifset.2015.12.022

[67] Ramazzina I, Berardinelli A, Rizzi F, Tappi S, Ragni L, Sacchetti G, et al. Effect of cold plasma treatment on physico-chemical parameters and antioxidant activity of minimally processed kiwifruit. Postharvest Biology and Technology. 2015 May;**107**:55-65. DOI: 10.1016/j.postharvbio.2015.04.008

8

Anthocyanins-Smart Molecules for Cancer Prevention

Zorița M. Diaconeasa, Alexandra D. Frond,
Ioana Ştirbu, Dumitrița Rugina and Carmen Socaciu

Abstract

Anthocyanins are one of the most widespread natural pigments in the plant kingdom. Being surrounded by so many fruits and vegetables rich in anthocyanins, it is recommended to consume a relatively large amount of them. A daily intake of anthocyanins has a certain demonstrated benefits: lowers the risk of cardiovascular disease, diabetes, arthritis, and cancer due, at least in part, to their antioxidant and anti-inflammatory activities. Lately, great attention is paid to their anticancer properties due to the need for user-friendly approaches to improve the treatment. So far, cancer had been nominated to be the second in top 10 diseases of the twenty-first century. Those colorful pigments have the ability to modulate the activity of multiple targets involved in carcinogenesis through direct interaction or modulation of gene expression and can also inhibit the growth of cancer cells. However, the main concern related to the use of anthocyanins as anticancer agents is their poor bioavailability, more specific poor absorption, and biodistribution. In this chapter, the anticancer activities of anthocyanins or anthocyanin-rich extracts *in vitro* or *in vivo* were reviewed.

Keywords: anthocyanins, berries, cancer

1. Introduction

Anthocyanins are cell vacuole components, abundant flavonoid constituents, which are responsible for the varied colors (red, purple, and blue) of flowers, vegetables, or fruits. Apart from fruits and flowers, anthocyanins also are also accumulated in vegetative tissues where they are considered to confer protection against various biotic and abiotic stresses [1–4]. They are the largest and the most important group of water-soluble plant pigments. Berries, grapes, apples, purple cabbage, black soybean, and black rice are some examples of rich anthocyanins fruits and vegetables. In their natural environments, plants are vulnerable because of multiple attacks by many different species of herbivores and also pathogens [5]. A vast spectrum of secondary metabolites have been demonstrated to act against their predators [6]. Among them are the phenolics, a large group of structurally diverse compounds, as well as certain flavonoids such as the anthocyanins. There are several ways anthocyanins assist plants in their defense against other organisms, such as chemical repellents and visual signals [7]. Along with other flavonoids, certain anthocyanins have demonstrable antiviral, antibacterial, and fungicidal activities. Also, it is generally accepted that the colors of flowers and fruits enhance reproductive success by facilitating communication between plants, their pollinators, and seed-dispersers [8]. Another positive propriety of anthocyanins is that they have demonstrated to exhibit antioxidant potential *in vitro* and *in vivo*. The antioxidant potential of anthocyanins have been demonstrated *in vitro* using several cell culture lines including ovarian, colon, endothelial liver, breast, leukemic cells, and keratinocytes [9–17]. Applied *in vitro* as treatment, anthocyanins have exhibited multiple antiproliferative and anticarcinogenic effects [18, 19]. The antioxidant activity of anthocyanins is a great property and was demonstrated that their chemical structure seems to be responsible for that [20–23].

2. Chemical structure of anthocyanins

Anthocyanins occur naturally in fruits and vegetables as glycosides, having one or more sugar attached to an aglycone nucleus (anthocyanidin). Their aglycones share a C6-C3-C6 carbon skeleton, characterized by the presence of two benzyl rings (A and B) and a heterocyclic ring (C) [24].

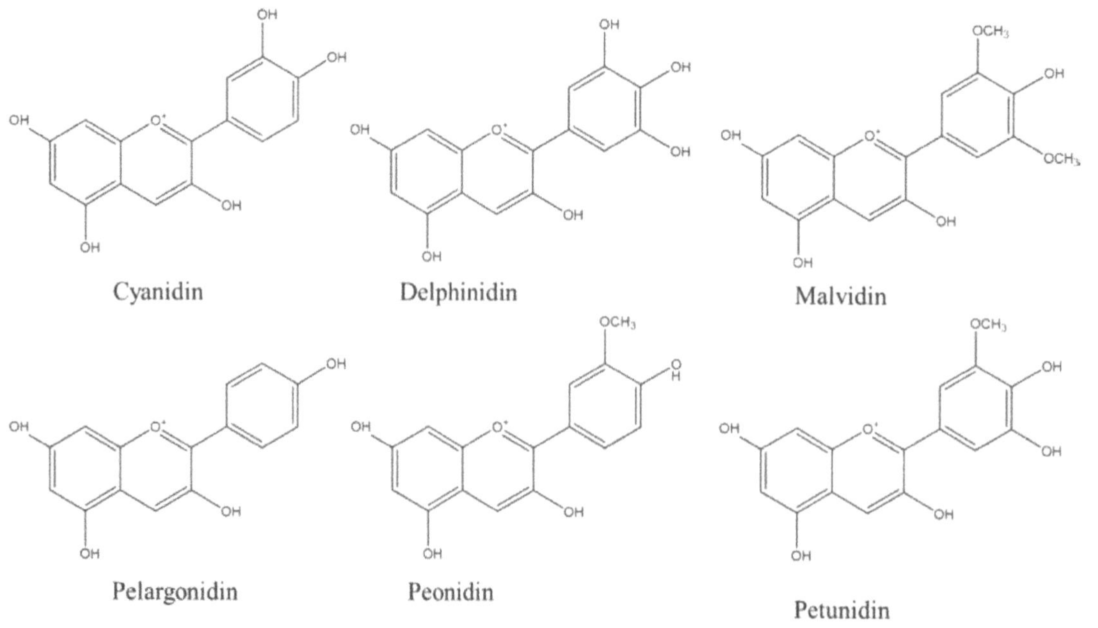

Figure 1. Chemical structure of the six most common anthocyanidins.

According to hydroxylation and methylations on the different positions of the rings, there are close to 25 different aglycones [25]. They exist in natural products, mainly in a form combined with glucose, galactose, and rhamnose, the more common sugar moieties attached to the aglycone but others sugars are also frequently found, and can be divided into at least six common types, such as pelargonidin, cyanidin, delphinidin, peonidin, petunidin, and malvidin, according to the different substituent groups on flavylium B-ring (**Figure 1**) [26, 27]. The sugars attached to the aglycone may in turn be further linked to other sugars through glyosidic bonds or acylated with organic aromatic or aliphatic acids [28]. One of the most striking properties linked to their chemical structure is that their color changes depending on the pH. They are natural pH indicators; they appear pink at low pH, purple in neutral conditions, and greenish-yellow in basics but the most stable form dominates at low pH [26].

3. Anthocyanins' potential health benefits

Since we consume a great amount of fruits, the daily intake of anthocyanins is highly variable and dependent on eating habits. Residents of the United States consume about 12.5 mg/day while in Europe, a highest consumption was found in Italy, about 64.9 mg/day [29, 30]. Many studies have suggested that anthocyanins have antioxidant, anti-inflammatory, and anti-carcinogenic properties and lower the risk of cardiovascular disease, diabetes, arthritis, and cancer due, at least in part, to their antioxidant and anti-inflammatory activities (**Figure 2**) [19, 26, 31, 32].

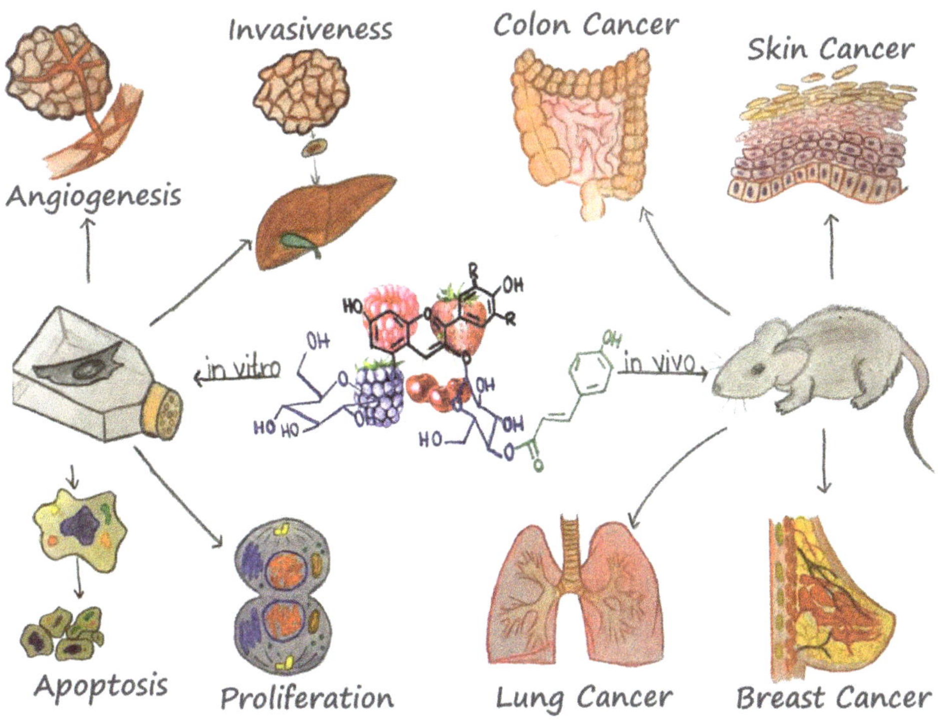

Figure 2. Anticancer properties of anthocyanins.

Reactive oxygen species (ROS) are produced by all aerobic cells and are important to the immune system, cell signaling, and many other normal body functions. They can elicit cellular damage, leading to degenerative diseases such as inflammation, cardiovascular disease, cancer, and aging if ROS are excessively produced [33–35]. As we mention previously, anthocyanins are potent antioxidants and their effectiveness has been tested *in vitro* and *in vivo*. They quench free radicals and terminate the chain reaction that is responsible for the oxidative damage. Because of the pH in the human body, their antioxidant activity at a neutral pH has a particular importance [36]. To assess the *in vivo* antioxidant activity of anthocyanins, an anthocyanin mixture was administered to mice/rats that were subjected to psychological stress [37, 38]. It was noticed that anthocyanins have similar antioxidant potency as vitamin E (α-tocopherol). Dietary anthocyanins have the potential to increase serum antioxidant capacity and thereby protect against LDL oxidation and prevent cardiovascular diseases as demonstrated in a human trial [39]. Deposits oxidized cholesterol into the artery wall can lead to atherosclerosis and eventually cardiovascular diseases [40]. Several studies have shown that anthocyanins have anti-obesity effect on high-fat diets and consequently may contribute to the prevention of type 2 diabetes. One of the studies demonstrates that black soybean anthocyanins were found to effectively reverse the weight gain of high-fat diet group rats [41]. Moreover, a number of different reports indicate that consumption of fruits and vegetables, especially rich in polyphenols, decrease the incidence of type-2 diabetes, a condition associated with insulin resistance [42, 43]. Nevertheless, evidence in the use of anthocyanins to improve night vision was also revealed in other scientific articles [44, 45].

4. Anticancer properties of anthocyanins

The uncontrolled growth of cells which can invade and spread to distant sites of the body is a global health problem, called cancer, with high mortality. Prevention and routine monitoring are critical to early and accurate diagnosis. Most therapeutic options do not offer cure but rather a deceleration of cancer progression. They not only aim at life extension and the improvement of patients' life quality but also often they have multiple side effects. In recent years, fruit and vegetables, including soft fruits such as berries, may represent a valid alternative than drugs with undesirable side and adverse effects, because of their chemopreventive or chemotherapeutic properties against certain diseases, such as cancer. Recent studies on the cancer preventative activities of the anthocyanins include results from *in vitro* cell culture and *in vivo* animal model tumor systems, as well as data from human epidemiological studies. Cancer cells differ from normal cells by a number of characteristics, thus being different in morphology and function. Anthocyanins can attack cancer cells due to these differences and cause a number of effects. A significant characteristic of cancer cells is their uncontrolled cell cycle, which leads to continuous division and proliferation. Pure anthocyanins and anthocyanin-rich extracts have demonstrated to inhibit cell proliferation by the ability of anthocyanins to block various stages of the cell cycle [46, 47]. Moreover, they can selectively inhibit the proliferation of cancer cells, but have little influence on the proliferation of normal cells [48, 49]. Anthocyanins have demonstrated to induce the apoptosis of cancer cells through the internal mitochondrial pathway and the external death receptor pathway. Usually, apoptosis, the programed cell death, in tumor cells is not present; therefore, dead cells cannot be eliminated normally. Cancer cells have deregulated several genes to avoid the apoptosis, such as p53, and these cells have high resistance to death compared with normal cells. In the intrinsic pathway, cytochrome *c* release and modulation of caspase-dependent anti- and proapoptotic proteins appear as an increase in mitochondrial membrane potential, because of anthocyanin treatment on cancer cells. In the extrinsic pathway, the expression of FAS and FASL is modulated by anthocyanins resulting apoptosis in cancer cells [50–52]. Lately, anthocyanins have been shown to suppress angiogenesis through several mechanisms such as: inhibition of H_2O_2 and tumor necrosis factor alpha (TNF-α)-induced VEGF expression in epidermal keratinocytes and by reducing VEGF and VEGF receptor expression in endothelial cells [53]. Angiogenesis is the physiological process of forming new blood vessels from the existing vascular network for the growth and metastasis of malignant tumors. The process of angiogenesis is controlled by multiple cytokines, of which the most important factor is vascular endothelial growth factor (VEGF); therefore, inhibiting the receptor of angiogenesis vascular endothelial growth factor receptor (VEGFR) could inhibit the metastasis of tumors effectively [18]. Anthocyanins were found to inhibit cancer cell invasion by reducing the expression of matrix metalloproteinase (MMP) and urokinase plasminogen activator (u-PA), both of which degrade extracellular matrix as part of the invasive process and, by stimulating the expression of inhibitors, both of which counteract the action of MMP and uPA [54]. There are two main aspects of cancer cells that threaten patient's health and life: invasion and metastasis. Successful tumor cell extravasation is successful by facilitating degradation of the extracellular matrix barriers. The balance of activated proteases and their naturally occurring inhibitors determine the degradation of the basement membrane [55].

5. *In vivo* studies

In carcinogen-treated animals and also animals with a hereditary predisposition to cancer, anthocyanins have been shown to inhibit the development of cancer. Moreover, they have been proven effective in: esophageal cancer, colon cancer, skin cancer, and lung cancer. After treatment, administration in different forms, such as anthocyanin-rich tart cherry extract, black raspberry powder, lyophilized black raspberries or ethanol: H_2O extract from berries, certain effects, were observed. All diets were equally effective in preventing the development of tumors, reducing tumor numbers by 42–47%, suggesting that anthocyanins in the fruits are important for their chemopreventive activity. A small summary of several types of cancer will be discussed further.

5.1. Colon cancer

Colon cancer is one of the most prevalent diseases across the world. In the United States, colon cancer is the second most prevalent cause of death from cancer in men and women after lung cancer, with approximately 50,310 causes of death [56]. In Europe, colorectal cancer is the second most common cancer, with 50,000 new cases diagnosed in 2012 [57]. The development of colon cancer is associated with high alcohol consumption, high-fat diet poor in fiber, red meat, obesity, smoking, lack of physical exercise, diabetes, inflammatory bowel disease, and some genetic and epigenetic alterations as: microsatellite instability, chromosomal instability, mutation of p53 gene is one of the familiar genetic changes in the development of colon cancer, and several others [58]. A very recent study published in 2017, used a mouse model, which treated them comparatively with azoxymethan (AOM)/dextran sodium sulfate (DSS) and anthocyanin-rich extract from bilberries for colon cancer development [59]. The anthocyanin extract administered to mice resulted in less inflammation of the colon and a reduced number of tumors than the control group. The formation and the growth of colorectal cancer in AOM/DSS-treated Balb/c mice were prevented by anthocyanins. Another *in vivo* study investigated the chemopreventive activity of commercially available anthocyanin-rich extracts of bilberry, chokeberry, and grape prepared for the food industry [60] Colon cancer male rats treated with a colon carcinogen, azoxymethane, had multiple biomarkers investigated such as: the number and multiplicity of colonic aberrant crypt foci, colonic cell proliferation, urinary levels of oxidative DNA damage, and expression of cyclooxygenase (COX) genes. Compared to the control group, rats fed with different extracts showed several changes. In rats fed with bilberry, chokeberry, and grape extracts, the number of large aberrant crypt foci was reduced. The bilberry and chokeberry diet decreased the colonic cellular proliferation, and the grape and bilberry diets had lower COX-2 mRNA expression of gene. These results clearly support the chemopreventive activity of tested extracts.

5.2. Breast cancer

Breast cancer is the second most common cause of cancer-associated mortalities in women. The American Cancer Society estimated that 60,290 new cases of breast carcinoma *in situ* were expected to be diagnosed among women in the United States during 2015 [61]. Understanding the biology of the human epidermal growth factor receptor 2 (HER2) helps with the classification, prognosis, and treatment of breast cancer because of the overexpression of HER2 identified in 15–20% cases. HER2 is involved in proliferation, angiogenesis, invasion, and metastasis [62]. A group of scientists have used injection of cyaniding-3-glucoside and peonidin-3-glucoside to evaluate the effect on the tumors of the rats used in the experiments [63]. Compared with the control group, the tumors treated with cyanidin-3-glucoside and peonidin-3-glucoside expressed lower levels of HER2 as well as Ki67, a proliferation marker, demonstrated with histopathological studies. Also, the treated tumors expressed higher levels of caspase 3, showing the apoptotic effect of the treatment. A recent published study [64] evaluated the cytotoxicity of an anthocyanin-rich extract from black rice (AEBR) on breast cancer cells *in vitro* and *in vivo*. This study demonstrated that black rice extract has promising roles against breast cancer. The oral administration of anthocyanin-rich extract from black rice (100 mg/kg/day) on nude mice bearing MDAMB-453 cell xenografts, significantly suppressed tumor growth and angiogenesis, as well as antagonized VEGF activity.

5.3. Lung cancer

Lung cancer emerged as the most common cancer worldwide, with 1.8 million new cases in 2012 [57]. The treatment and prevention for lung cancer remains scarce, comparing too many other types of cancer (e.g., breast and prostate). Also, there are no standard practices for the prevention of lung cancer recurrence and metastasis, so there is a great need for some unconventional, user-friendly approaches to improve the treatment and prevent or delay the recurrent lung disease. A recent study published in 2016, investigated the tumor inhibitory activity of diet supplemented with blackberry, alone and in combination with black raspberry, against lung tumor xenograft using nude mice [65]. Their findings indicated that the mixture of blackberry and black raspberry resulted in higher inhibition of tumor growth vs. blackberry alone. Also, the combination between delphinidin (bioactive in blackberries) and punicalagin (bioactive in black raspberry, which gets converted to ellagic acid *in vivo*) determined a higher tumor growth inhibition than delphinidin alone. In another study, two bioactive compounds, peonidin 3-glucoside and cyanidin 3-glucoside, were isolated and identified the from *Oryza sativa* L. Moreover, those compounds were used to treat various cancer cells. They have demonstrated the inhibition on the growth of Lewis lung carcinoma cells *in vivo* [66].

5.4. Skin cancer

Malignant melanoma of skin accounted for 232,000 new cases, and the regions affected are largely those with white populations [57]. Melanoma skin cancer originates in melanocytes, specialized pigment-producing cells found in both the basal layer of the epidermis. Solar UVB radiation has been implicated as the main cause for skin cancer [67]. Early diagnosis is the key for curing this potentially deadly disease. Also prevention is playing a crucial role in spotting melanomas at earlier and more curable stages [68]. Biochemotherapy, the coadministration of traditional chemotherapeutic drugs and biological agents, show a higher response rate for patients than classical treatments that are based only on chemotherapy alone [69–72]. Most anticancer treatments are derived from natural resources such as marine, microbial, and botanical sources [72]. Natural supplements, a rich diet in antioxidants used as a complementary medication, become a common field of research in order to develop new products originating from natural sources with antioxidant and chemopreventive properties. The ability of anthocyanins to influence parameters of skin tumor development on mice was demonstrated in various studies. SKH-1 hairless mouse was used in order to investigate the photo-chemopreventive effect of delphinidin on UVB-induced biomarkers of skin cancer development [17]. After the treatment, the results suggest that delphinidin inhibited UVB-mediated oxidative stress and reduced DNA damage, thereby protecting the cells from UVB-induced apoptosis. The antitumor activity of the anthocyanins extract from *Fructus Sorbi aucupariae* on B-16 melanoma in C57BI/6 mice was also demonstrated [73]. The study revealed an increase in the counts of stromal progenitor cells in the tumor node and their accelerated maturation. The potentiation of the antimetastatic activity of the cytostatic was demonstrated as well. The inhibitory effects of mulberry anthocyanins on the metastasis of B16-F1 cells under noncytotoxic concentrations were investigated. The findings of the study have demonstrated that mulberry anthocyanins have strong anticancer effects by inhibiting the metastasis ability of B16-F1 cells. Further investigations revealed that the antimetastatic effect of these compounds was also evident in a C57BL/6 mice model.

5.5. Prostate cancer

Prostate cancer is the most common malignancy in men and affects most men over the age of 50 and also presents one of the main causes of mortality. For the *in vivo* study, athymic nude mice are used. To highlight the effects of anthocyanins on tumor growth *in vivo*, DH145 tumor xenograft have been established in these mice. The group of animals treated with anthocyanins received an oral dose of 8 mg/kg per day. The effects of treatment were analyzed every 4 weeks. In the first 4 weeks after incubation, the difference between the control and the treated group was insignificant. In the second set of analyses (8 weeks), the difference between the groups was very clear, the control group tumors being much bigger. These differences were observed until the end of the experiment, demonstrating the ability of anthocyanins to reduce tumor growth [74]. Another study has found that delphinidin is effective *in vitro* on PC3 cells and has determined whether these results are also visible in *in vivo* models. The delphinidin doses were not toxic to the animals because they did not lose weight and did not affect the amount of food they consumed. After measurements for 12 weeks, the differences between the tumors of the two groups (control and treated) each week were significant, suggesting an antiangiogenic effect on tumor cells. At the end of the experiment, tumors were extirpated and analyzed, where effects similar to *in vitro* studies were observed [75].

5.6. Leukemia

Acute myeloid leukemia is a hematological malignancy that has numerous causes such as chromosomal abnormalities and various gene mutations. Fifty years ago, this type of cancer was incurable, but now around 35–40% of the cases is treatable [85]. Mice Balc/c has been used to identify *in vivo* benefits of mulberry anthocyanins. Leukemia mice treated with anthocyanins had a higher survival rate than the untreated ones, this survival being correlated with the concentration of treatment. All leukemia-induced mice had the spleen and liver measured at autopsy, indicating splenomegaly and hepatomegaly. The size of these organs was significantly reduced for those treated compared to the control group. The organs were evaluated histopathologically as well and again the treated group had less infiltrated tissue with leukemic cells. Taken all this into consideration, we can say that mulberry anthocyanins can improve or eliminate the leukemic mice disorder [86].

6. *In vitro* studies

6.1. Colon cancer

Based on the substitution pattern of anthocyanidins, a recent study reported that growth inhibition of HT29 cells (human colon cancer) was highly affected by delphinidin and malvidin, while pelargonidin exhibited the lowest growth inhibitory potential. Moreover, same study reported that malvidin could inhibit the activity of phosphodiesterase (PDE) and the hydrolysis of cAMP effectively in HT29 cells thereby inhibiting the MAPK signaling pathway [76]. Another research paper [77] investigated anthocyanin-rich extracts from grape (*Vitis vinifera*), bilberry (*Vaccinium myrtillus* L.), and chokeberry (*Aronia melanocarpa* E.) for their potential chemopreventive activity against colon cancer. The growth of colon-cancer-derived HT-29 and nontumorigenic colonic NCM460 cell lines exposed to semipurified anthocyanin-rich extracts (AREs) was monitored for up to 72 h. All extracts inhibited the growth of HT-29 cells, chokeberry extract being the most potent inhibitor. Most importantly, the growth of NCM460 cells was not inhibited at lower concentrations of all three extracts, illustrating better inhibition of colon cancer, as compared to nontumorigenic colon cells. Lately, another study [78] investigated and observed the effects of extracts from five cultivars of strawberries on the proliferation of colon cancer cells HT29 and breast cancer cells MCF-7. Using strawberry as a source of anthocyanins, they demonstrated that strawberry extracts decreased the proliferation of two cell lines in a dose-dependent manner.

6.2. Breast cancer

Human epidermal growth factor 2 (HER2) is a member of the epidermal growth factor receptor family which is overexpressed in breast cancer, and to study the *in vitro* effect of anthocyanins, the cell lines in breast cancer are usually HER2 positive; unfortunately, there are many other types of breast cancer that occur due to other causes. Regarding potential chemopreventive effects of anthocyanins, recently, it was demonstrated that black rice anthocyanins reduce the adhesion, migration, and invasion of HER2 MDA-MB-453 cells. The morphology of these cells was significantly altered, moving from a mesenchymal to an epithelial state. The western blot analysis shows an increase of the epithelial marker, E-cadherin, and decreased the expression of the mesenchymal markers, fibronectin and vimentin; this shows the effect that BRAC has on epithelial mesenchymal transition (EMT). EMT is a process by which epithelial cells lose their cell polarity and cell-cell adhesion, and gain migratory and invasive properties which occurs in the initiation of metastasis in cancer progression [4]. An important role in the metastasis of MDA-MB-453 cells is the focal adhesion kinase (FAK)-signaling pathway. FAK promotes the increased expression of transcription factors associated with EMT. The cells used in certain analysis were treated with Y15 (FAK inhibitor) that inhibits the autophosphorylation site of FAK. The study shows that BRAC has a similar effect to Y15, and also BRAC decreases the activation and transduction of FAK signaling [79].

6.3. Lung cancer

Inhibitory effect of anthocyanins on the migration and invasion of lung cancer was also studied. A previous study reported that glycosylated cyanidins isolated from mulberry exerted a dose-dependent inhibitory effect on the migration and invasion of metastatic A549 human lung carcinoma cells. Their results showed that the applied treatments could decrease the expressions of matrix matalloprotinase-2 (MMP-2) and urokinase plasminogen activator (u-PA) in a dose-dependent manner and also enhance the expression of tissue inhibitor of matrix matalloprotinase-2 (TIMP-2) and plasminogen activator inhibitor (PAI). Moreover, Western blot analysis revealed that anthocyanins treatment to A549 cells inhibited the activation of c-Jun (p48) and NF-kB (p65). Further, another study using anthocyanins from fruits of *Vitis coignetiae Pulliat* (AIMs) reported their anticancer effects on lung cancer cells. AIMs inhibited the growth; migration and invasion of A549 cells; and also some proteins involved with cancer effects are inhibited. AIMs suppressed MMP-2 (gelatinase-A) and MMP-9 (gelatinase-B), both involved in the proteolytic digestion of the ECM (extracellular matrix) and cell migration through the basement membranes to reach the circulatory system. Through the immunoblotting results, a large number of proteins have been demonstrated to be suppressed by AIMs. A couple of these proteins are involved in cancer proliferation (COX-2, cyclin D1), migration and invasion (MMP-2, MMP-9), as mentioned before, anti-apoptosis (XIAP), adhesion, and angiogenesis (VEGF). However, they were not able to identify in which signaling pathway is AIMs mainly involved. This study identifies that AIMs might have anticancer effects on human lung cancer [80].

6.4. Skin cancer

Several studies have demonstrated that flavonoids are one of the candidates for prevention of the adverse effects of UV radiation due to their UV absorbing property, and antioxidant properties. In this context, a published study revealed that grape seed proanthocyanidins (GSP) inhibits cell growth, induces G1-phase arrest, promotes apoptosis in human epidermoid carcinoma A431 cells through alterations in Cdki-Cdk-cyclin cascade, and caspase-3 activation via loss of mitochondrial membrane potential [81]. Many other studies have also proved the antiproliferative and proapoptotic effects of anthocyanins on melanoma or others skin diseases [82–84]. Our latest published revealed that anthocyanins may inhibit melanoma cell proliferation, increase the level of oxidative stress, and diminished mitochondrial membrane potential [84].

6.5. Prostate cancer

Cyanidin-3-O-β-glucopyranoside (C3G) is well known to be found in a lot of anthocyanin-rich fruits, like berries. To study its effect on cancer, two cells lines were used, LnCap and DU145. These cell lines were chosen because DU145 is a tumor cell line androgen-independent and LnCap is androgen-dependent. Androgen-dependent prostate cancer is characterized by the absence of the androgen receptor due to promoter methylation. In this case, the treatment is based on hormone elimination, yet other approaches are needed if the amount of hormones does not affect the development of cancer [79]. C3G causes a decrease in cell viability in both cell lines, and apoptosis is also induced, DU145 being more responsive in this aspect. The positive effect of treatment is demonstrated by the activation of caspase 3 and a significant increase in expression of p21 protein, evidence that cells undergo apoptosis [80]. Another study focuses on proteins that indicate the presence of apoptosis such as p53 and Bax. P53, or "the guardian of the genome" is a suppressor tumor protein that initiates apoptosis in degraded DNA cells, and Bax is a pro-apoptotic protein of the Bcl-2 family [81].

6.6. Leukemia

An bilberry extract (Antho 50) was used to determine its effect on Jurkat cells. The main interest of this study is the result of Antho 50 on certain proteins, polycomb group (PcG), which are epigenetic regulators. These proteins reduce the expression of suppressor tumor genes, promoting the survival of tumor cells [81]. The aim is to see if the extract is able to inhibit these PcG proteins. The extract was able to downregulate the PcG and related proteins and induces apoptosis. All these events have an effect on the intracellular ROS formation, causing an increase, resulting in the death of tumor cells [82]. In another study, delphinidin and cyanidin, two major compounds in *Hibiscus sabdariffa*, were investigated. They are able to induce cell cycle arrest in human leukemia cell line HL-60. This effect occurs because of their action on signaling pathways whose role is to induce cell cycle arrest. This indicates promising anticarcinogenic effects [83].

7. Conclusions

Interests in anthocyanins have increased substantially during the past two decades. In this review, we discussed at what level anthocyanins act when talking about anticancer effects. *In vitro*, we saw that anthocyanins affect: the proliferation of the cancer cells, inhibiting of the ability of cancer cells to divide uncontrollably, the induction of apoptosis, the process of angiogenesis where tumors form new blood vessels, and the cancer cells invasion through healthy tissue. Also, a few of the *in vivo* studies demonstrate that dietary anthocyanins inhibit the growth of different types of tumors, angiogenesis, and show apoptotic effect against the cancer cells. It remains to be determined whether the anticancer activity of anthocyanins is due to anthocyanins or their metabolites.

Conflicts of interest

The authors indicate no potential conflicts of interest. "The authors declare no conflict of interest"; "the founding sponsors had no role in the design of the study; in the collection, analyses, or interpretation of data; in the writing of the manuscript, and in the decision to publish the results."

Funding statement

This work was published under the frame of a national grant financed by Romanian National Authority for Scientific Research (UEFISCDI) project number PN-III-P2-2.1-PED-2016-1002, 186PED, 01/09/2017. The work of Dumitrița Rugină is sustained by the National Fellowship Program L'Oréal-UNESCO-For Women in Science.

Abbreviations

ROS	reactive oxygen species
PDE	phosphodiesterase
ARE	anthocyanin-rich extract

LC-MC	chromatography: liquid chromatography-mass spectrometry
VEGF	vascular endothelial growth factor
VEGFR	vascular endothelial growth factor receptor
TNF-α	tumor necrosis factor alpha
MMP	matrix metalloproteinase
u-PA	urokinase plasminogen activator
AOM	azoxymethan
DSS	dextran sodium sulfate
COX	cyclooxygenase
HER2	human epidermal growth factor receptor 2
UVB	ultraviolet B
BRAC	black rice anthocyanins
EMT	epithelial mesenchymal transition
FAK	focal adhesion kinase
Y15	FAK inhibitor
AIMs	anthocyanins from fruits of *Vitis coignetiae Pulliat*
ECM	extracellular matrix
GSP	grape seed proanthocyanidins
C3G	cyaniding-3-O-β-glucopyranoside
Antho 50	bilberry extract
PcG	polycomb group
MAC	mulberry anthocyanins

Author details

Zorița M. Diaconeasa*, Alexandra D. Frond, Ioana Ştirbu, Dumitrița Rugină and Carmen Socaciu

*Address all correspondence to: zorita.sconta@usamvcluj.ro

University of Agricultural Sciences and Veterinary Medicine, Cluj-Napoca, Romania

References

[1] Lev-Yadun S, Gould KS. Role of anthocyanins in plant defence. In: Winefield C, Davies K, Gould K, editors. Anthocyanins: Biosynthesis, Functions, and Applications. New York, NY: Springer; 2009. pp. 22-28

[2] Chalker-Scott L. Environmental significance of anthocyanins in plant stress responses. Photochemistry and Photobiology. 1999;**70**:1-9

[3] Gould KS. Nature's swiss army knife: The diverse protective roles of anthocyanins in leaves. Journal of Biomedicine and Biotechnology. 2004;**2004**:314-320

[4] Heerboth S, Housman G, Leary M, Longacre M, Byler S, Lapinska K, Willbanks A, Sarkar S. Emt and tumor metastasis. Clinical and Translational Medicine. 2015;**4**:6

[5] Wink M. Plant breeding: Importance of plant secondary metabolites for protection against pathogens and herbivores. Theoretical and Applied Genetics. 1988;**75**:225-233

[6] Falcone Ferreyra ML, Rius SP, Casati P. Flavonoids: Biosynthesis, biological functions, and biotechnological applications. Frontiers in Plant Science. 2012;**3**:222

[7] Mason JR, Bullard RW, Dolbeer RA, Woronecki PP. Red-winged blackbird (*Agelaius phoeniceus* L). Feeding response to oil and anthocyanin levels in sunflower meal. Crop Protection. 1989;**8**:455-460

[8] Saito N, Harborne JB. Correlations between anthocyanin type, pollinator and flower colour in the labiatae. Phytochemistry. 1992;**31**:3009-3015

[9] Renis M, Calandra L, Scifo C, Tomasello B, Cardile V, Vanella L, Bei R, La Fauci L, Galvano F. Response of cell cycle/stress-related protein expression and DNA damage upon treatment of $CaCo_2$ cells with anthocyanins, The British Journal of Nutrition. 2008;**100**:27-35

[10] Parry J, Su L, Moore J, Cheng Z, Luther M, Rao JN, Wang JY, Yu LL. Chemical compositions, antioxidant capacities, and antiproliferative activities of selected fruit seed flours. Journal of Agricultural and Food Chemistry. 2006;**54**:3773-3778

[11] Roy S, Khanna S, Alessio HM, Vider J, Bagchi D, Bagchi M, Sen CK. Anti-angiogenic property of edible berries. Free Radical Research. 2002;**36**:1023-1031

[12] Shin DY, Lee WS, Kim SH, Kim MJ, Yun JW, Lu JN, Lee SJ, Tsoy I, Kim HJ, Ryu CH, et al. Anti-invasive activity of anthocyanins isolated from vitis coignetiae in human hepatocarcinoma cells. Journal of Medicinal Food. 2009;**12**:967-972

[13] Takikawa M, Inoue S, Horio F, Tsuda T. Dietary anthocyanin-rich bilberry extract ameliorates hyperglycemia and insulin sensitivity via activation of amp-activated protein kinase in diabetic mice. The Journal of Nutrition. 2010;**140**:527-533

[14] Singletary KW, Jung KJ, Giusti M. Anthocyanin-rich grape extract blocks breast cell DNA damage. Journal of Medicinal Food. 2007;**10**:244-251

[15] Olsson ME, Gustavsson KE, Andersson S, Nilsson A, Duan RD. Inhibition of cancer cell proliferation in vitro by fruit and berry extracts and correlations with antioxidant levels. Journal of Agricultural and Food Chemistry. 2004;**52**:7264-7271

[16] Del Pozo-Insfran D, Percival SS, Talcott ST. Acai (*Euterpe oleracea* Mart.) polyphenolics in their glycoside and aglycone forms induce apoptosis of hl-60 leukemia cells. Journal of Agricultural and Food Chemistry. 2006;**54**:1222-1229

[17] Afaq F, Syed DN, Malik A, Hadi N, Sarfaraz S, Kweon MH, Khan N, Zaid MA, Mukhtar H. Delphinidin, an anthocyanidin in pigmented fruits and vegetables, protects human hacat keratinocytes and mouse skin against uvb-mediated oxidative stress and apoptosis. The Journal of Investigative Dermatology. 2007;**127**:222-232

[18] Chen X-Y, Zhou J, Luo L-P, Han B, Li F, Chen J-Y, Zhu Y-F, Chen W, Yu X-P. Black rice anthocyanins suppress metastasis of breast cancer cells by targeting ras/raf/mapk pathway. BioMed Research International. 2015;**2015**:11

[19] Diaconeasa Z, Ayvaz H, Rugina D, Leopold L, Stanila A, Socaciu C, Tabaran F, Luput L, Mada DC, Pintea A, et al. Melanoma inhibition by anthocyanins is associated with the reduction of oxidative stress biomarkers and changes in mitochondrial membrane potential. Plant Foods for Human Nutrition (Dordrecht, The Netherlands). 2017;**72**:404-410

[20] Yi L, Chen C-Y, Jin X, Mi M-T, Yu B, Chang H, Ling W-H, Zhang T. Structural requirements of anthocyanins in relation to inhibition of endothelial injury induced by oxidized low-density lipoprotein and correlation with radical scavenging activity. FEBS Letters. 2010;**584**:583-590

[21] Glover BJ, Martin C. Anthocyanins. Current Biology. 2012;**22**:R147-R150

[22] Chen Y, Zheng R, Jia Z, Ju Y. Flavonoids as superoxide scavengers and antioxidants. Free Radical Biology and Medicine. 1990;**9**:19-21

[23] Wang LS, Stoner GD. Anthocyanins and their role in cancer prevention. Cancer Letters. 2008;**269**:281-290

[24] Harborne JB. Phenolic compounds. In: Harborne JB, editor. Phytochemical Methods—A Guide to Modern Techniques of Plant Analysis. 3rd ed. New York: Chapman & Hall; 1998. pp. 66-74

[25] Andersen OM, Jordheim M. The anthocyanins. In: Andersen OM , Markham KR, editors. Flavonoids: Chemistry, Biochemistry and Applications. Boca Raton, FL: CRC Press; 2006. pp. 471-552

[26] He J, Giusti MM. Anthocyanins: Natural colorants with health-promoting properties. Annual Review of Food Science and Technology. 2010;**1**:163-187

[27] Tsao R. Chemistry and biochemistry of dietary polyphenols. Nutrients. 2010;**2**:1231-1246

[28] Schwartz SJ, von Elbe JH, and Giusti MM. Colorants. In: Damodaran S, Parkin K, Fennema OR, editors. Fennema's Food Chemistry. 4th ed. Boca Raton, FL: CRC Press/Taylor and Francis, Inc.; 2008. pp. 571-638

[29] Wu X, Beecher GR, Holden JM, Haytowitz DB, Gebhardt SE, Prior RL. Concentrations of anthocyanins in common foods in the United States and estimation of normal consumption. Journal of Agricultural and Food Chemistry. 2006;**54**:4069-4075

[30] Zamora-Ros R, Knaze V, Lujan-Barroso L, Slimani N, Romieu I, Touillaud M, Kaaks R, Teucher B, Mattiello A, Grioni S, et al. Estimation of the intake of anthocyanidins and their food sources in the european prospective investigation into cancer and nutrition (epic) study. The British Journal of Nutrition. 2011;**106**:1090-1099

[31] Prior RL, Wu X. Anthocyanins: Structural characteristics that result in unique metabolic patterns and biological activities. Free Radical Research. 2006;**40**:1014-1028

[32] Gerardi C, Frassinetti S, Caltavuturo L, Leone A, Lecci R, Calabriso N, Carluccio MA, Blando F, Mita G. Anti-proliferative, anti-inflammatory and anti-mutagenic activities of a *Prunus mahaleb* L. anthocyanin-rich fruit extract. Journal of Functional Foods. 2016;**27**:537-548

[33] Allen RG, Tresini M. Oxidative stress and gene regulation. Free Radical Biology & Medicine. 2000;**28**:463-499

[34] Rugina D, Hanganu D, Diaconeasa Z, Tabaran F, Coman C, Leopold L, Bunea A, Pintea A. Antiproliferative and apoptotic potential of cyanidin-based anthocyanins on melanoma cells. International Journal of Molecular Sciences. 2017;**18**(5):949

[35] Rugina D, Diaconeasa Z, Coman C, Bunea A, Socaciu C, Pintea A. Chokeberry anthocyanin extract as pancreatic β-cell protectors in two models of induced oxidative stress. Oxidative Medicine and Cellular Longevity. 2015;**2015**:10

[36] Wang H, Cao G, Prior RL. Oxygen radical absorbing capacity of anthocyanins. Journal of Agricultural and Food Chemistry. 1997;**45**:304-309

[37] Rahman MM, Ichiyanagi T, Komiyama T, Sato S, Konishi T. Effects of anthocyanins on psychological stress-induced oxidative stress and neurotransmitter status. Journal of Agricultural and Food Chemistry. 2008;**56**:7545-7550

[38] Ramirez-Tortosa C, Andersen OM, Cabrita L, Gardner PT, Morrice PC, Wood SG, Duthie SJ, Collins AR, Duthie GG. Anthocyanin-rich extract decreases indices of lipid peroxidation and DNA damage in vitamin e-depleted rats. Free Radical Biology & Medicine. 2001;**31**:1033-1037

[39] Day AP, Kemp HJ, Bolton C, Hartog M, Stansbie D. Effect of concentrated red grape juice consumption on serum antioxidant capacity and low-density lipoprotein oxidation. Annals of Nutrition & Metabolism. 1997;**41**:353-357

[40] Aviram M. Review of human studies on oxidative damage and antioxidant protection related to cardiovascular diseases. Free Radical Research. 2000;**33**(Suppl):S85-S97

[41] Kwon SH, Ahn IS, Kim SO, Kong CS, Chung HY, Do MS, Park KY. Anti-obesity and hypolipidemic effects of black soybean anthocyanins. Journal of Medicinal Food. 2007;**10**:552-556

[42] Anderson RA, Broadhurst CL, Polansky MM, Schmidt WF, Khan A, Flanagan VP, Schoene NW, Graves DJ. Isolation and characterization of polyphenol type-a polymers from cinnamon with insulin-like biological activity. Journal of Agricultural and Food Chemistry. 2004;**52**:65-70

[43] Landrault N, Poucheret P, Azay J, Krosniak M, Gasc F, Jenin C, Cros G, Teissedre PL. Effect of a polyphenols-enriched chardonnay white wine in diabetic rats. Journal of Agricultural and Food Chemistry. 2003;**51**:311-318

[44] Zadok D, Levy Y, Glovinsky Y. The effect of anthocyanosides in a multiple oral dose on night vision. Eye. 1999;**13**:734

[45] Muth ER, Laurent JM, Jasper P. The effect of bilberry nutritional supplementation on night visual acuity and contrast sensitivity. Alternative Medicine Review: A Journal of Clinical Therapeutic. 2000;**5**:164-173

[46] Rugina D, Sconta Z, Leopold L, Pintea A, Bunea A, Socaciu C. Antioxidant activities of chokeberry extracts and the cytotoxic action of their anthocyanin fraction on hela human cervical tumor cells. Journal of Medicinal Food. 2012;**15**:700-706

[47] Diaconeasa Z, Leopold L, Rugină D, Ayvaz H, Socaciu C. Antiproliferative and antioxidant properties of anthocyanin rich extracts from blueberry and blackcurrant juice. International Journal of Molecular Sciences. 2015;**16**:2352-2365

[48] Malik M, Zhao C, Schoene N, Guisti MM, Moyer MP, Magnuson BA. Anthocyanin-rich extract from aronia meloncarpa e induces a cell cycle block in colon cancer but not normal colonic cells. Nutrition and Cancer. 2003;**46**:186-196

[49] Wang L-S, Stoner GD. Anthocyanins and their role in cancer prevention. Cancer Letters. 2008;**269**:281-290

[50] Reddivari L, Vanamala J, Chintharlapalli S, Safe SH, Miller Jr JC. Anthocyanin fraction from potato extracts is cytotoxic to prostate cancer cells through activation of caspase-dependent and caspase-independent pathways. Carcinogenesis. 2007;**28**:2227-2235

[51] Chang YC, Huang HP, Hsu JD, Yang SF, Wang CJ. Hibiscus anthocyanins rich extract-induced apoptotic cell death in human promyelocytic leukemia cells. Toxicology and Applied Pharmacology. 2005;**205**:201-212

[52] Hientz K, Mohr A, Bhakta-Guha D, Efferth T. The role of p53 in cancer drug resistance and targeted chemotherapy. Oncotarget. 2017;**8**:8921-8946

[53] Bagchi D, Sen CK, Bagchi M, Atalay M. Anti-angiogenic, antioxidant, and anti-carcinogenic properties of a novel anthocyanin-rich berry extract formula. Biochemistry. Biokhimiia. 2004;**69**:75-80. (71 p preceding 75)

[54] Lamy S, Lafleur R, Bedard V, Moghrabi A, Barrette S, Gingras D, Beliveau R. Anthocyanidins inhibit migration of glioblastoma cells: Structure-activity relationship and involvement of the plasminolytic system. Journal of Cellular Biochemistry. 2007;**100**:100-111

[55] Brandstetter H, Grams F, Glitz D, Lang A, Huber R, Bode W, Krell HW, Engh RA. The 1.8-a crystal structure of a matrix metalloproteinase 8-barbiturate inhibitor complex reveals a previously unobserved mechanism for collagenase substrate recognition. The Journal of Biological Chemistry. 2001;**276**:17405-17412

[56] Siegel RL, Miller KD, Jemal A. Cancer statistics, 2018. CA: A Cancer Journal for Clinicians. 2018;**68**:7-30

[57] Ferlay J, Soerjomataram I, Dikshit R, Eser S, Mathers C, Rebelo M, Parkin DM, Forman D, Bray F. Cancer incidence and mortality worldwide: Sources, methods and major patterns in globocan 2012. International Journal of Cancer. 2015;**136**:E359-E386

[58] Afrin S, Giampieri F, Gasparrini M, Forbes-Hernandez TY, Varela-Lopez A, Quiles JL, Mezzetti B, Battino M. Chemopreventive and therapeutic effects of edible berries: A focus on colon cancer prevention and treatment. Molecules (Basel, Switzerland). 2016; **21**:169

[59] Lippert E, Ruemmele P, Obermeier F, Goelder S, Kunst C, Rogler G, Dunger N, Messmann H, Hartmann A, Endlicher E. Anthocyanins prevent colorectal cancer development in a mouse model. Digestion. 2017;**95**:275-280

[60] Lala G, Malik M, Zhao C, He J, Kwon Y, Giusti MM, Magnuson BA. Anthocyanin-rich extracts inhibit multiple biomarkers of colon cancer in rats. Nutrition and Cancer. 2006;**54**:84-93

[61] Cancer Facts & Figures American Cancer Society. Atlanta, GA. 2015

[62] Li X, Xu J, Tang X, Liu Y, Yu X, Wang Z, Liu W. Anthocyanins inhibit trastuzumab-resistant breast cancer in vitro and in vivo. Molecular Medicine Reports. 2016;**13**: 4007-4013

[63] Liu W, Xu J, Liu Y, Yu X, Tang X, Wang Z, Li X. Anthocyanins potentiate the activity of trastuzumab in human epidermal growth factor receptor 2-positive breast cancer cells in vitro and in vivo. Molecular Medicine Reports. 2014;**10**:1921-1926

[64] Hui C, Bin Y, Xiaoping Y, Long Y, Chunye C, Mantian M, Wenhua L. Anticancer activities of an anthocyanin-rich extract from black rice against breast cancer cells in vitro and in vivo. Nutrition and Cancer. 2010;**62**:1128-1136

[65] Farrukh Aqila JJ, Kausarb H, Munagalaa R, Singhd IP, Guptab R. Lung cancer inhibitory activity of dietary berries and berry polyphenolics. Journal of Berry Research. 2016;**62**: 105-114

[66] Chen PN, Chu SC, Chiou HL, Chiang CL, Yang SF, Hsieh YS. Cyanidin 3-glucoside and peonidin 3-glucoside inhibit tumor cell growth and induce apoptosis in vitro and suppress tumor growth in vivo. Nutrition and Cancer. 2005;**53**:232-243

[67] Hurst EA, Harbour JW, Cornelius LA. Ocular melanoma: A review and the relationship to cutaneous melanoma. Archives of Dermatology. 2003;**139**:1067-1073

[68] Hirst NG, Gordon LG, Scuffham PA, Green AC. Lifetime cost-effectiveness of skin cancer prevention through promotion of daily sunscreen use. Value in Health. 2012;**15**:261-268

[69] Aquilato A, Lopez V, Doonan B, Hsieh T-C, Pinto JT, Wu E, Wu JM. Chapter 102 – Braf mutation in melanoma and dietary polyphenols as adjunctive treatment strategy. In: Polyphenols in Human Health and Disease. San Diego: Academic Press; 2014. pp. 1353-1365

[70] Ives NJ, Stowe RL, Lorigan P, Wheatley K. Chemotherapy compared with biochemotherapy for the treatment of metastatic melanoma: A meta-analysis of 18 trials involving 2621 patients. Journal of Clinical Oncology: Official Journal of the American Society of Clinical Oncology. 2007;**25**:5426-5434

[71] Siddiqui IA, Tarapore RS, Chamcheu JC, Mukhtar H. Bioactive Food Components for Melanoma: An Overview, Skin Cancer Overview Yaguang Xi, IntechOpen, DOI: 10.5772/25830

[72] Chinembiri TN, du Plessis LH, Gerber M, Hamman JH, du Plessis J. Review of natural compounds for potential skin cancer treatment. Molecules (Basel, Switzerland). 2014;**19**:11679-11721

[73] Razina TG, Zueva EP, Ulrich AV, Rybalkina OY, Chaikovskii AV, Isaikina NV, Kalinkina GI, Zhdanov VV, Zyuz'kov GN. Antitumor effects of *Sorbus aucuparia L.* extract highly saturated with anthocyans and their mechanisms. Bulletin of Experimental Biology and Medicine. 2016;**162**:93-97

[74] Ha US, Bae WJ, Kim SJ, Yoon BI, Hong SH, Lee JY, Hwang TK, Hwang SY, Wang Z, Kim SW. Anthocyanin induces apoptosis of du-145 cells in vitro and inhibits xenograft growth of prostate cancer. Yonsei Medical Journal. 2015;**56**:16-23

[75] Hafeez BB, Siddiqui IA, Asim M, Malik A, Afaq F, Adhami VM, Saleem M, Din M, Mukhtar H. A dietary anthocyanidin delphinidin induces apoptosis of human prostate cancer pc3 cells in vitro and in vivo: Involvement of nuclear factor-kappab signaling. Cancer Research. 2008;**68**:8564-8572

[76] Marko D, Puppel N, Tjaden Z, Jakobs S, Pahlke G. The substitution pattern of anthocyanidins affects different cellular signaling cascades regulating cell proliferation. Molecular Nutrition & Food Research. 2004;**48**:318-325

[77] Zhao C, Giusti MM, Malik M, Moyer MP, Magnuson BA. Effects of commercial anthocyanin-rich extracts on colonic cancer and nontumorigenic colonic cell growth. Journal of Agricultural and Food Chemistry. 2004;**52**:6122-6128

[78] Olsson ME, Andersson CS, Oredsson S, Berglund RH, Gustavsson KE. Antioxidant levels and inhibition of cancer cell proliferation in vitro by extracts from organically and conventionally cultivated strawberries. Journal of Agricultural and Food Chemistry. 2006;**54**:1248-1255

[79] Zhou J, Zhu Y-F, Chen X-Y, Han B, Li F, Chen J-Y, Peng X-L, Luo L-P, Chen W, Yu X-P. Black rice-derived anthocyanins inhibit her-2-positive breast cancer epithelial-mesenchymal transition-mediated metastasis in vitro by suppressing fak signaling. International Journal of Molecular Medicine. 2017;**40**:1649-1656

[80] Lu JN, Panchanathan R, Lee WS, Kim HJ, Kim DH, Choi YH, Kim GS, Shin SC, Hong SC. Anthocyanins from the fruit of vitis coignetiae pulliat inhibit tnf-augmented cancer proliferation, migration, and invasion in a549 cells. Asian Pacific Journal of Cancer Prevention. 2017;**18**:2919-2923

[81] Meeran SM, Katiyar SK. Grape seed proanthocyanidins promote apoptosis in human epidermoid carcinoma a431 cells through alterations in cdki-cdk-cyclin cascade, and caspase-3 activation via loss of mitochondrial membrane potential. Experimental Dermatology. 2007;**16**:405-415

[82] Rugină D, Hanganu D, Diaconeasa Z, Tăbăran F, Coman C, Leopold L, Bunea A, Pintea A. Antiproliferative and apoptotic potential of cyanidin-based anthocyanins on melanoma cells. International Journal of Molecular Sciences. 2017;**18**:949

[83] Bunea A, Rugină D, Sconţa Z, Pop RM, Pintea A, Socaciu C, Tăbăran F, Grootaert C, Struijs K, VanCamp J. Anthocyanin determination in blueberry extracts from various cultivars and their antiproliferative and apoptotic properties in b16-f10 metastatic murine melanoma cells. Phytochemistry. 2013;**95**:436-444

[84] Diaconeasa Z, Ayvaz H, Rugină D, Leopold L, Stănilă A, Socaciu C, Tăbăran F, Luput L, Mada DC, Pintea A. Melanoma inhibition by anthocyanins is associated with the reduction of oxidative stress biomarkers and changes in mitochondrial membrane potential. Plant Foods for Human Nutrition. 2017;**72**:404

[85] Medinger M, Lengerke C, Passweg J. Novel therapeutic options in acute myeloid leukemia. Leukemia Research Reports. 2016;**6**:39-49

[86] Fan MJ, Yeh PH, Lin JP, Huang AC, Lien JC, Lin HY, & Chung JG. Anthocyanins from black rice (Oryza sativa) promote immune responses in leukemia through enhancing phagocytosis of macrophages in vivo. Experimental and Therapeutic Medicine. 2017;**14**(1): 59-64

9

Qualitative Analysis of Phytochemicals from Sea Buckthorn and Gooseberry

Ana-Alexandra Sorescu, Alexandrina Nuta,
Rodica-Mariana Ion and Lorena Iancu

Abstract

This chapter describes in detail recent research results obtained from the qualitative screening of different phytochemicals found in aqueous extracts of sea buckthorn and gooseberry, fruits with important pharmacological effects due to their high content in vitamin C. Phytochemical investigations reveal the presence of active principles (e.g., saponins, flavonoids, alkaloids, carbohydrates, terpenoids, etc.) in sea buckthorn and gooseberry and are accomplished by using well-established standard methods. All these qualitative determinations rely on the visual color change reaction as a basic response to the presence of a specific phytochemical compound. The active principles from sea buckthorn and gooseberry are extracted according to a well-settled extraction method, which involves infusing the fruits in an aqueous medium, for 24 h, at a constant temperature of 4°C.

Keywords: phytochemicals, qualitative screening, sea buckthorn, gooseberry, aqueous extracts

1. Introduction

Phytochemistry, basically described as the chemistry of plants and different plant parts, is generally considered an early subdivision of organic chemistry and is very important in the identification of plant compounds with medicinal properties [1].

Phytochemistry is associated with numerous species of secondary metabolites produced in plants by biosynthesis and the natural combination of all these secondary metabolites gives the general beneficial therapeutic effects of that specific plant [2, 3].

Plants biosynthesize phytochemicals to protect themselves from insect attacks and plant diseases. Phytochemicals ("Phyto" is the Greek word for plant) are plant chemicals with no nutritional value, non-essential nutrients, and with disease preventive properties. Some of the most common phytochemicals are lycopene (found in tomatoes), flavonoids (found in fruits), and isoflavones (found in soy) [4, 5].

Species belonging even to the same genus can differ one from another in different proportions and sometimes these differences are subtle and extremely difficult to determine. Therefore, new phytochemical methods quickly developed coming in addition to those that were already known and applied [6, 7].

There are many known phytochemicals, and each has its own possible action [8–10]:

- *antioxidant*: protect human cells from oxidative stress thus considerably reducing the risk of developing numerous types of cancer;
- *hormonal action*: isoflavones are able to imitate human estrogens, reducing the symptoms of osteoporosis;
- *antibacterial*: can be used as alternative therapy against infections caused by different bacteria;
- *physical action*: many phytochemicals physically attach to cell walls thus preventing the adhesion of pathogens.

Sea buckthorn (*Hippophae rhamnoides* L.), an ancient plant with modern attributes, has numerous pharmacological effects: cardioprotective, inhibits platelet aggregation, lowers the levels of cholesterol and blood pressure, and provides antioxidant activity. The berries have an orange-yellowish color (see **Figure 1a**) and are an important source of vitamin C and A, phenolic compounds (especially flavonoids), and phytosterols [11, 12]. The mineral content (whether it's the fruit itself or the juice) is another important factor, which comes to complete all the beneficial properties of sea buckthorn: five essential minerals (calcium, iron, magnesium, sodium, and manganese) and four trace elements (chromium, vanadium, selenium, and cobalt) [13].

Gooseberries (*Ribes grossularia*) are generally divided into two groups, namely European (*Ribes grossularia* var. *uva-crispa*) and American (*Ribes hirtellum*) [14]. The fruits (**Figure 1b**) contain

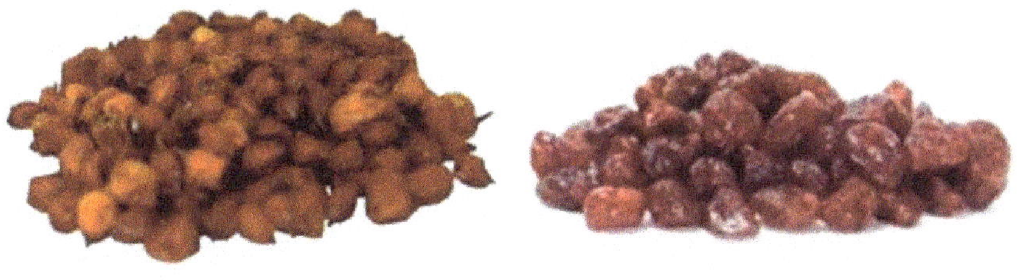

(a) (b)

Figure 1. (a) Sea buckthorn and (b) gooseberry.

more than 80% water and important amounts of proteins, fibers, phenolic compounds, minerals, and vitamins [15]. Most species of the *Ribes* genus are rich in prodelphinidin, contain no ellagitannins, and are low in carotenoid content [16].

Although both sea buckthorn and gooseberry are used in traditional medicine for the treatment of various diseases, no clear scientific evidence exists to prove their therapeutic benefits and, therefore, it is very important to determine the qualitative content of these two fruits.

In this chapter, sea buckthorn and gooseberry dried fruits are used to prepare aqueous extracts using a method that involves the cold infusion at a constant temperature of 4°C for 24 h. The two aqueous extracts are further used for the qualitative screening of phytochemicals, and the most important bioactive chemical constituents that are studied are carbohydrates, flavonoids, alkaloids, glycosides, steroids, tannins, proteins, amino acids, and terpenoids. All these qualitative studies use standard analytical methods and the results are clearly detailed in the present chapter.

2. Preparation of aqueous extracts from sea buckthorn and gooseberry

Sea buckthorn (*Hippophae rhamnoides* L.) and gooseberry (*Ribes grossularia*) are bought readily dried from local natural shops and are further used to prepare aqueous extracts using a method that involves the following steps (**Figure 2**): grinding the dried fruits into a fine powder, weighting an exact amount of powder, and extracting it using a determined volume of distilled water at a constant temperature of 4°C.

The cold infusion takes place in sealed "French press" type coffee filters (**Figure 3**), one for every fruit involved in this research [17].

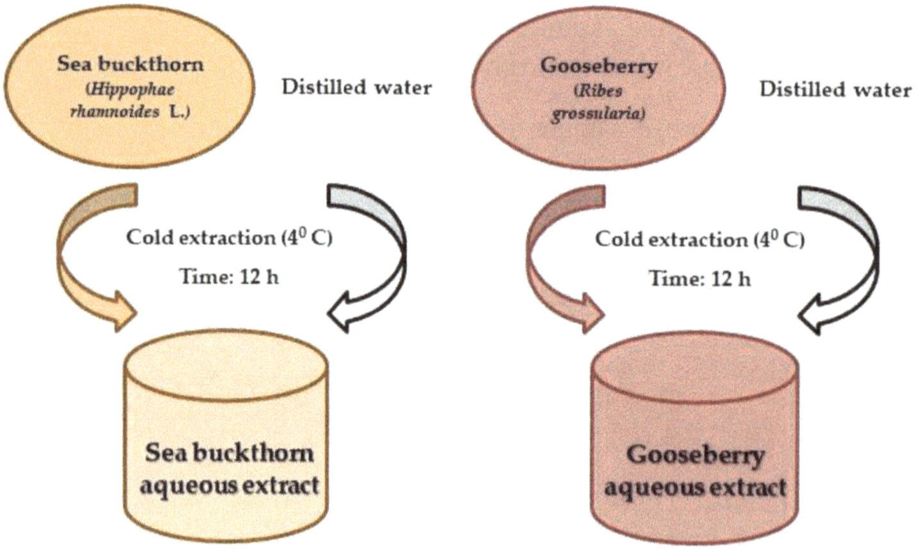

Figure 2. Preparation of sea buckthorn and gooseberry aqueous extracts.

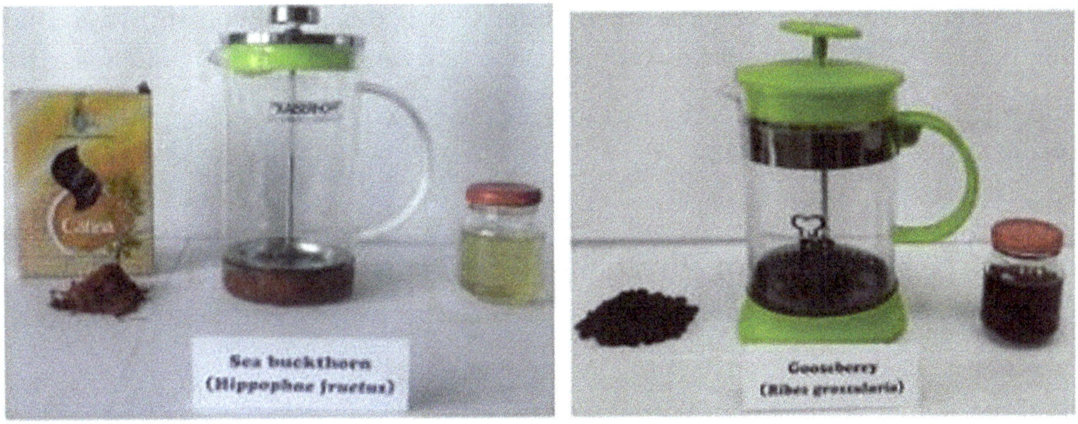

Figure 3. "French press" type coffee filters used to prepare the aqueous extracts.

The two extracts were left to incubate for 24 h so that as much of sea buckthorn and gooseberry as possible could be transferred to the aqueous extracts. The aqueous extracts thus prepared were separated, filtered, and the volumes of the resulted aqueous extracts were measured. An additional vacuum filtration was carried out so that all debris were removed from the aqueous extracts.

The sea buckthorn aqueous extract and the gooseberry extract were kept in the refrigerator for more than 12 weeks for further use, without any alteration.

The extractive value (yield percentage) of the sea buckthorn and gooseberry samples were weighted before and after the preparation of the aqueous extracts and the results are presented in **Table 1** [18]:

$$\text{Extract yield } \% = [W_1/W_2] \times 100 \tag{1}$$

Crt. no.	Aqueous extract	Weight before extraction (g)	Weight after extraction (g)	Yield (%)
1	Sea buckthorn	25	18.66	74.64
2	Gooseberry	25	16.78	67.12

Table 1. Quantities of dry fruit before and after the aqueous extractions.

Crt. no.	Aqueous extract	Distilled water (mL)	Aqueous extract (mL)
1	Sea buckthorn	100	84
2	Gooseberry	100	92

The pH was measured for the two aqueous extracts and the value was 6.5 for sea buckthorn as well as for gooseberry aqueous extracts.

Table 2. Volume of resulted aqueous extracts.

where W_1 = net powder weight (g) resulted after the aqueous extraction and W_2 = total powder weight (g) used for the preparation of sea buckthorn and gooseberry aqueous extracts.

The volume of the resulted aqueous extracts was measured (mL) and compared to the initial volume of distilled water (**Table 2**).

3. Qualitative screening of phytochemicals from sea buckthorn and gooseberry

Different qualitative phytochemical analyses are known that allow, by using standard analytical techniques, the determination of chemical groups, or compounds in aqueous extracts from different plants. These qualitative tests are based on color or precipitation reactions as a positive response to the presence of those specific chemical compounds [19, 20]. All the color reactions allow only determining the presence or absence of various chemical groups and not the amount in which they are present in different aqueous extracts.

Standard qualitative methods are used to analyze qualitatively the aqueous extract prepared from sea buckthorn and gooseberry [21, 22].

3.1. Qualitative screening of carbohydrates

In nature, there are numerous carbohydrate materials that can be generally classified as follows [23]:

a. *Monosaccharides*: glucose, fructose, and galactose;

b. *Oligosaccharides*: sucrose, lactose, and maltose;

c. *Polysaccharides*: starch, glycogen, and dextrin.

Carbohydrates are usually neutral, water-soluble chemical compounds, but there are some exceptions and some, such as pectic acid, gluconic acid, or alginic acid, are acidic in the living world.

There are different standard phytochemical methods used for the qualitative screening of carbohydrates found in aqueous extracts [24]. The results obtained for sea buckthorn and gooseberry aqueous extracts are fully described in **Table 3**.

3.1.1. General screening of carbohydrates

Experimental: 1 ml Molisch reagent (a solution of α-naphthol in ethanol) is added to 2 ml aqueous extract and few drops of concentrated sulfuric acid are slowly dripped and the resulted solution is shaken carefully. The appearance of a violet ring at the interface of the two liquids indicates the presence of carbohydrates in the aqueous extracts.

In the case of sea buckthorn aqueous extract, the solution turns purple-red and a brown precipitate is obtained from gooseberry aqueous extract.

Phytochemical test	Sea buckthorn	Gooseberry
Carbohydrates (general)—Molisch	Purple red solution	Purple coloration
Carbohydrates (reducing sugars)—Benedict	Brick-red precipitate	Brick-red precipitate
Carbohydrates (reducing sugars)–Fehling A	Khaki solution	Green-yellow solution
Carbohydrates (reducing sugars)—Fehling B	Brown-yellow solution	Brown solution
Carbohydrates (monosaccharides)—Barfoed	Blue-green solution	Brick-red precipitate
Carbohydrates (reducing sugars)—Trommer	Red precipitate	Red-brown precipitate
Carbohydrates (reducing sugars)—Tollens	Black precipitate	Silver mirror
Carbohydrates (reducing sugars)—Moore	Red-brown solution	Red-brown solution

Table 3. Qualitative screening of carbohydrates.

3.1.2. Detection of reducing sugars

The general definition of reducing sugars is any type of sugar that can act as a reducing agent due to the free aldehyde or ketone groups. All monosaccharides are reducing sugars, along with some di-, oil- and polysaccharides. Several tests are available for detecting reducing sugars in aqueous extracts (**Figures 4** and **5**) (**Table 3**) [25].

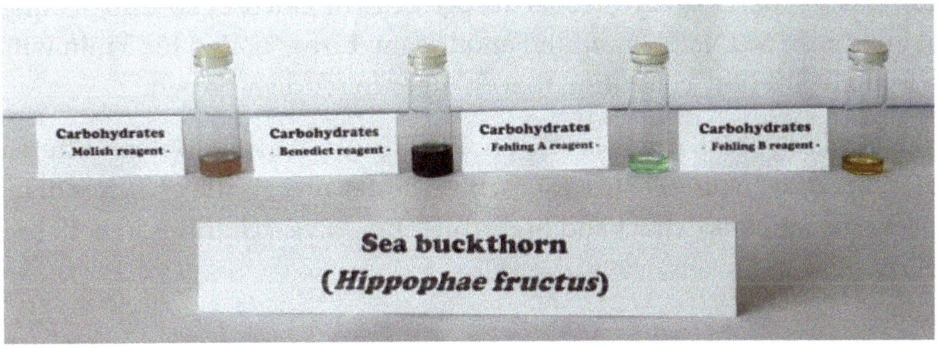

Figure 4. Carbohydrates in sea buckthorn aqueous extract.

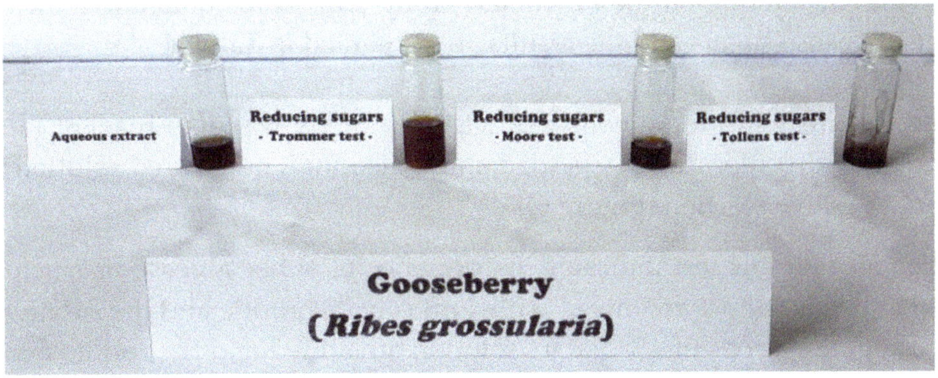

Figure 5. Reducing sugars from gooseberry aqueous extract.

a. *Benedict test*: to 1 ml of aqueous extract 5 ml Benedict's reagent (a complex solution of sodium carbonate, sodium citrate, and copper sulfate pentahydrate) was added and the resulted mixture is boiled for 5 min. Initially, the solution turns green and upon boiling a red, yellow, or green precipitate is formed.

b. *Fehling A test*: to 1 ml aqueous extract few drops of Fehling A reagent (aqueous solution of copper sulfate) are added; a green coloration indicates the presence of reducing sugars.

c. *Fehling B test*: to 1 ml aqueous extract few drops of reagent (a solution of potassium sodium tartrate in sodium hydroxide) are added and the formation of a brown coloration is a positive response.

d. *Barfoed test*: this test reveals the presence of reducing monosaccharides. To 1 ml aqueous extract, 3 ml Barfoed's reagent (solution of copper acetate) are added, boiled for 2 min and then cooled. A red precipitate is formed.

e. *Trommer test*: to 3 ml of aqueous extract an ml of 2.5% copper sulfate and 2 ml of 5% sodium hydroxide is added and the mixture is boiled for 3 min. Initially, a blue precipitate appears which turn red upon heating, thus indicating the presence of reducing sugars.

f. *Tollens test*: to 4 ml of aqueous extract a drop of dilute NH_4OH is added and then a solution of 0.1 M silver nitrate is poured to the resulted solution. After 5–10 min of boiling a silver mirror is formed (silver precipitates in the presence of reducing sugars).

g. *Moore test*: this test particularly reveals the presence of glucose. To 2 ml of aqueous extract an equal volume of 5% NaOH is added and the mixture is boiled for 5 min with. The solution has initially a yellow coloration that changer to reddish-brown.

By performing Molisch's test, it reveals that both aqueous extracts contain different classes of carbohydrates. Specific qualitative test for carbohydrates reveals the presence of monosaccharides in gooseberry aqueous extract and of di-, oil- and polysaccharides in both sea buckthorn and gooseberry extracts.

3.1.3. Detection of hexose sugars

Hexoses are monosaccharides that contain six carbon atoms and are divided into aldohexoses and ketohexoses depending on the functional group [26]. Three qualitative methods reveal the presence of hexose sugars and the results are presented in **Table 4**.

a. *Seliwanoff test*: to 1 ml of aqueous extract, 3 ml of Seliwanoff's reagent (a mixture of resorcinol in hydrochloric acid) is added and boiled for 2 min. A red solution is obtained indicated a positive reaction (**Figure 6**).

b. *Cobalt chloride test*: this test indicates the presence of either glucose or fructose or both. Three ml aqueous extract are mixed with 2 ml cobalt chloride and the solution in boiled. After cooling, few drops of 4% NaOH solution are added and the results are as follows: a greenish-blue solution (glucose), purplish-violet solution (fructose), or the upper layer turns greenish-blue, while the lower layer purplish (both glucose and fructose).

c. *Ammonium molybdate test*: this test reveals the presence of ketohexozes as follows: to 2 ml aqueous extract, 2 ml ammonium molybdate solution are added, the solution is then heated to form a bluish-green solution.

As it is clear from the **Table 4**, hexose sugars are present in both sea buckthorn aqueous extract as well as in gooseberry aqueous extract.

3.2. Qualitative screening of tannins and phlobatannins

Most of the tannins, a group of phenol compounds usually found in plants, are soluble in water. Phlobatannins are considered a novel class of ring-isomerized condensed tannins [17].

The test for tannins is generally described as [27]: to 1 ml aqueous extract 2 ml of 5% ferric chloride are added and a dark-blue or greenish-black color appears.

Phlobatannins are tested following a standardized method: to 1 ml aqueous extract of sea buckthorn and gooseberry few drops of diluted HCl (1%) is added and a red precipitate should appear (**Table 5**).

Tannins are present in both aqueous extracts, while small traces of phlobatannins can be found in gooseberry aqueous extract.

3.3. Qualitative screening of saponins

The general method involved in the qualitative analyze of saponins is: 2 ml of aqueous extract and 2 ml of distilled water are shaken for 15 min in a graduated cylinder. A 1 cm foam layer is a positive response to the presence of saponins (see **Table 6**).

Qualitative screening of saponins in aqueous extracts from sea buckthorn and gooseberry revealed that only the second one contains saponins.

3.4. Qualitative screening of flavonoids and phenolic flavonoids

Flavonoids have important functions in plants: attract pollinating insects, fight against different microbial infections, and control cell growth [28].

Flavonoids are tested according to the following method: 2 ml aqueous extract and 1 ml of 2N sodium hydroxide are mixed. A yellow color indicates the presence of flavonoids.

Phytochemical test	Sea buckthorn	Gooseberry
Carbohydrates (hexose sugars)—Seliwanoff	Cognac-red solution	Red solution
Carbohydrates (hexose sugars)—cobalt chloride	Lower layer-blue precipitate, upper layer-pink solution	Reddish solution, yellow-white precipitate
Carbohydrates (hexose sugars)—ammonium molybdate	Blue-green solution	Blue-green solution

Table 4. Qualitative screening of hexose sugars.

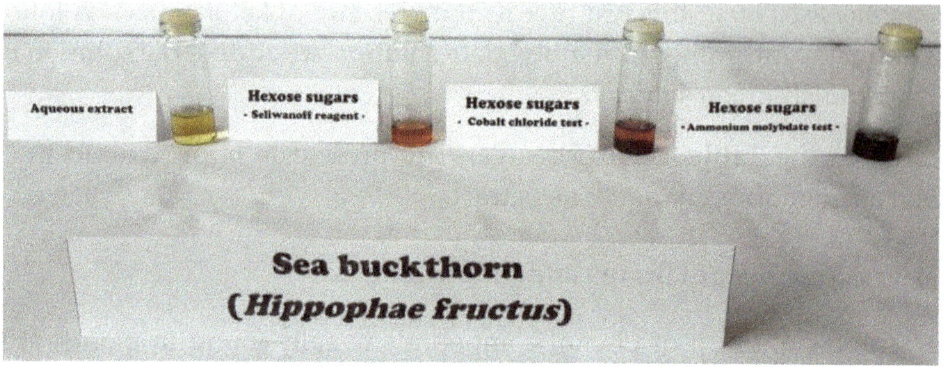

Figure 6. Hexose sugars in sea buckthorn aqueous extract.

Phytochemical test	Sea buckthorn	Gooseberry
Tannins	Green-black solution	Green-black solution
Phlobatannins	Pale pink solution	Red-orange solution

Table 5. Qualitative screening of tannins and phlobatannins.

Phytochemical test	Sea buckthorn	Gooseberry
Saponins	0.2 cm foam layer	1.5 cm foam layer

Table 6. Qualitative screening of saponins.

The test for phenolic flavonoids (**Figure 7**): 1 ml aqueous extract is mixed with 2 ml of 10% lead acetate solution and a brown precipitate indicates a positive response (see **Table 7**).

Flavonoids are present in both aqueous extracts (sea buckthorn and gooseberry), while phenolic flavonoids are present as small traces in gooseberry aqueous extract.

3.5. Qualitative screening of alkaloids

Alkaloids are a group of basic plant bioactive compounds that possess an N-containing heterocycle, are generally colorless, crystalline, insoluble in water but soluble in many organic solvents [29].

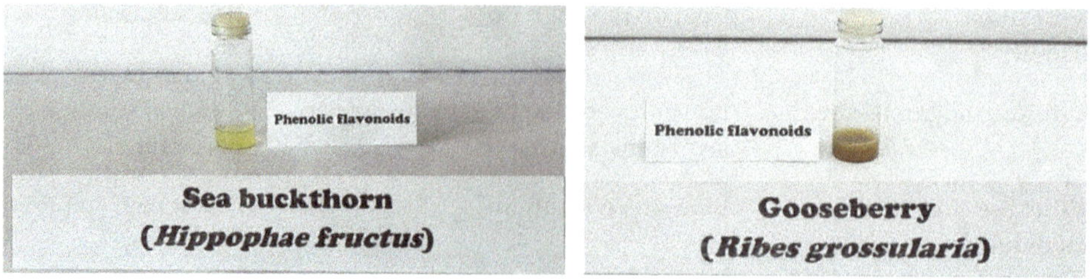

Figure 7. Phenolic flavonoids in sea buckthorn and gooseberry.

Phytochemical test	Sea buckthorn	Gooseberry
Flavonoids	Green-yellow solution	Light brown yellow solution
Phenolic flavonoids	Light yellow solution	Opalescent brown-yellow solution

Table 7. Qualitative screening of flavonoids and phenolic flavonoids.

There are three different standard phytochemical methods used to determine the presence of tannins in aqueous extracts from sea buckthorn and gooseberry:

a. *Wagner test*: 1 ml aqueous extract and 1 ml Wagner's reagent (iodine in potassium iodide solution) react and if a reddish-brown precipitate is formed it indicates a positive reaction.

b. *Mayer test*: to 1 ml aqueous extract, 2 ml concentrated HCl is added followed by few drops of Mayer's reagent (a solution of mercuric chloride and potassium iodide in water); a green color or white precipitate indicates the presence of alkaloids (the results are presented in **Table 8**).

c. *Hager test*: 2 ml aqueous extract and 2 ml Hager's reagent (a saturated aqueous solution of picric acid) are mixed together and a yellow precipitate indicates a positive test.

According to the results presented in **Table 8**, alkaloids are absent from all the aqueous extracts.

3.6. Qualitative screening of anthraquinones and anthocyanosides

The method used for the qualitative screening of anthraquinone compounds involves the reaction of 1 ml aqueous extract with a few drops of 10% ammonia solution with the formation of a pink precipitate.

Anthocyanosides are present when a pink color appears after the reaction between 1 ml aqueous extract with 5 ml dilute hydrochloric acid (1%). The results are detailed in **Table 9**.

Phytochemical test	Sea buckthorn	Gooseberry
Alkaloids—Wagner	Red-brown solution	Red-brown solution
Alkaloids—Mayer	Light-yellow solution	Red-brown solution
Alkaloids—Hager	Clear yellow solution	Red-brown solution

Table 8. Qualitative screening of alkaloids.

Phytochemical test	Sea buckthorn	Gooseberry
Anthraquinones	Green-yellow solution	Brown-yellow solution
Anthocyanosides	Light yellow solution	Brown-yellow solution

Table 9. Qualitative screening of anthraquinones and anthocyanosides.

According to the results presented in **Table 9**, anthraquinones and anthocyanosides are absent from both aqueous extracts.

3.7. Qualitative screening of proteins and amino acids

Proteins are involved in all physiological processes that take place in all living cells. Proteins are colloidal, do not diffuse through the plasma membrane, are irreversible coagulated upon heating and are insoluble in neutral salts [30].

Amino acids are amphoteric phytocompounds, highly reactive, with an amino and carboxylic acid moiety, therefore, being mostly water soluble.

3.7.1. General screening of proteins and amino acids

Experimental: 1 ml aqueous extract reacts with 5–6 drops of Millon's reagent (mixture of mercuric nitrate, mercurous nitrate, concentrated nitric acid, and distilled water) and a white precipitate is formed that changes its color to red upon heating. Millon's test is a non-specific test for detecting proteins and amino acids (tyrosine) and, therefore, it must be confirmed by other qualitative tests.

The results obtained after the two aqueous extracts react with Millon reagent are as follows: an opalescent orange solution in the case of Sea buckthorn and a red-brownish precipitate in the case of Gooseberry, therefore confirming the presence of small amounts of proteins and/or aminoacids in Gooseberry aqueous extract.

3.7.2. Detection of amino acids

There are two different standard methods used (see results in **Table 10**):

a. *Ninhydrin test*: take 3 ml aqueous extract and mix it with three drops of 5% lead acetate solution then heat the resulted solution. A purple or blue coloration indicates a positive reaction (**Figure 8**).

b. *Test for cysteine*: 5 ml aqueous extract is boiled with a small amount of 40% NaOH and few drops of 5% lead acetate solution are added. A black precipitate is formed.

The test for cysteine gives a positive reaction in the case of sea buckthorn, while ninhydrin test is negative for both aqueous extracts.

Phytochemical test	Sea buckthorn	Gooseberry
Proteins and amino acids—Millon	Opalescent orange solution	Red-brownish precipitate
Amino acids—ninhydrin test	Opalescent white-yellow solution	Opalescent orange solution, gray precipitate
Amino acids—test for cysteine	Red-brown solution, black precipitate	Opalescent dark-brown solution

Table 10. Qualitative screening of amino acids.

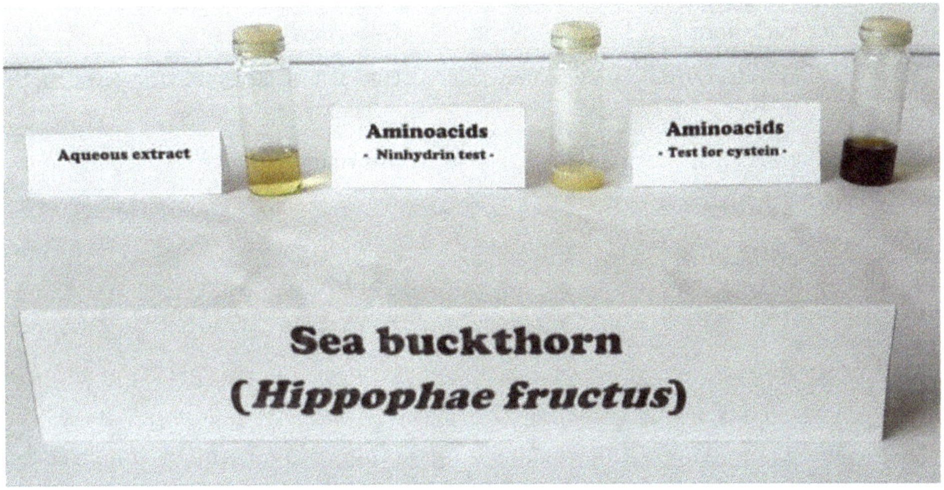

Figure 8. Amino acids in sea buckthorn.

3.7.3. Detection of proteins

There are two different standard methods used (see results in **Table 11**):

a. *Biuret test:* to 3 ml aqueous extract, 3 ml 4% sodium hydroxide solution, and few drops of 1% copper sulfate are added to form a purple solution.

b. *Xanthoproteic test*: to 3 ml aqueous extract, 1 ml of concentrated H_2SO_4 is slowly dropped. A white precipitate appears that turns yellow upon boiling and orange after 1 ml of NH_4OH solution is added.

3.8. Qualitative screening of steroids and terpenoids

The general procedure to test the presence of steroids is: to 1 ml aqueous extract, 10 ml chloroform is added and then slowly 10 ml sulfuric acid is dripped. Upper layer turns red and sulfuric acid layer turns yellow-green.

Terpenoids are analyzed by reacting 1 ml aqueous extract with 2 ml of chloroform and then, slowly, few drops of concentrated sulfuric acid. An interface with a reddish-brown coloration appears (**Table 12**). The change in color can be observed in **Figure 9**.

The qualitative screening of steroids revealed that these phytochemicals are absent from all the extracts while very small traces of terpenoids could be visually observed in gooseberry aqueous extract.

Phytochemical test	Sea buckthorn	Gooseberry
Proteins and amino acids—Millon	Opalescent orange solution	Red-brownish precipitate
Proteins—biuret test	Green solution	Brown solution
Proteins—xanthoproteic test	Opalescent brown solution	Dark-brown precipitate

Table 11. Qualitative screening of proteins.

Phytochemical test	Sea buckthorn	Gooseberry
Steroids	Colorless layer, brown ring, colorless upper layer	Pale-yellow layer, thick brown ring, pale-yellow upper layer
Terpenoids	Colorless	Brown interface

Table 12. Qualitative screening of steroids and terpenoids.

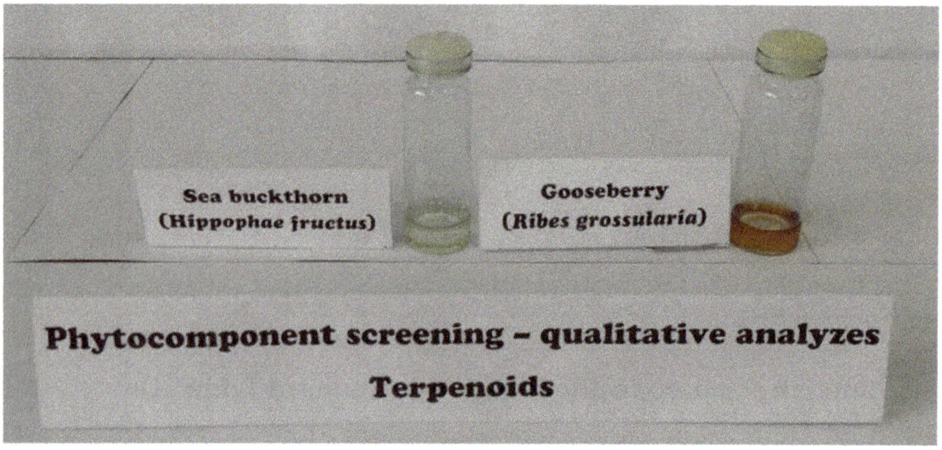

Figure 9. Terpenoids in sea buckthorn and gooseberry.

3.9. Qualitative screening of glycosides

There are three different standard phytochemical methods:

a. *$FeCl_3$ reagent*: the test is for cardiac glycosides: 1 ml aqueous extract, 1 ml $FeCl_3$ reagent (1 ml 5% $FeCl_3$ solution mixed with 99 ml glacial acetic acid) and few drops of concentrated H_2SO_4 gives a greenish-blue color that appears in time.

b. *Keller-Killiani test*: the test is for cardiac glycosides: 5 ml aqueous extract, 2 ml glacial acetic acid, a drop of $FeCl_3$ solution, and 1 ml concentrated H_2SO_4 form a brown ring and often a purple ring appears below (see results in **Table 13**).

c. *Borntrager test*: this test reveals the presence of anthraquinonic glycosides: 2 ml aqueous extract react upon boiling with 2 ml H_2SO_4. The solution is filtered, and equal volumes of chloroform are added and shaken vigorously, and two layers can be clearly observed. The organic layer is separated, and ammonia is added to form a pinkish-red color as a sign of positive reaction.

Phytochemical test	Sea buckthorn	Gooseberry
Glycosides (cardiac)—$FeCl_3$ reagent	Orange-yellow solution	Red-brown solution
Glycosides (cardiac)—Keller-Killiani test	Brown ring at the interface	Brown ring at the interface
Glycosides (anthraquinonic)—Borntrager test	Colorless lower layer, opalescent white upper layer	Colorless lower layer, light-yellow upper layer

Table 13. Qualitative screening of glycosides Keller-Killiani test is positive for both aqueous extracts.

4. Conclusions

This chapter describes the qualitative phytochemical screening of two aqueous extracts prepared from dried fruits of sea buckthorn and gooseberry, plants with the important pharmacological properties and rich in nutrients. The qualitative screening consists of standard methods that are able to determine whether a phytochemical is present or not in the aqueous extracts.

The two aqueous extracts are obtained after a cold infusion at a constant temperature of 4°C for 24 h and are kept at the refrigerator for more than 12 weeks without alteration.

The general screening of carbohydrates revealed that, in the case of sea buckthorn aqueous extract, the solution turns purple-red and a brown precipitate is obtained from gooseberry aqueous extract. Molisch's test revealed that both aqueous extracts contain different classes of carbohydrates. Specific qualitative test for carbohydrates reveal the presence of monosaccharides in gooseberry aqueous extract and of di-, oil- and polysaccharides in both sea buckthorn and gooseberry aqueous extracts.

Alkaloids are absent from both extracts, while cardiac glycosides are present. The test for cysteine gives a positive reaction in the case of sea buckthorn, while ninhydrin test is negative for both aqueous extracts.

The results obtained when aqueous extract from sea buckthorn reacts with Millon reagent is an opalescent orange solution and, in the case of gooseberry aqueous extracts, a red-brownish precipitate is formed, thus confirming that small amounts of proteins and/or amino acids are present in gooseberry.

Acknowledgements

This chapter received the financial support of the projects: PN 120BG/2016, PN-III-P1-1.2-PCCDI2017-0476, and PN 18.22.04.01.01.

Conflict of interest

The authors declare no potential conflicts of interest with respect to the research, authorship, and publication of this article.

Author details

Ana-Alexandra Sorescu[1,2*], Alexandrina Nuta[1,3], Rodica-Mariana Ion[1,2] and Lorena Iancu[1]

*Address all correspondence to: anaalexandrasorescu@yahoo.com

1 The National Research and Development Institute for Chemistry and Petrochemistry—ICECHIM, Evaluation and Conservation of Cultural Heritage, Bucharest, Romania

2 Materials Engineering Doctoral School, Valahia University, Târgoviște, Romania

3 The Romanian Academy, "Stefan S. Nicolau" Institute of Virology, Bucharest, Romania

References

[1] Oszahin AD, Kirecci OA. Antioxidant properties, characterization of nutrients, and phytochemistry of seven medicinal plants. Chemistry of Natural Compounds. 2016;**52**(6):1081-1083. DOI: 10.1007/s10600-016-1866-2

[2] Kharchouf S, Bouchador A, Drioiche A, Khiya Z, Hilali FE, Zair T. Étude phytochimique et évaluation de l'activité antioxydante de *Stevia rebaudiana*. Phytothérapie. 2nd ed. Lavoisier. 2017:1-7. DOI: 10.1007/s10298-017-1163-7

[3] Verpoorte R, Choi YH, KIM HK. NMR-based metabolomics at work in phytochemistry. Phytochemistry Reviews. 2017;**6**(1):3-14. DOI: 10.1007/s11101-006-9031-3

[4] Phytochemicals [Internet]. Available from: http://www.phytochemicals.info [Accessed: April 1, 2018]

[5] Phytochemicals [Internet]. Available from: https://www.sciencedirect.com/topics/agricultural-and-biological-sciences/phytochemical [Accessed: April 1, 2018]

[6] Caroling G, Vinodhini E, Mercy Ranjitham A, Shanti P. Biosynthesis of copper nanoparticles using Phyllanthus Embilica (gooseberry) extract—Characterisation and study of antimicrobial effects. International Jorunal of Nanomaterials and Chemistry. 2015;**1**:53-63

[7] Veerachari U, Bopaiah AK. Preliminary phyto-chemical evaluation of the leaf extract of five *Cassia Species*. Journal of Chemical and Pharmaceutical Research. 2011;**5**:574-583

[8] Jonas Sagbo I, Afolayan AJ, Bradley G. Antioxidant, antibacterial and phytochemical properties of two medicinal plants against the wound infecting bacteria. Asian Pacific Journal of Tropical Biomedicine. 2017;**7**(9):817-825. DOI: 10.1016/j.apjtb.2017.08.009

[9] Chah KF, Eze CA, Emuelosi CE, Esimone CE. Antibacterial and wound healing properties of methanolic extracts of some Nigerian medicinal plants. Journal of Ethnopharmacology. 2006;**104**(1-2):164-167. DOI: 10.1016/j.jep.2005.08.070

[10] Kisseih E, Lechtenberg M, Petereit F, Sendker F, Zacharski D, Brandt S, Agyare S, Hensel A. Phytochemical characterization and *in vitro* wound healing activity of leaf extracts from *Combretum mucronatum* Schum. & Thonn.: Oligomeric procyanidins as strong inductors of cellular differentiation. Journal of Ethnopharmacology. 2015;**174**:628-636. DOI: 10.1016/j.jep.2015.06.008

[11] Olas B. Sea buckthorn as a source of important bioactive compounds in cardiovascular diseases. Food and Chemical Toxicology. 2016;**97**:199-204. DOI: 10.1016/j.fct.2016.09.008

[12] Suryakumar G, Gupta A. Medicinal and therapeutic potential of sea buckthorn (*Hippophae rhamnoides* L.). Journal of Ethnopharmacology. 2011;**2**:268-278. DOI: 10.1016/j.jep.2011.09.024

[13] Sidor AM. The intake of minerals in the diet brought by the consumption of sea buckthorn (*Hippophae rhamnoides* L.) berries and juice. Food and Environment safety—Journal of Faculty of Food Engineering. 2015;**XIV**(3):327-330

[14] Pluta S. Gooseberry – *Ribes uva-crispa, sin. R. grossularia* L. Exotic fruits. 2nd ed. London: Academic Press. 2018. 211 p. DOI: 10.1016/B978-0-12-803138-4.00027-7

[15] Olivares-Tenorio ML, Dekker M, Verkerk R, van Boekel MAJS. Health-promoting compounds in cape gooseberry (*Physalis peruviana* L.): Review from a supply chain perspective. Trends in Food Science & Techonlogy. 2016;**57**(A):83-92. DOI: 10.1016/j.tifs.2016.09.009

[16] Gross J. Chlorophyll and carotenoid pigments in *Red fruits*. Scientia Horticulturae. 1982;**18**(2):131-136. DOI: 10.1016/0304-4238(82)90127-3

[17] Sorescu AA, Nuta A, Ion RM. Qualitative screening of phytochemicals found in aqueous extracts of *Prunus domestica* stone. In: Proceedings of the International Conference "Agriculture and Food for the XXI Century" (AGRIFOOD '17); 11-13 May 2017; Sibiu, Romania; 2017. pp. 121-126

[18] Gong R, Zhang X, Liu H, Sun Y, Liu B. Uptake of cationic dyes from aqueous solution by biosorption onto granular kohlrabi peel. Bioresource Technology. 2007;**98**(6):1319-1323. DOI: 0.1016/j.biortech.2006.04.034

[19] Fahey JW. Reference Module in Food Science. Encyclopedia of Food and Health. 1st ed. Oxford: Elsevier Ltd.; 2016. 469 p. DOI: 10.1016/B978-0-12-384947-2.00083-0

[20] Choi S, Beuchat LR, Kim H, Ryu JH. Viability of sprout seeds as affected by treatment with aqueous chlorine dioxide and dry heat, and reduction of *Escherichia coli* O157:H7 and *Salmonella enterica* on pak choi seeds by sequential treatment with chlorine dioxide, drying and dry heat. Food Microbiology. 2016;**54**:127-132. DOI: 10.1016/j.fm.2015.10.007

[21] Kosewski G, Gorna I, Boleslawska I, Kowalowka M, Wieckowska B, Glowska AK, Morawska A, Jakubowski K, Dobrzynska M, Miszczuk P, Przyslawski J. Comparison of antioxidative properties of raw vegetables and thermally processed ones using the conventional and sous-vide methods. Food Chemistry. 2018;**240**:1092-1096. DOI: 10.1016/j.foodchem.2017.08.048

[22] Muhamad II, Hassan ND, Mamat SNH, Nawi NM, Rashid WA, Tan NA. Extraction technologies and solvents of phytocompounds from plant materials: Physicochemical characterization and identification of ingredients and bioactive compounds from plant extracts using various instrumentation. Ingredients Extraction by Physicochemical Methods in Food. Handbook of Food Bioengineering. Oxford: Elsevier Ltd.; 2017. 523 p. DOI: 10.1016/B978-0-12-811521-3.00014-4

[23] Detection of carbohydrates in plants [Internet]. Available from: http://www.biology-discussion.com/plants/detection-of-carbohydrates-in-plants-practical-botany/57156 [Accessed: March 29, 2018]

[24] Safina G. Application of surface plasmon resonance for the detection of carbohydrates, glycoconjugates, and measurement of the carbohydrate-specific interactions: A comparison with conventional analytical techniques. A critical review. Analytica Chimica Acta. 2012;**712**:9-29. DOI: 10.1016/j.aca.2011.11.016

[25] Test for Reducing Sugars [Internet]. Available from: https://sciencing.com/test-reducing-sugars-5529759.html [Accessed: April 1, 2018]

[26] Gabius HJ. The sugar code: Why glycans are so important. Bio Systems. 2018;**164**:102-111. DOI: 10.1016/j.biosystems.2017.07.003

[27] Loman AA, Ju LK. Enzyme-based processing of soybean carbohydrate: Recent developments and future prospects. Enzyme and Microbial Technology. 2017;**106**:35-47. DOI: 10.1016/j.enzmictec.2017.06.013

[28] Wang TY, Li Q, Bi KS. Bioactive flavonoids in medicinal plants: Structure, activity and biological fate. Asian Journal of Pharmacological Sciences. 2018;**13**(1):12-23. DOI: 10.1016/j.ajps.2017.08.004

[29] Ilkei V, Hazai L, Antus S, Bőlcksei H. Flavonoid alkaloids: Isolation, bioactivity and synthesis. Studies in Natural Products Chemistry. 2018;**56**:247-285. DOI: 10.1016/B978-0-444-64058-1.00008-X

[30] Li-Beisson Y, Neunzig J, Lee Y, Philippar K. Plant membrane-protein mediated intracellular traffic of fatty acids and acyl lipids. Current Opinion in Plant Biology. 2017;**40**:138-146. DOI: 10.1016/j.pbi.2017.09.006

10

Evaluation of Nutritional and Medicinal Properties of *Opuntia elatior* Mill

Krishna N. Patel and Kalpeshkumar B. Ishnava

Abstract

Medicinal plant *Opuntia elatior* Mill., family Cactaceae, was studied for its nutritional value and health benefited properties from fruit. The fruit of the plants was extracted in sequential manner using methanol, hexane and distilled water. Out of these, maximum extract yield present in the methanolic extract was 36.84%. Nutritional value present in the 100 g of methanolic extracts of fruit was 1.02, 0.60, 63.26, and 0.11 mg of carbohydrates, protein, vitamin C and fat, respectively. Methanolic extract exhibits the highest antioxidant activity that is 54.10% and the lowest antioxidant activity is exhibited by the hexanoic extract at 45.66% and the distilled water at 50.40% of antioxidant activity. The anti-inflammation activity, the ability of protein denaturation in different fruit extracts of the maximum percentage of inhibition of 37.49% was observed from methanol extract followed by distilled water at 34.15% and then hexane at 30.38%. Phytochemical constituents present in the methanolic extract are alkaloids and phytosterols compound. High-performance thin-layer chromatography (HPTLC) analysis of methanolic extract showed the presence of three bands. Gas Chromatography-Mass Spectroscopy (GC-MS) analysis of methanolic extracts 19 characterization of bioactive compound. The methanolic extracts of fruits containing high content of protein, vitamin-C and carbohydrates provide good nutritional potential value and antioxidant activity and antiinflammation activity that may be possibly contribute to the treatment of arthritic disease.

Keywords: *Opuntia elatior*, nutritive elements, antioxidant activity, anti-inflammation activity, phytochemical constituents, bioactive compounds, HPTLC, GC-MS

1. Introduction

Traditionally useful medicinally important plants and health benefits foods related material last few years have more focused by common human population. The prevention of disease and medical professionals very great demand for improving overall life. In this line, all types of wild fruits and vegetables have been recognized as valuable sources of nutraceuticals. The large number of natural product presents the chemically useful active compound and their multifunctional properties present. Opunitia *sp.* fruits and cladodes perfect member of traditionally useful for the health-prevention. The present research data show the high content of natural chemical constituents, which can give more added values to this fruit. High levels of some of chemical compounds like betalains, taurine, calcium, magnesium, and antioxidants present are very useful [1].

1.1. Nutrition

Human body requires the proper nutrition for growth, maintenance of body, reproduction, and health of organism is the science that interprets the interaction of nutrients and other substances [2]. It includes food intake, absorption, assimilation, biosynthesis, catabolism and excretion. Essential nutrient includes protein, carbohydrate, fat, vitamins, minerals and electrolytes. Human body normally requires 85% of energy for daily use from fat and carbohydrates and 15% from protein. In humans, nutrition is mainly achieved by the process of taking foods into our mouths, chewing, swallowing and digesting it. Nutrition is an essential component for marinating the immune system, proper growth and development of cell, tissue and organ of human body. Eating a nutritional diet contributes to prevent the future disease, improves the quality of life and provides long lasting life. Your nutritional status is the state of your health determined by what you eat. Some of the minerals necessary for health are as follows: (1) Calcium: Calcium is a very important mineral in the diet. The major function of calcium is to build and help maintain strong bones. It is involved in blood clotting. (2) Iron: Iron in food exists as haem and nonhaem iron. In red meat, the haem iron is found, and 20–30% of this is relatively well absorbed. In cereals, pulses, certain vegetables and eggs, nonhaem iron is mostly found and is generally less well absorbed. (3) Zinc: It is essential for synthesizing protein, DNA and RNA in human body. Only 0.003% of zinc is present in the human body. It is required for growth in all stages of life. (4) Sodium: Sodium helps to maintain fluid volume outside of the cells and helps cells to function normally. (5) Potassium: Potassium maintains fluid volume inside and outside of cells and prevents the excess rise of blood pressure with increased sodium intake.

1.2. Essential nutrient requirements

In human body, essential element is not synthesized in the adequate amount and body cannot synthesize on its own and must be provided by the nutritional diet. The chemical components present in the food are classified into six major groups like protein, fats, carbohydrates, minerals, vitamins and water. Utilization of nutrients as an essential component requires water. In our body, nutrients are required for the various functions like respiration, digestion, growth and development. The amounts of the essential nutrients required differ by age and the state of the body [3].

1.3. Use of fruits as nutritional and medicinal source

Fruits are considered in dietary guidance because of their high concentration of dietary fibers, vitamins, minerals, electrolytes, phytochemicals, and especially antioxidants. Various reviews have been associated with the low intake of fruits include chronic diseases such as cardiovascular diseases, blood pressure, hypercholesterolemia, many cancers, respiratory problems as well as mental health. Traditionally many fruits reported have been useful in many non-communicable diseases and reduce the risk of epidemiologically. Nowadays, people are more interested in the prevention of health-related diseases which is that vital role of antioxidants. This fruit of bright color act as scavengers clean up free radicals before they cause any health effects.

In this fruit, more amount of the fibers are present and are helpful in reducing intestinal passage rates resulting in a more amount of nutrient absorption and hence prevent the constipation. It increases the concentration of short chain fatty acids because of fermented in colon that having maintained gut health and anti-carcinogenic properties. Recent report shows that fruits containing high number of anthocyanins, flavanols, and procyanidins, such as berries, grapes, and pomegranate are effective at decreasing cardiovascular risks while citrus fruit and apples had a moderate effect on blood pressure and blood lipid level [4].

Fruits have also been suggested to prevent osteoporosis in adults mainly due to their rich source of calcium and other vitamins present in them, which are vital for bone health. The high fiber content of fruit may play a major role in the reduction of acid load of the diet and in enhancing bone formation through calcium absorption. Interestingly, phytochemicals in fruits have been found to act as antiobesity agents because they also play a role in suppressing growth of adipose tissue. Fruits have been suggested to prevent obesity since they add up to dietary variety.

1.4. *Opuntia elatior Mill.* Fruit

1.4.1. Classification

Kingdom: plantae; Division: Magnoliophyta (Angiosperms); Class: Magnoliopsida (Dicotyledons); Subclass: Archichlamydeae; Order: Caryophyllales (cactales); Family: Cactaceae; Subfamily: Opuntiodeae; Tribe: Opuntieae; Genus: *Opuntia;* Species: *elatior* Mill.

Opuntia elatior plant is scrubby, 3–4 m height (**Figure 1**). Leaves 6–7 mm long, recurved and reddish at the tops. Joints are 18–30 cm size in height by 10–18 cm in width, obovate, thin and dull bluish green color. Small area spike bearing is about 4–5 cm and increase up to 10 cm, rather slender straight prickles which are, grey and opaque except when quite young, the largest of around 3–5 cm long. Flower is 5 cm across, yellow or orange in color. The perianth rotate, with the outer segments short, ovate, acute, they are red in the center, yellow at the edges, and the inner spatulate is acute. Stamens are a little shorter than the perianth. Style exceeds the stamens; stigmas six in numbers. Berry pyriform are, bearing tufts of glochidia and a few prickles, reddish purple color when ripe [5].

1.5. Medicinal properties

Cactus have been used in treating several diseases, such as rheumatic disease, hypertension, diabetes, asthma and gastric mucosa diseases traditionally use as medicine in many countries over the world. This plant contains bioactive molecules that are well known for their health-related properties present in the cactus fruits and cladodes that is the reason for the more focus of many studies. It has been shown that there is a positive correlation between a nutritional rich in prickly pear cactus and a reduced risk of diseases associated with such as diabetes, cancer, cardiovascular and neurodegenerative diseases [6].

Opuntia traditionally used as a valuable health supporting nutrient, the vegetative parts of *Opuntia* spp. is scarcely used in modern nutrition and medicine. It is suggested that Opuntia spp. could be considered as a new approach in treating noninsulin dependent diabetes mellitus. Prickly pear is widely used as folk medicine for burned wound and indigestion and it is found that the effect of fruit extract is better than those of stem extract. Fruits are recommended as an expectorant and remedy for whooping cough, asthma, gonorrhea, ulcers, tumors, treatment of diarrhea and syphilis [7].

The presence of potentially active nutrients and their multifunctional properties make fruits and cladodes of *Opuntia* spp. ideal candidates to produce nutraceutical products. In India, traditionally acceptable for its pharmacological properties of prickly pear, but insufficient scientific information and knowledge on these plants is still rarely available. *Opuntia* species in the last several years have been used as antidiabetic, antihyperlipidemic, antioxidant, anti-ulcer, antiviral, diuretic, immunomodulatory, analgesic and anti-inflammatory, anticancer and neuroprotective. It is also used to improve platelet function, promote wound healing and is nutritionally important [8–11]. A novel food product which is a mixture of both soluble and insoluble fibers made from dehydrated leaves of the cactus *Opuntia is* found to have hypolipaemic properties and hence useful for patients with lipid metabolism disorders.

Opuntia elatior (prickly pear) uses as a highly nutritive food. These people are interested in healthy, prevention disease, natural life-style often promote prickly pear fruit used as a nutritional fruit. The fruit reported the anticlotting, anti-inflammatory and antiviral properties. In India, ethno- medicine, the cactus pulp and juice are used to treat the urinary tract infection, skin wounds, digestive problem and stomach swelling. The natural extract is a useful for alcohol hangovers, and the plant's gel-like sap is often used as a hair conditioner.

This fruit is used commonly by tribal people of the Kachchh region of Gujarat, India. This fruit has high medicinal properties. But information about this fruit regarding the chemical constitutes, nutritional value of fruit and medicinal properties, primary and secondary metabolites unknown is lacking. Thus, this fruit was analyzed for its nutritional value and medicinal properties.

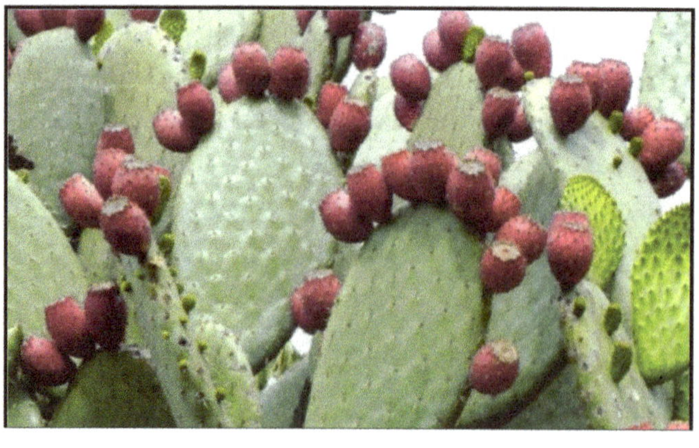

Figure 1. *Opuntia elatior* Mill. plant.

2. Materials and Methods

2.1. Collection of raw material

Opuntia elatior Mill plant species fruits were selected and collected between May and June 2017, from the surrounding areas Jamnagar city of Gujarat (**Figure 2**). These fruits were healthy and disease free and were used to check nutritional value and medicinal properties.

2.2. Drying and grinding the plant material

The fruits were collected and sliced into small pieces and distributed evenly for homogeneous drying. They were kept to dry at ambient temperature with adequate ventilation. Dry condition is required to prevent microbial contamination and subsequent degradation of metabolites. These fruits were kept away from direct sunlight to minimize chemical reaction which is caused by ultraviolet rays. After drying the fruits, they were grounded into a fine powder and passed through 60 mm mesh, this is then stored in an air tight container, in a dry and cool place. Grinding the fruits into a fine powder, for the extraction procedure, helps increase the surface area thus making it more homogeneous, and therefore making it easy for the solvent to penetrate the cells.

2.3. Preparation of fruit extract

2.3.1. Soxhlet extraction method

An extract is prepared using the soxhlet extraction method. In this method, "thimble" made up of cellulose or cloth placed put up the material to be extracted is placed in a central compartment, lower compartment connected with a siphon device and side-arm both. The solvent is placed in the lower compartment, and a reflux condenser is attached above the central sample compartment. It is made sure that all the components of the setup are assembled together with appropriate contents to complete the apparatus [12]. For the extraction procedure, three different solvents were used, one after another, they were methanol, hexane and distilled water, respectively. Each extraction procedure took around 6 h. For each extraction, 230 ml of the solvent was placed in the lower compartment. A sample of 25 g of the fruit

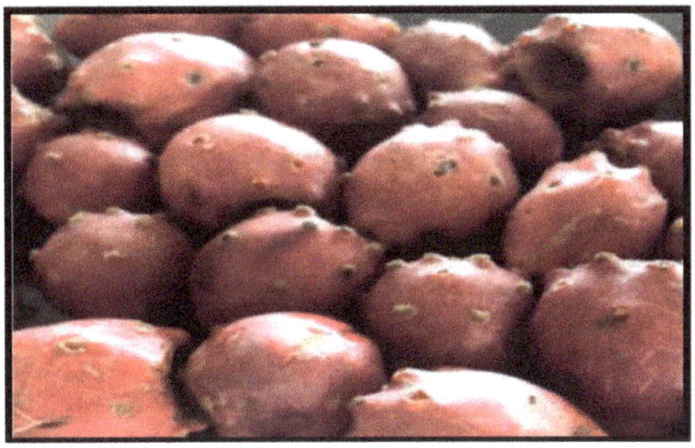

Figure 2. *Opuntia elatior* Mill. fruits.

powder was placed in a porous thimble and kept in the middle compartment. For the procedure, the solvent in the lower container is heated to its boiling temperature (different solvents have different boiling temperature to maintain), and reflux condenser vapor passes through the side arm up. The thimble containing the material to be extracted using the vapor liquefies and drips. Here, central compartment extract gradually collects from warm water percolates through the material and the wall of the thimble. The entire liquid in the central compartment flows through the side tube and back into the lower solvent container of the height of the extract reaches to the top of the siphon. The extract removed in a petri dish and left aside to evaporate. After evaporation of solvent, the leftover extract was filled in the eppendorf tube. This process is then repeated with the other solvents.

2.4. Analysis of nutritional value

2.4.1. *Sample preparation and nutritive analysis*

Stock solution is prepared by dissolving 30 mg of methanolic, hexanoic and distilled water extract in to 30 ml of methanol, hexane and distilled water respectively to give the concentration of 1 mg/1 ml [13].

2.4.2. *Estimation of moisture*

(1) Ten grams of fruit sample were taken in a Petri dish and kept in a hot air oven at 90–100°C for 5–6 h. (2) Weight of the fruit was measured after it was completely dry. (3) Loss in weight was regarded as a measure of moisture content.

2.4.3. *Estimation of fat content*

(1) A mixture of 50 ml of methanol and diethyl ether were taken in 1:1 concentration. (2) From 30 ml of stock solution, 1 ml of test sample was added in the mixture and few drops of phenolphthalein as an indicator. (3) The solution was titrated with 0.1 N NaOH. (4) The change in color was observed from light yellow to a brownish coffee color.

Calculation

$$\text{Acid value (mg/L)} = \frac{(Test - Blank)X0.1X254}{Sampled\ used\ (ml)}$$

2.4.4. *Estimation of crude protein*

The biuret test is a chemical test used to detect the presence of peptide bonds. In the presence of peptides (–CO-NH- groups), a copper (II) ion forms violate coordination complexes in an alkaline solution. Copper (II) reduces to copper (I). The intensity of the color complex is measured by colorimetrically at 520 nm.

Reagents: (1) Biuret reagent: Dissolve 3 g of CuSO4.5H2O and 9 g of sodium potassium tartrate in 500 ml of 0.2 N NaOH solutions. To this solution, add 5 g of potassium iodide and make about 1 L with 0.2 N NaOH. (2) Standard protein solution: 5 mg of bovine serum albumin/ml water. Prepare fresh.

Method: (1) From 30 ml of stock solution, take 1 ml of sample and make volume of up to 4 ml with distilled water. (2) Add 6 ml of biuret reagent to it and mix well. (3) Heat the mixture at 37°C for 10 min. (4) Cool the tubes and read the absorbance at 520 nm against a reagent blank. (Prepare similarly with 4 ml of distilled water). (5) Draw the standard graph by pipetting out 0.1, 0.2, 0.4, 0.6, 0.8 and 1.0 ml, of standard protein solution into a series of test tubes and make volume of up to 4 ml with distilled water in each. Carry out steps 2 to 4. (6) Calculate the protein content in the sample using a standard graph.

2.4.5. Estimation of carbohydrate by Anthrone method

Carbohydrates are first hydrolyzed into simple sugars using hydrochloric acid to form furfural. This compound condenses with anthrone to form a green colored complex which can be measured by using colorimetrically at 620 nm.

Procedure: (1) From 30 ml of stock solution, take 0.5 ml of test sample in a test tube. (2) Make up volume of 1 ml with distilled water then add 4 ml of Anthrone reagent. (3) Heat the tubes in a boiling water bath for 10 min, the color changes from blue to green after boiling. (4) Prepare the working standards by taking 0, 0.2, 0.4, 0.6, 0.8 and 1 ml, where '0' serves as blank. (5) All the tubes including the sample tubes by adding distilled water and make up the total volume to 1 ml. (6) After adding the 4 ml of anthrone reagent. (7). Ten minutes of heat is provided in a boiling water bath. (8) After the tube is cooled rapidly and read the absorbance at 620 nm the green to dark green color. (9) The plotting concentration of the standard on the X-axis versus absorbance on the Y-axis and draw the standard graph. (10) The amount of carbohydrates present in the sample tube find out from the graph calculate.

2.4.6. Determination of vitamin-C

Preparation of standard solution: 5 mg of ascorbic acid was taken and dilute in 5 ml of distilled water to give concentration of 1 mg/1 ml.

Procedure: (1) Take 25 ml of test sample and add 25 ml of 20% Meta phosphoric acid. (2) Dilute it to 100 ml with distilled water. (3) Take 10 ml of aliquot from the above solution and add 2.5 ml of acetone. (4) Titrate it with 0.05% dye solution till a pink color persist for 15 s (V1). (5) For the standard readings take 0.05 g of vitamin C (ascorbic acid) (A). (6) Add 60 ml of 20% Metaphosphoric acid and dilute it to 50 ml with distilled water. (7) Titrate the known volume of the above solution with 0.05% dye solution till a pink color persist for 15 s (V2).

Calculation:

$$\text{Amount of ascorbic acid (mg/100ml)} = \frac{(\text{A mg})\text{X}\,(V2)\text{X}250\ \text{X}100}{(\text{V1 ml})\text{X}\,(\text{B})\text{X}\,(\mathit{wt\ of\ Sampled})}$$

A mg = Std. vitamin C taken; V1 ml = Vol. of dye taken to titrate the sample; V2 ml = Vol. of dye taken to titrate std. vitamin C; B = Total vol. of std. solution taken which is to be titrated against 0.05% dye; 250 = Total vol. of std. solution made after dilution.

2.5. Antioxidant activity by DPPH method

This method is simple and sensitive. The assay is based on the theory of hydrogen donor is an antioxidant. It measures compounds that are total radicle scavengers. DPPH accept hydrogen from an antioxidant. The antioxidant effect is proportional to disappearance of DPPH in the test sample. These methods involve measurement of decrease in absorbance of DPPH at its absorption maxima of 516 nm, which is proportional to concentration of free radicle scavenger added to DPPH reagent solution [14].

2.5.1. Preparation of standard solution, test sample and DPPH solution

Standard solution is prepared by dissolving 10 mg of ascorbic acid in 10 ml of methanol to give the concentration of 1 mg/1 ml. Stock solution is prepared by dissolving 5 mg of methanolic, hexanoic and distilled water extract in to 5 ml of methanol, hexane and distilled water respectively to give the concentration of 1 mg/1 ml. 0.1 mM DPPH is prepared by dissolving 11 mg of DPPH in 8.46 ml of distilled water. It is protected from light by covering the tubes by aluminum foil. **Procedure:** (1) In 3 ml of methanol, 150 μl DPPH is added and reading is taken at 516 nm as control. (2) 0.2, 0.4, 0.6, 0.8, and 1.0 ml aliquots are taken from the test sample. (3) The test sample is diluted by adding methanol up to 3 ml. (4) 150 μl DPPH is added to each of the tubes. (5) Absorbance is taken by UV–visible spectrophotometer at 516 nm. (6) The % of antiradical activity is calculated by using the following equation.

Calculation

$$\% \ of \ antiradical \ activity = \frac{Control \ absorbance - Sample \ absorbancex}{Control \ absorbance!} \times 100$$

2.6. Anti-inflammatory activity by antidenaturation activity

The anti-inflammatory activity of *Opuntia elatior* was studied by using inhibition of albumin denaturation technique [15].

2.6.1. Preparation of test sample and standard solution

Stock solution is prepared by dissolving 5 mg of methanolic, hexanoic and distilled water extract in to 5 ml of methanol, hexane and distilled water respectively to give the concentration of 1 mg/ 1 ml. From this stock solution 100, 200, 300, 400, 500 μl of each solution was taken and added in to 900, 800, 700, 600, 500 μl of their respective solvents, to make 1 ml of working standard solution. 5 mg of Diclofen tablet was dissolved in 5 ml of methanol water to make 1 mg/ 1 ml of concentration. From this stock solution 100, 200, 300, 400, 500 μl of solution was taken and added in to 900, 800, 700, 600, 500 μl of methanol respectively to make 1 ml of working standard. **Procedure:** 0.05 μl of test samples were taken from working stand and 0.45 ml of 5% BSA solution was added to it. The tubes were incubated for 30 min at 37°C in an incubator. A 2.5 ml of PBS buffer was then added and the O.D was taken at 660 nm. Distilled water was served as a blank. Distilled water and BSA solution was taken as a control.

Calculation

$$\% \ of \ anti - denaruration \ activity = \frac{Control \ absorbance - Sample \ absorbancex}{Control \ absorbance!} \times 100$$

2.7. Qualitative phytochemical analysis

The qualitative phytochemical analysis of test for alkaloids, test for flavonoids, test for phytosterols, test for saponin, test for phenol and test for tannin perform by standard method reported by Parekh and Chanda (2008) [16].

2.8. Thin Layer chromatography

The separate chemical mixtures using the thin layer chromatography (TLC). TLC is performed on a sheet of aluminum foil, thin layer coated with of adsorbent material use the silica gel. This thin layer of adsorbent is known as the stationary phase. The solvent mixture (mobile phase) is drawn up the plate via capillary action and after the sample has been applied on the plate. Separation is achieved based on the different ascends the TLC plate at different rates [17]. **Procedure:** 10 ml of Methanol: chloroform (6: 4) was taken in glass beaker as a stationary phase. Test sample was applied on thin layer of absorbent material using capillary tube. This absorbent sheet was placed in beaker containing methanol: chloroform solvents and allowing it to run. After running of sample with solvent mixture absorbent sheet was removed from the beaker and was allowed it to dry. After drying of sheet, it was observed in UV light at high and short wavelength. Spray of concentrated sulfuric acid was applied to it to detect presence of alkaloids in the sample.

Calculation

$$Rf \text{ value} = \frac{\text{Distance travelled by solute}}{\text{Distance travelled by solvent}}$$

2.9. HPTLC analysis

HPTLC analysis based on the principles of adsorption the separation of compound. The mobile phase solvent flows based upon the principle of capillary action. The chemical components separation according to their affinities toward the absorbent. The stationary phase travels slower because component with more affinity. Travels faster the chemical molecule component with lesser chemical charge toward the stationary phase. Thus, the component separated on a chromatographic plate. A 10 mg of methanolic extract was dissolved in 1 ml of methanol. This test solution was used for HPTC analysis. HPTLC aluminum sheet precoated with silica gel was used as the adsorbent. The chromatographic development chamber was saturated with mobile phase to place the plates. The plates were run and derivatized. The derivatized plates were heated, bands were observed and scanned at 254 nm and photographs were taken for record.

2.10. Gas chromatography-mass spectroscopy

The GC-MS method separates different chemical compound and correct identifies the component of chemical constitute. It is one of the most accurate tools for analyzing environmental samples. The GC works on the principle that a mixture will separate in to individual substances when heated. Mass spectroscopy identifies the compound by the mass of the analyte compounds is stored on a computer. A 1 ml of test sample of methanolic extract of *Opuntia elatior* fruit was analyzed by GC-MS. Concentration of the test sample was 10 mg/ml. The GC-MS analysis was done by electron impact ionization (EI) method on Auto system XL gas chromatography, coupled to a Turbo Mass Spectrophotometer at, Sophisticated and Instrumentation Centre for Applied Research and Training (SICART), Vallabh Vidyanagar, Gujarat. The column was a fused silica capillary column.

3. Result and discussion

Medicinal plants due to therapeutic values have long been used to address human diseases. From as early as 800 Before Common Era, plants and herbs were used for their medicinal properties. In ancient Indochina culture, herbal remedies were part of the day to day usage. India has a long history of safe and continuous usage of plant originated drugs. Officially recognize systems of medicine such as Ayurveda, unani, homeopathy and so on. Constantly use herbal drugs to cure illnesses. Today, these ancient practices of Southern Asia are widely growing and highly valued field of the medical industry.

Opuntia elatior (prickly pear) uses as a highly nutritional rich food. These people are interested in healthy body and illness from disease often uses the prickly pear fruit. This fruit present the many medicinal properties in the fruit. In Mexican and India folk medicine, the cactus pulp and juice are used to treat many diseases like skin wounds, stomach swelling and digestive problems. The natural extract is a useful for alcohol hangovers, and the plant's gel-like sap is often used as a hair conditioner.

This fruit is widely used in America, Mexico and many other counties. This fruit is part of their daily diet as it is highly nutritious but, not many people are aware about this fruit in India. It grows best in hot and dry regions and therefore can be easily cultivated in the north-western regions of India. Thus, this fruit was used to analyze its nutritional and medicinal properties.

3.1. Extract yield (%) of *Opuntia elatior* Mill

Pharmaceutical industries prefer plants that yield higher extract and are rich in their potency. Therefore, the work was carried out with yield calculation. We have selected hexane, methanol and distilled water solvent for extracting the plant constituents. A 36.84% of extract was produced by methanol, 15.79% extract was produced by distilled water and 3.40% of extract was produced by hexane from 25 g of powder by using 230 ml of solvents shown in **Figure 3**. Maximum extract was produced by methanol and minimum extract was produced by hexane.

3.2. Nutritive value of *Opuntia elatior* fruit extract

Appropriate knowledge about the nutritive value of fruit may enhance utility of the fruit. With the aim of increasing the utility, we have selected this fruit based on the ethno-botanical information and medicinal properties. For determination of nutritive value, various parameters were studied using fruit extract. *Opuntia elatior* fruit contained 84% moisture, as compared to *Opuntia ficus-indica* which had 87.07% moisture [18]. This shows that both the fruits have close moisture content and therefore are both great sources for reducing dehydration. This plant an indication of the stems adapted the storing water nature of the fruit pericarp. The small variation may result from difference in season whether wet or dry. Sample was collected during the driest month of the region when temperatures were over 35°C during May and June.

The percentage of various nutritional parameters that are analyzed in methanolic extract, distilled water extract and hexanoic extract of fruit are summarized in **Table 1**. Nutritive value of methanolic extract is higher than distilled water and hexanoic extract. As compared to Feugang *et al.* report *Opuntia spp.* contained 0.21–1.6% of protein, 0.09–0.7% of fat and 12–17% of carbohydrates whereas *Opuntia elatior* has 0.60%, 0.11% and 1.02% of protein, fat and carbohydrates respectively [19]. This shows that *Opuntia elatior* has an average protein and fat content and very low carbohydrate content.

Opuntia elatior fruit extract showed highest presence of vitamin C in distilled water extract that is 63.29 mg/ml. Hydrophilic extract of purple cactus pear fruit contains 36.6 mg/100 g of vitamin C [20]. From this we can say that *Opuntia elatior* is a rich source of vitamin C; this can help to reduce the oxidative stress in the human body. From the abovementioned, it can be seen that *Opuntia elatior* is a good source of nutrients.

3.3. Antioxidant activity of different extracts of *Opuntia elatior* fruit

3.3.1. DPPH Method (1, 1diphenyl 2, picryl hydrazyl)

In a living organism, free radicals are constantly generated; few amongst those remain as the unregulated radicals, which can cause extensive damage to tissue and biomolecules leading to various disease conditions, especially degenerative diseases and extensive lysis. This is the most widely reported method for screening of antioxidant activity. The lipophilic radical uses the model of DPPH radical. The lipid autoxidation was initiated by chain of lipophilic radicals. The stable free radical of DPPH at room temperature and stable diamagnetic molecule accepts an electron or hydrogen radical. The DPPH reducing capacity was observed by the decrease in its absorbance at 516 nm, which is induced by antioxidants. The suggested that the samples were free radical scavengers the DPPH test positive.

The best antioxidant activity was exhibited by the methanolic extract compared to hexanoic and distilled water extract. Methanolic extract exhibit the highest antioxidant activity that is 54.10% and the lowest antioxidant activity was exhibit by the hexanoic extract at 45.66% and the distilled water at 50.40% of antioxidant activity. The data obtained for different solvent

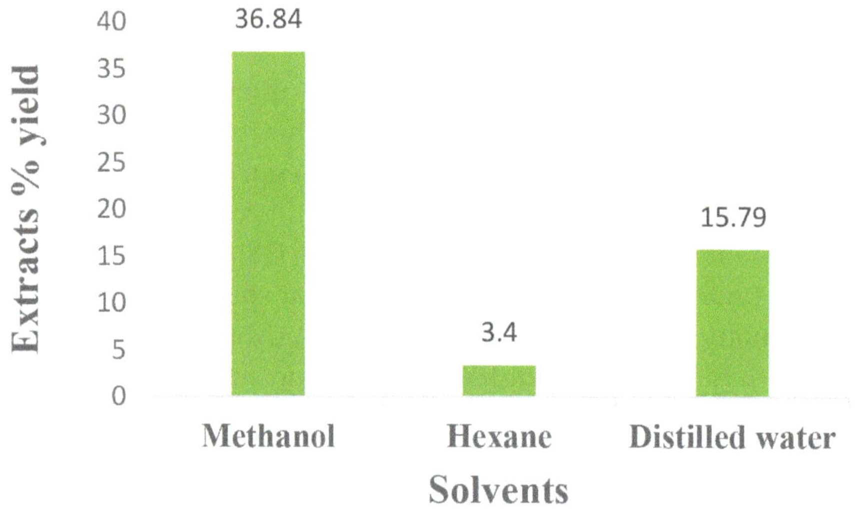

Figure 3. Extract yielded (%) of *Opuntia elatior* fruit.

Nutrients	Methanolic extract	Hexanoic extract	Distilled water extract
Protein (%)	0.60	0.42	0.40
Carbohydrate (%)	1.02	0.66	0.91
Fat (%)	0.11	0.08	0.05
Vitamin C (mg/100 g)	63.29	31.64	45.21

Table 1. Nutritional value of ***Opuntia elatior*** fruit extract.

extracts using DPPH method are shown in **Figure 4**. DPPH radical scavenging activity of methanolic extract of *Cantaloupe* (muskmelon) pulp shows 48.55% [18] (Ibrahim *et al.*, 2016), and *Opuntia shows* 57.37% activity. This shows that *Opuntia* has a good antioxidant potential.

Itankar *et al.* reported that *Opuntia elatior* fruit has 64.14% of activity which is close to methanolic extract of *Opuntia elatior* [21]. *Opuntia* is a good source of vitamin C this helps increase antioxidant properties and reduces the risk of diseases such as atherosclerosis and cancer. Vitamin C is an electron donor. As an electron donor, it helps stabilize unpaired electrons in the body and reduces oxidative stress.

3.4. Anti-inflammatory properties of *Opuntia elatior* extract

Inflammation in the body acts as a defense mechanism. When a foreign substance enters in the body, it causes infection and injury. To protect our body from this, the infected area swells. The purpose of inflammation is to localize and eliminate the foreign substances so that the body can heal itself. Inflammation prevents excess blood flow to rich the site of damage.

The anti-inflammatory activity of *Opuntia elatior* was studied using inhibition of protein denaturation method. Protein denaturation means the loss of biological properties of protein molecules. Denaturation of proteins is responsible for the cause of inflammation and its conditions like rheumatoid, arthritis, diabetes, cancer, and so on. Hence, prevention of protein denaturation may also help in preventing inflammatory conditions.

As a part of the investigation on the mechanism of the anti-inflammation activity, the ability of protein denaturation in different fruit extracts with different solvents was studied. The maximum percentage of inhibition of 37.49% was observed from methanol extract followed by distilled water at 34.15% and then hexane at 30.38%. All the solvent extract inhibited the albumin denaturation. The methanol extract shows the highest inhibition and distilled water extract shows the lowest inhibition. Diclofen, a standard anti-inflammatory drug, showed the maximum inhibition of 63.33%.

Several anti-inflammatory drugs have shown dose-dependent ability to inhibit protein denaturation. *Opuntia* fruit has more than 50% of protein denaturation inhibition properties present in anti-inflammation drugs. This shows that *Opuntia* can be used as a natural source of anti-inflammatory activities. The ability of *Opuntia elatior* extract to bring down denaturation of protein is a contributing factor for its anti-inflammatory activity. The data of this study suggest that *Opuntia elatior* shows significant anti-inflammatory activity with the tested in vitro methods. The data collected by protein denaturation method for inflammation are given in **Figure 5**.

3.5. Qualitative phytochemical analysis of *Opuntia elatior* fruit extract

The phytochemical constituents present in the methanolic extract of *Opuntia elatior* are phytosterols and alkaloid compounds. The presence of yellow color precipitates of test sample by Mayer's reagent shows the presence of alkaloids. The presence of golden yellow color of test sample by adding conc. H_2SO_4 shows the presence of phytosterols. Flavanoids, saponin, phenol and tannin are absent in methanolic extract of *Opuntia elatior*. Phytochemical constituents of the methanolic extract of *Opuntia elatior* were qualitatively tested for their presence as depicted in **Table 2**.

The presence of these phytochemicals in the plants extract enhances their pharmaceutical and therapeutic potentials. Alkaloid is reported to carry antimicrobial activities [22]. The presence of alkaloids in the investigated plants of the wild cucurbits indicates that they have medicinal values. Alkaloids have a powerful effect on the physiology of animals [23]. Sterols in modern clinical studies have shown that they play an important role as anti-inflammatory and analgesic agents [24].

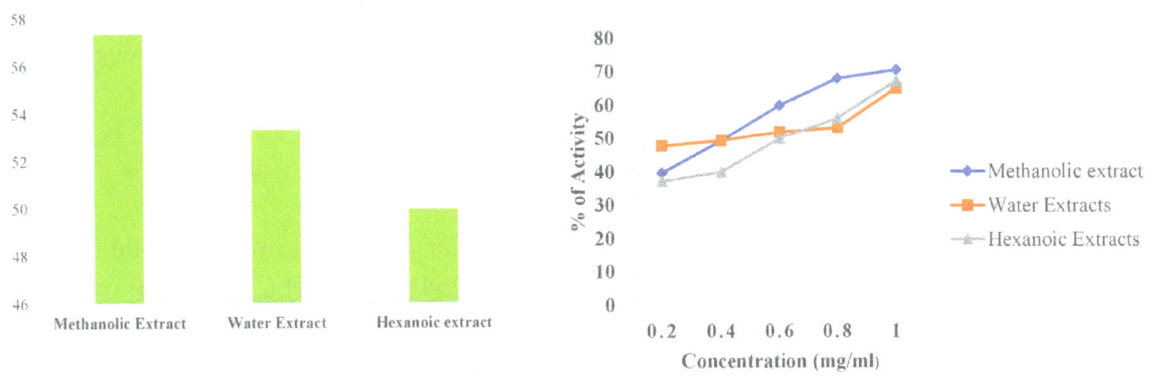

Figure 4. Antioxidant activity of different extract of *Opuntia elatior* fruit.

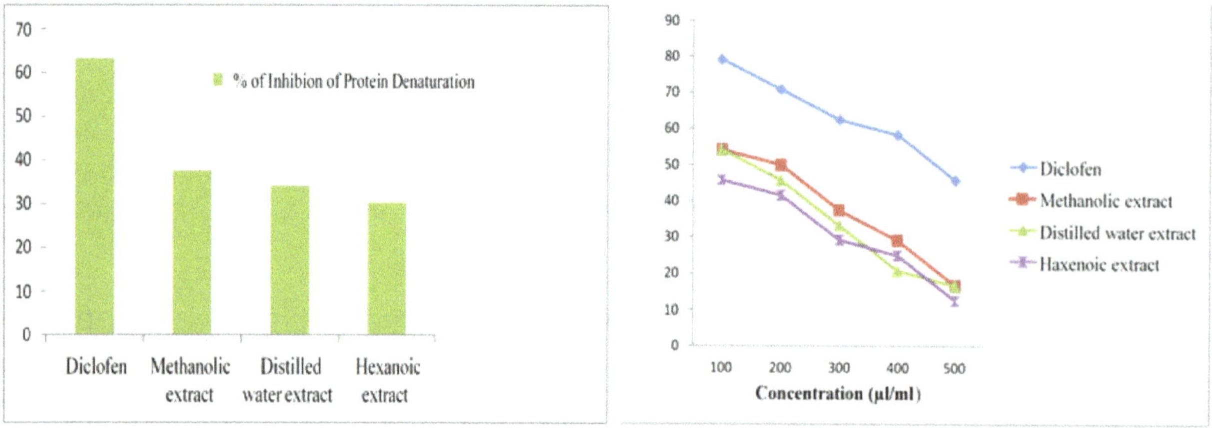

Figure 5. Inhibition of protein denaturation, of different extract of *Opuntia elatior* fruit.

Phytochemical constituent	Color observed	Methanolic extract	Distilled water extract	Hexanoic extract
Alkaloids	Yellow color ppt	+	–	+
Flavanoids	Purple to cherry red	–	–	–
Saponin	Presence of foam	–	–	–
Phytosterols	Golden yellow	+	+	+
Phenol	Blue green	–	–	–
Tannin	White ppt	–	–	–

Table 2. Phytochemical constituents of ***Opuntia elatior*** fruit extract.

3.6. Thin layer chromatography of *Opuntia elatior* fruit extract

Methanolic extract obtained from *Opuntia elatior* fruit was carried out to thin layer chromatography to establish the purity and composition of materials. The component present in methanolic fruit extract was identified by the concentrated H_2SO_4 test. After separation of methanolic fruit extract, one band was observed. The band observed under UV light is shown in figure–3.8. R*f* value of the band was measured that is 0.85. After application of H_2SO_4 band, H_2SO_4 was applied to the band to check the presence of compound. Brownish color of the band was observed after applying of H_2SO_4. This brownish color of the band shows the presence of alkaloid in the methanolic extract of *Opuntia elatior*.

3.7. HPTLC analysis of methanolic extract of *Opuntia elatior* fruit

For the HPTLC analysis the extract of *Opuntia elatior* was run in a mobile phase of methanol:chloroform (8:2). The plate was visualized at 254 nm. HPTLC profile of methanolic extract of *Opuntia elatior* shows three bands at 254 nm, it is shown in **Figure 6**. Maximum R*f* values were obtained by track 1. Different peak spectral comparison of methanolic extract is shown in **Figure 5**. This shows the different compounds present in the sample. Each compound has its own unique pattern. Determination of the peak height of chromatographic peak

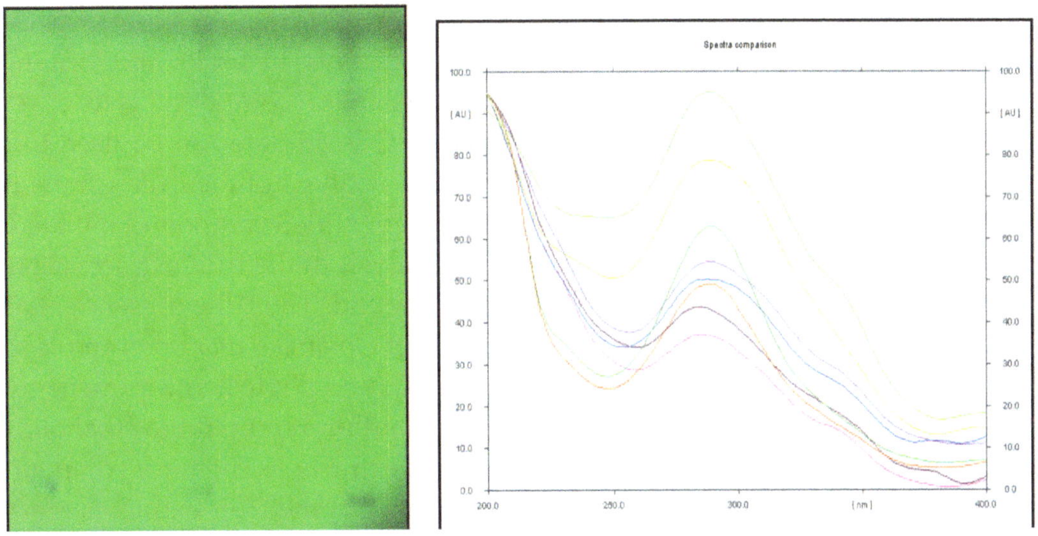

Figure 6. HPTLC profile and chromatogram of methanolic extract of *Opuntia elatior* fruit.

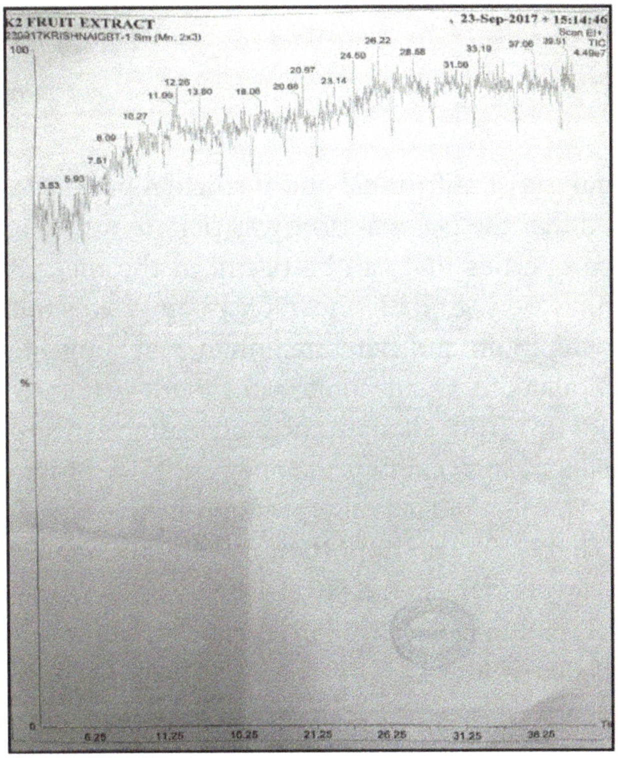

Figure 7. GC-MS chromatogram of methanolic extracts of *Opuntia elatior*.

gives quantitative assessment of a compound. Peak size of the area is nearly equal to the amount of the substance present in the mixture. For the identification of the chemical profile, the sample was subjected to further characterization and isolation of compound. In this study, total nine bands were obtained in the sample.

3.8. GC-MS analysis of methanolic extract of *Opuntia elatior* fruit

GC-MS analysis of methanolic extract of *Opuntia elatior* is shown in **Figure 7**. The separation techniques coupled with GC-MS allowed separation of constituents as shown in the GCMS trace in **Figure 7**. Compounds are not separated properly because of its higher background value. Because of higher background peaks are not seen clearly. The peaks start forming at 70% and continued for minutes. The identifications of phytochemical compound were based on the peak area, retention time and molecular formula. The GC-MS data can be used to identify major bioactive, phytochemical constituent. The GC-MS analysis of the fruit sample revealed the presence of 19 compounds. Thus, the presence of unidentified compound initiated further investigation on the fruits of *Opuntia elatior*. Further analysis of the fruit extract is being done for the NMR studies for structural analysis of the compound. Thus, the presence of alkaloids and phytosterols present in the methanolic fruit extract of *Opuntia elatior* open ample scope for further investigations. Thus, chemical present of alkaloids and phytosterols present give activity of antioxidant and anti-inflammatory. The different author reported the ethanolic extracts present the 14 compounds compared to the methanolic extracts 19 chemical compound presents. This indication more support to the further analysis of the fruit extract is required for the NMR studies for structural analysis of the compound identification. It gives better idea of which chemical compound is responsible for the antioxidant and anti-inflammatory activity.

4. Conclusion

This study shows the analysis of nutritional and medicinal properties of *Opuntia elatior* fruit. From the study, it is seen that the *Opuntia* fruit was rich in nutrients. It also has antioxidant and anti-inflammatory properties that can be useful in the medical stream. The intake of proper nutrients helps increase your daily metabolism, improves the strength of your bones, increases blood flow to the brain and helps maintain a healthy life style. To date, around 25% of drugs that have alkaloid agent come from plant origin. Through the Qualitative phytochemical analysis of this fruit, alkaloids and phytosterols were found. TLC analysis of methanolic extract of *Opuntia elatior* exhibits the one band. The brownish color of band shows the presence of alkaloid. The alkaloid acts as a phytoprotective agent against invading microorganisms. These phytosterols play an important role in cell membrane function. This helps reduce blood cholesterol levels in the body. HPTLC analysis of methanolic extract showed the presence of three bands. From this result we can conclude that three different components are present in the *Opuntia elatior* fruit extract. By the analysis of GC-MS of *Opuntia*, fruit extract peaks were not shown clearly. It may be because of high background values that the peaks of the compounds were not seen.

Acknowledgements

The authors are thankful to SICART (Sophisticated Instrument Centre for Applied Research and Testing), DST, India for GC-MS analyses. Charutar Vidya Mandal (CVM), Vallabh Vidyanagar, Gujarat, India and Director of Ashok and Rita Patel Institute of Integrated Studies and Research in Biotechnology and Allied Sciences (ARIBAS), New Vallabh Vidyanagar 388,121, Gujarat, India, thankful for providing necessary support research and laboratory facility.

Author details

Krishna N. Patel and Kalpeshkumar B. Ishnava*

*Address all correspondence to: ishnavakb203@yahoo.com

Ashok and Rita Patel Institute of Integrated Study and Research in Biotechnology and Allied Sciences, New Vallabh Vidyanagar, India

References

[1] Jana S. Nutraceutical and functional properties of cactus pear and its utilization for food application. Journal of Engineering Research and Studies. 2012;**3**(2):60-66

[2] National Institutes of Health, Department of Health & Human Services. National Institutes of Health Public Access: Overview [Internet]. 2014. Available from: http://publicaccess.nih.gov

[3] Johanna D. Nutritional requirements and dietary assessment. In: Longo et al., editors. Harrison's Principles of internal medicine. 18th ed. 2006. Vol. 1. pp. 172-181. Chapter 73

[4] Pem D, Jeewon R. Fruits and vegetable intake: Benefits and progress of nutrition education interventions-narrative review article. Iranian Journal Public Health. 2015;**44**(10):1309-1321

[5] Kirtikar KR, Basu BD. Indian Medicinal Plants. 2nd ed. India: International Book Distributors, Dehradun; 1999. pp. 1173-1178

[6] Ulises Osuna-Martínez, Jorge Reyes-Esparza, Lourdes Rodríguez-Fragoso. Cactus (*Opuntia ficus-indica*): A review on its antioxidants properties and potential pharmacological use in chronic diseases. Natural Products Chemistry & Research. 2014;**2**(6):1-8

[7] Shetty AA, Rana MK, Preetham SP. Cactus: A medicinal food. Journal of Food Science Technology. 2012;**49**:530-536

[8] Luo C, Zhang W, Sheng C, Zheng C, Yao J, et al. Chemical composition and antidiabetic activity of Oputina Milpa Alta extracts. Chemistry & Biodiversity. 2010;**7**:2869-2879

[9] Fernández-López JA, Almela L, Obón JM, Castellar R. Determination of antioxidant constituents in cactus pear fruits. Plant Foods for Human Nutrition. 2010;**65**:253-259

[10] Osorio-Esquivel O, Ortiz-Moreno A, Garduño-Siciliano L, Alvarez VB, Hernández-Navarro MD. Antihyperlipidemic effect of methanolic extract from Opuntia joconostle seeds in mice fed a hypercholesterolemic diet. Plant Foods for Human Nutrition. 2012;**67**:365-370

[11] Zhao LY, Lan QJ, Huang ZC, Ouyang LJ, Zeng FH. Antidiabetic effect of a newly identified component of Opuntia dillenii polysaccharides. Phytomedicine. 2011;**18**:661-668

[12] Luque de Castro MD, García-Ayuso LE. Soxhlet extraction of solid materials: An outdated technique with a promising innovative future. Analytica Chimica Acta. 1998;**36**:1-10

[13] Thimmaiah SR. Nutritional analysis. Standard Methods of Biochemical Analysis. 2009;**1**(2):455-465

[14] Goyal AK, Middha SK, Sen A. Evaluation of the DPPH radical scavenging activity, total phenols and antioxidant activities in Indian wild Bambusa vulgaris "Vittata" methanolic leaf extract. Journal of Natural Pharmaceutical Products. 2010;**1**:40-45

[15] Karthik K, Bharath Rathna Kumar P, Venu Priya R, Sunil Kumar K, Rathore RSB. Evaluation of anti-inflammatory activity of Canthium parviflorum by in-vitro method. Indian Journal of Research in Pharmacy and Biotechnology. 2013;**1**(5):729-730

[16] Parekh J, Chanda SV. Phytochemical analysis of dome Indian medicinal plants. Tukish Journal of Biotechnology. 2008;**31**:53-58

[17] Bele AA, Khale A. An overview on thin layer chromatography. International Journal of Pharmacutical sciences and Research. 2011;**2**(2):256-267

[18] Chiteva R. Norman Wairagu: Chemical and nutritional content of *Opuntia ficus-indica* (L.). African Journal of Biotechnology. 2013;**12**(1):3309-3312

[19] Feugang JM, Konarski P, Zou D, Stintzing FC, Zou C. Nutritional and medicinal use of cactus pear (Opuntia spp.) cladodes and fruits. Frontiers in Bioscience. 2006;**11**:2574-2589

[20] Albano C, Negro C, Tommasi N, Gerardi C, Mita G, Miceli A, De Bellis L, Blando F. Betalains, phenols and antioxidant capacity in cactus pear [*Opuntia ficus-indica* (L.) Mill.] fruits from Apulia (south Italy) genotype. Antioxidant. 2015;**4**:269-280

[21] Itankar PR, Sontakke VA, Tauqeer M, Charde SS. Antioxidant potential and its relationship with polyphenol content and degree of polymerization in *Opuntia elatior* Mill. Fruits. Pharmaceutical standardization. 2014;**35**(4):423-427

[22] Ebana RU, Essian AT, Ekpo OD. Nutritional and potentially medicinal value of the leaves of *Lasisnthera africiana* (Breaur). Global Journal of Pure Applied Science. 1995;**1**:1-8

[23] Edeoga HO, Eriata DO. Alkaloid,tannin and saponin contents of some Nigeria medicinal plants. Journal of Medicinal and Aromatic Plant Sciences. 2001;**23**:344-349

[24] Singh G, Wu O, Langhorne P, Madhok R. Risk of acute myocardial infarction with non-selective non-steroidal anti-inflammatory drugs: A meta-analysis. Arthritis Research and Therapy. 2006;**8**:R153

11

Free Radicals and the Role of Plant Phytochemicals as Antioxidants Against Oxidative Stress-Related Diseases

Godwill Azeh Engwa

Abstract

Free radicals or reactive oxygen species (ROS) generated from various sources in the environment as well as from cellular processes in the body are of serious health challenges. Overwhelming levels of these free radicals disrupt the antioxidant defense system in the body thereby damaging cell membranes and cellular macromolecules such as proteins, lipids and nucleic acids leading to cell death or causing mutations leading to uncontrolled cell division. Once the cellular antioxidant system is disrupted and becomes deficient, oxidative stress emerges thereby promoting several diseases such as diabetes, arthrosclerosis, cancer, cardiovascular diseases, etc. Better management of oxidative stress requires antioxidants from external sources to supplement the body's antioxidant defense system. Because of their natural origin and therapeutic benefits, plants have been considered as a major source of antioxidants. Certain non-enzymatic plant phytochemicals such as glutathione, polyphenols, bioflavonoids, carotenoids, hydroxycinnamates as well as some vitamins have shown to possess antioxidant properties in vitro and in vivo. These plant phytochemicals are now been used in the prevention and management of oxidative stress-related diseases.

Keywords: free radicals, oxidative stress, reactive oxygen species (ROS), plants, phytochemicals, antioxidants, diseases

1. Introduction

Man as a living creature has always indulged himself into several activities to ensure his survival and well-being. In so doing, he has induced the production or release of various reactive substances or free radicals which are either consumed or inhaled. Also, certain physiological processes in the body generate free radicals or proxidants. These free radicals or reactive species, because of their deficiency in electron and instability, attack electron rich centers such as lipid membranes, proteins and nucleic acids thereby damaging cells and tissues in the body. Eventual, the human body is adapted to remove these unstable molecules by a myriad of molecules including certain enzymes collectively known as antioxidants. This antioxidant defense system reduces the level of these free radicals in the body and maintains the homeostatic balance for proper functioning of the body. However, when these reactive species are overwhelming high in the body, it surpasses the capacity of the antioxidant defense system leading to a condition known as oxidative stress. This imbalance between antioxidant and proxidants is characteristic of certain disease conditions such as diabetes, atherosclerosis, cardiovascular diseases, cancer etc. One of the possible remedy for this condition is to supplement the endogenous antioxidant defense system with exogenous antioxidants. Plants have gained considerable interest in recent time in managing oxidative stress related diseases; firstly, because of their ethnopharmacological uses in managing diseases and secondly, due to their richness in phytochemicals which possess antioxidant properties. Hence, this chapter is aimed to give an overview of free radicals, their sources of origin and processes of generation in the environment and body. Also, it will highlight on the various mechanisms of free radical induced cellular damage and the associated diseases due to oxidative stress. The various mechanisms of the antioxidant defense system; both enzymatic and non-enzymatic antioxidants will be described as well as the contribution of plant phytochemicals as antioxidants. Emphasis will be laid on some plants and phytochemicals with antioxidant activities stating their mode of scavenging free radicals and prevention of oxidative stress-related diseases.

2. Free radicals

Free radicals are molecular species with unpaired electrons in their atomic orbital capable of independent existence. As such, these radicals are highly reactive and can either extract an electron from molecules or donate an electron to other molecules thus acting as a reductant or an oxidant. Though free radicals have high reactivity, most of them have a very short half-life of less than 10^{-6} s in biological systems [1]. Some oxygen species known as reactive oxygen species (ROS) are non-reactive in their natural state but are capable of generating free radicals.

The idea of free radicals began in chemistry around the beginning of the twentieth century, where chemists initially described them as intermediate organic and inorganic compounds with several suggested definitions. A clear understand of these radicals was then proposed based on the work of Daniel Gilbert and Rebecca Gersham in 1954 [2] in which these radicals were suggested to play important roles in biological environments but also responsible for certain deleterious processes in the cell. Thereafter by 1956, Herman Denham further suggested that these reactive species may play critical roles in physiological process particularly aging process [3]. This hypothesis on the theory of free-radical on aging, inspired numerous research and studies which significantly contributed to the understanding of radicals and other related species such as ROS, reactive nitrogen species (RNS) and non-radical reactive species [4].

2.1. Types of free radicals or reactive oxygen species

ROS are classified into two major categories of compounds which includes the free radicals and the non-reactive radicals. The free radical includes nitric oxide radical ($NO^{\bullet}$), hydroxyl radical ($OH^{\bullet}$), superoxide ion radical ($O^{\bullet}_2$), peroxyl ($ROO^{\bullet}$), alkoxyl radicals ($RO^{\bullet}$), and one form of singlet oxygen ($^1O_2$) as shown in **Table 1** [5]. These species are considered as free radicals since they contain at least one unpaired electron in the shells around the atomic nucleus which makes them unstable and therefore can easily donate or obtain another electron to attain stability. As such, they are highly reactive and capable of independent existence [6, 7]. On the other hand, the non-reactive radicals are a group of compounds which are not radicals but are extremely reactive or can easily be converted to reactive species. Examples of these substances include hypochlorous acid (HClO), hydrogen peroxide (H_2O_2), organic peroxides, aldehydes, ozone (O_3), and O_2 as shown in **Table 1**.

2.2. Sources of free radicals

As reviewed from Sultan [8], free radicals can originate either from the environment, physiological processes or endogenous sources.

External sources: Certain organic compounds in the atmosphere can react non-enzymatically with oxygen to generate free radicals. Also, reactions initiated by ionizing radiations in the environment can generate free radicals. Thus, some external sources of free radicals include environmental pollutant, cigarette smoke, alcohol, radiations, ozone, ultraviolet light, pesticides, anesthetic, certain drugs, industrial solvents etc.

Endogenous sources: This includes processes in living organisms that necessitates enzymatic reactions to generate free radicals. These include reactions involved in the respiratory chain,

Free radicals	Name	Symbol
Oxygen radicals		
	Oxygen (bi-radical)	$O^{\bullet}_2$
	Superoxide ion	$O^{\bullet}_2$
	Hydroxyl	$OH^{\bullet}$
	Peroxyl	$ROO^{\bullet}$
	Alkoxyl	$RO^{\bullet}$
	Nitric oxide	$NO^{\bullet}$
Non-reactive oxygen radical		
	Hydrogen peroxide	H_2O_2
	Organic peroxide	ROOH
	Hypochlorous acid	HOCL
	Ozone	O_3
	Aldehydes	HCOR
	Singlet oxygen	$^1O_2$
	Peroxynitrite	ONOOH

Table 1. Free radicals and non-reactive radicals of oxygen species.

cytochrome P450 system, phagocytosis and prostaglandin synthesis. Some of these endogenous sources of free radicals generation include reactions in the mitochondria, phagocytes, inflammation, arachidonate pathways, etc. Also, reactions involving iron and other transition metals, peroxisomes, xanthine oxidase, etc. are also endogenous sources of free radicals.

Physiological sources: Certain physiological state or processes like stress, emotion, aging, etc. mental status and disease conditions are also responsible for the formation of free radicals. For example, hyperglycemia is a major source of free radicals in diabetes patients through various metabolic pathways which include increase flux of glucose through the polyol pathway, increase formation of advanced glycation end-products (AGEs) and activation of their receptors, activation of protein kinase C (PKC) isoforms, activation of overactivity of hexosamine pathway and decrease antioxidant defense [9].

2.3. Generation and chemical reactions of free radicals

Free radicals are generated through various physiological processes in living organisms. Once generated, they can react with other biomolecules to attain stability.

Superoxide ($O^{\bullet}_2$) is generally produced when a single electron is added unto oxygen. In living systems, superoxide can be generated through several mechanisms [10]. Several molecules such as flavine nucleotides, adrenaline, thiol compounds, glucose, etc. can be oxidized in the presence of oxygen to generate superoxide and these reactions are greatly accelerated by the presence of transition metals such as iron or copper. During the electron transport chain in the inner mitochondrial membrane, oxygen is reduced to water thereby producing free radical intermediates that subsequently reacts with free electrons to produce superoxide [11]. Certain reactions by enzymes such as cytochrome p450 oxidase in the liver releases free electrons that can react with oxygen to produce superoxide. Other enzymes can neutralize nitric oxide thereby producing superoxide [12]. Also, phagocytic cells during respiratory burst can generate superoxide [13].

Hydrogen peroxide (H_2O_2): Hydrogen peroxide is mostly produced from the spontaneous dismutation reaction of superoxide in biological systems. Also, several enzymatic reactions including those catalyzed by D-amino acid and glycolate oxidases can directly produce H_2O_2 [14]. Generally, H_2O_2 is not a free radical but it is considered as a reactive oxygen species (ROS) because it can be transformed to other free radicals such as hydroxyl radical which mediate most of the toxic effects ascribed to H_2O_2. Myeloperoxidase can decompose H_2O_2 into singlet oxygen and hypochlorous acid, a mechanism which phagocytes utilize to kill bacteria [15]. However, H_2O_2 is a weak oxidizing agent that might directly damage enzymes and proteins which contain reactive thiol groups. One of the most vital properties of H_2O_2 over superoxide is its ability to freely traverse cell membranes [16].

Hydroxyl radical ($OH^{\bullet}$) is one of the most important free radicals as it is extremely reactive with almost all type of biomolecules including amino acids, sugars, lipids and nucleotides. Most ROS are usually converted to hydroxyl radical. Thus, it is usually the final mediator of most free radical induced tissue damage [17]. Hydroxyl radical is generated by various mechanisms but the most important is the in vivo mechanism due to decomposition of superoxide and hydrogen peroxide catalyzed by transition metals [18]. Transition metals generally contain one or more unpaired electrons and thus are capable to transfer a single electron. Iron and copper are the most common transition metals capable of generating free radicals and much implicated in human diseases. As shown by Fenton [19], hydrogen peroxide can react with iron II (or copper I) to generate hydroxyl radical:

$$Fe^{2+} + H_2O_2 \rightarrow Fe^{3+} + OH^{\bullet} + OH^{-}. \quad (1)$$

At physiological pH, iron is usually oxidized to Fe^{3+} and chelates to biological molecules. Thus, for Fenton reaction to occur, iron must be converted to its reduced form Fe^{2+}. Superoxide radicals can reduce Fe^{3+} to Fe^{2+} ions thereby enabling the Fenton reaction.

$$Fe^{3+} + O_2^{-} \rightarrow Fe^{2+} + O_2. \quad (2)$$

net reaction (Haber-Weiss reaction):

$$O_2^{-} + H_2O_2 \rightarrow OH^{-} + OH^{\bullet} + O_2. \quad (3)$$

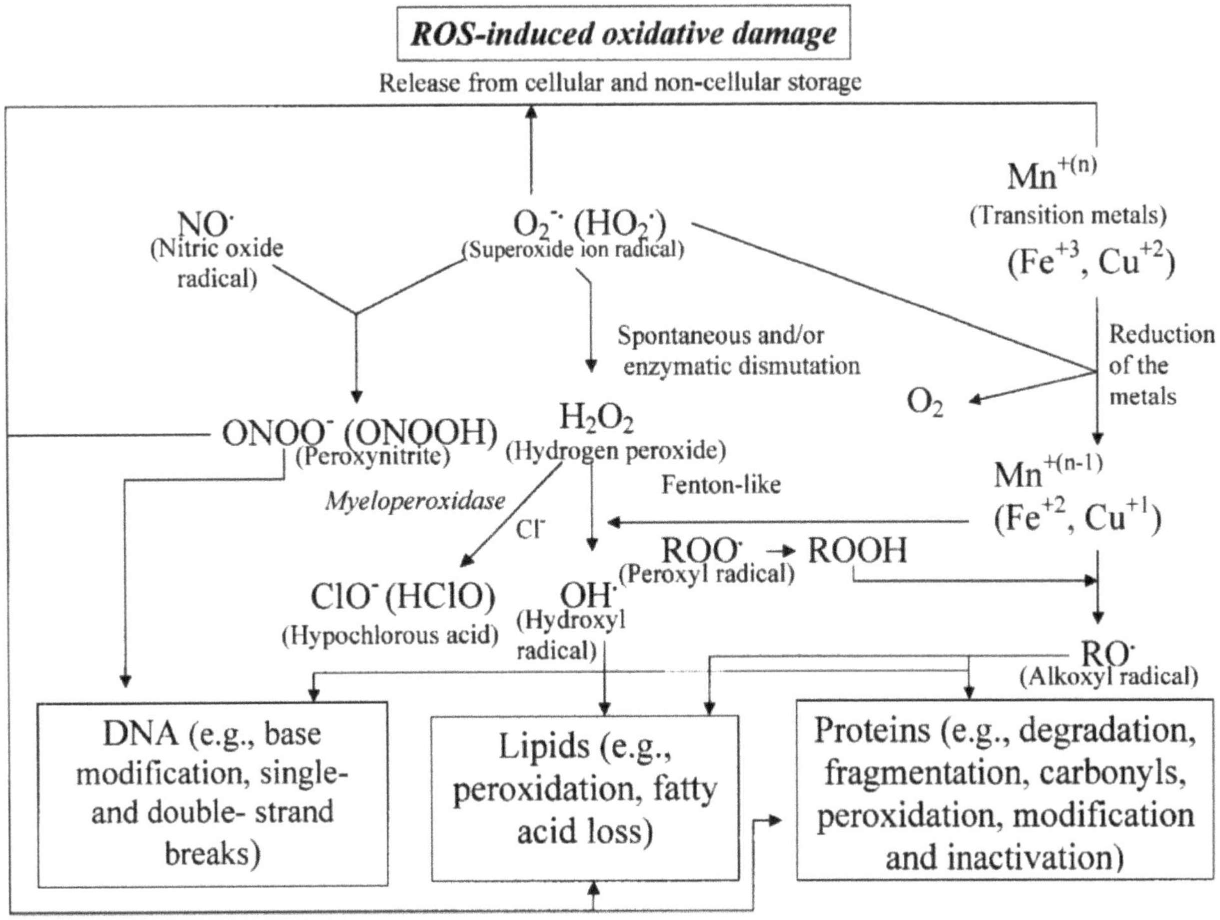

Figure 1. Reactive oxygen species (ROS)-induced oxidative damage. Source: Kohen and Nyska [21].

Nitric oxide ($NO^{\bullet}$) otherwise known as nitrogen monoxide is a radical produced by the oxidation of one of the terminal guanido nitrogen atoms of L-arginine catalyzed by the enzyme nitric oxide synthase (NOS) [6]. L-arginine and L-citrulline are both converted to nitric oxide. Nitric oxide can further react with superoxide to form peroxynitrite.

$$NO^{\bullet} + O^{\bullet}{}_2^{-} \rightarrow ONOO^{-}. \tag{4}$$

Protonated form of peroxynitrite (ONOOH) acts as a powerful oxidizing agent to sulfhydryl (SH) groups thereby causing oxidation of many molecules and proteins leading to cellular damage [20]. It can also cause DNA damage such as breaks, protein oxidation and nitration of aromatic amino acid residues in proteins. Reactive oxygen species and their oxidative stress induced damaged is summarized in **Figure 1**.

3. ROS induced oxidative damage

Continual influx and generation of ROS from endogenous and exogenous sources lead to oxidative damage of cellular components and may impair many cellular functions [22]. The most vulnerable biological targets to oxidative damage include proteins, enzymes, lipidic membranes and DNA [5].

Lipids: All cellular membranes are generally vulnerable to oxidative damage since they are highly rich in unsaturated fatty acid. The lipid damage due to ROS usually known as lipid peroxidation occurs in three stages [23]. The first stage, known as initiation involves the attack of a reactive oxygen metabolite capable of abstracting a hydrogen atom from a methylene group in the lipid due to the presence of a weak double bond. As such, the remaining fatty acid radical retains one electron and stabilizes by rearrangement of the molecular structure to form a conjugated diene. In the propagation stage, the fatty acid radical reacts with oxygen to form $ROO^{\bullet}$. The $ROO^{\bullet}$ is capable of abstracting another hydrogen atom from a neighboring fatty acid molecule, which again leads to the production of fatty acid radicals. These propagation reactions occur repeatedly leading to the peroxidation of several unsaturated lipid in the membrane. The $ROO^{\bullet}$ becomes a lipid hydroperoxide which can further be decomposed to an aldehyde or form cyclic endoperoxide, isoprotans, and hydrocarbons. The last stage which is chain termination occurs following interaction of one $ROO^{\bullet}$ with another radical or antioxidants.

Initiation:

$$RH + R^{\bullet} \rightarrow L^{\bullet} + RH \tag{5}$$

Propagation:

$$R^{\bullet} + O_2 \rightarrow LOO^{\bullet} \tag{6}$$

$$LOO^{\bullet} + LH \rightarrow LOOH + L^{\bullet} \tag{7}$$

$$LOOH \rightarrow LO^{\bullet} + LOO^{\bullet} + \text{aldehydes} \tag{8}$$

Termination by another radical:

$$LOO^{\bullet} + OH^{\bullet} \rightarrow LOOH + O^{\bullet} \tag{9}$$

Termination by an antioxidant:

$$LOO^{\bullet} + \alpha - \text{tocopherol} - OH \rightarrow LOOH + \alpha - \text{tocopherol} - O^{\bullet} \tag{10}$$

Proteins: Proteins are major targets for attack by ROS predominantly by the $OH^{\bullet}$, $RO^{\bullet}$ and nitrogen-reactive radicals causing damage. Hydrogen peroxide and superoxide radicals have weak effects on proteins except for proteins containing SH groups. Following interaction with ROS, proteins can undergo direct damages such as damaging specific amino acid residues and changing their tertiary structures and indirect damages such as peroxidation, degradation and fragmentation. The consequences of protein damage include loss of enzymatic activity and altered cellular functions. Protein oxidation products are usually keto, aldehydes and carbonyls compounds. Oxidation of tyrosine by $ONOO^{\bullet}$ and other nitrogen reactive radicals leads to the formation of 3-nitrotyrosine which is a detectable marker for protein oxidation. Oxidation of proline and glutamate by $OH^{\bullet}$ radicals usually leads to the formation of hydroxyproline and glutamyl semialdehyde. Following protein oxidation, proteins are susceptible to many changes in their function which include inactivation, chemical fragmentation and increased proteolytic degradation [24].

Nucleic acid: Though DNA is a stable molecule, ROS can interact with it to cause several types of damages which include double- and single- DNA breaks, modification of DNA bases, loss of purines (apurinic sites), DNA-protein cross-linkage, damage to the deoxyribose sugar and damage to the DNA repair system. Hydroxyl radical is the most detrimental ROS that affects nucleic acids [25]. For example, $OH^{\bullet}$ can attack guanine and adenine to yield an oxidation product, 8-hydroxydeoxyguanosine [26] and hydroxyadenine respectively. Also, hydroxyl radicals can attack pyrimidines leading to the formation of thymine peroxide, thymine glycols, 5-(hydroxymethyl) uracyl, and other such products. ROS such as $O^{\bullet}_2$ and H_2O_2 do not have direct interaction with DNA and hence do not lead to damage at their physiological concentrations. Transition metals such as iron that have high-binding affinity to DNA sites can catalyze the production of $OH^{\bullet}$ which in turns attack DNA.

4. Oxidative stress and human diseases

When the concentration of ROS exceeds those of antioxidant neutralizing species, a condition known as oxidative stress occurs. As reviewed from Rahman et al. [27], oxidative stress has been implicated in several diseases including atherosclerosis, cancer, malaria, rheumatoid arthritis, chronic fatigue syndrome, and neurodegenerative diseases such as Alzheimer's disease, Parkinson's disease and Huntington's disease [28]. Evidence via monitoring biomarkers such as the presence of ROS and RNS as well as antioxidant defense has indicated oxidative damage may be implicated in the pathogenesis of these diseases [29]. Elevated levels of free radicals such as 4-hydroxy-2,3-nonenal (HNE), acrolein, malondialdehyde (MDA) and F2-isoprostanes have been observed in Alzheimer's disease [30, 31]. Oxidative stress also contributes to tissue injury following hyperoxia and irradiation. Evidence from studies have shown oxidative stress to play an important role in the pathogenesis and development of metabolic syndrome related disorders such as obesity, hypertension, diabetes, dyslipidemia etc. as well as in cardiovascular related diseases such as myocardial infarction, aortic valve stenosis, angina pectoris, atherosclerosis and heart failure [32–35]. Cancer is another disease associated with ROS as ROS have been suggested to stimulate oncogenes such as Jun and Fos whose overexpression is directly associated with lung cancer [36]. In lung cancers, p53 can be mutated by ROS thereby losing its function of apoptosis and functioning as an oncogene [37]. Also, the development of gastric cancer has been thought to be due to increase production of ROS and RNS by *Helicobacter pylori* infection in human stomach [29]. Excess ROS in human kidney leads to urolithiasis [29]. ROS have also been reported to damage cellular components in cartilage leading to osteoarthritis [38] and has been shown to be involved in damaging the islets cells of the pancreas [39]. More so, hyperglycemia triggers ROS production in both tubular and mesangial cells of human kidney, making functional and structural changes in glomeruli causing diabetic nephropathy [40].

5. Defense mechanism against free radicals

In response to the prevailing level of free radicals both from exogenous and endogenous sources, the human body developed a defense mechanism for protection against cellular damages. These may involve direct and indirect mechanisms put in place by the body.

5.1. Indirect defense mechanisms

Firstly, the indirect mechanisms are those mechanisms that do not directly act on the free radicals to eliminate them or convert them to less reactive forms. Rather this indirect system can act in several ways. Certain regulatory mechanisms can control and regulate processes that lead to the endogenous production of ROS [41]. This may be transcriptional control of the enzymes that are involved in the generation of endogenous ROS. Another indirect approach consists of certain molecules and enzymes that are transported to oxidative-damage sites for repair of macromolecules. This may include repair of damage DNA, protein or lipids. For examples damage oxidized adducts of DNA such as 8-hydroxy-2-deoxyguanosine, thiamine glycol, and apurinic can be removed from a nucleotide sequence and replaced by a normal nucleotide base [42]. Also, certain molecules that can donate hydrogen atoms to damaged molecules are also considered as repair compounds. Molecules such as ascorbate or tocopherol can donate hydrogen atom to a fatty acid radical on cell membrane thereby repairing the membrane. Certain natural cellular or surface barriers such as the skin or cell membranes act as indirect defense system against ROS by preventing exogenous ROS from entering the body or preventing certain endogenous ROS from reaching the target macromolecules. Though these indirect defense mechanisms are helpful against ROS, they are usually non-specific and do not act directly on the ROS.

5.2. Direct defense mechanism

This category of defense system which constitutes the antioxidant system is the most important because they directly act on free radicals either by decomposing, scavenging or converting free radicals to less reactive forms. This defense mechanism constitute two groups; the enzymatic and non-enzymatic antioxidants.

5.2.1. Enzymatic antioxidants

The enzymatic antioxidants include superoxide dismutase (SOD), catalase, glutathione reductase (GRx) and glutathione peroxidase (GPx).

Superoxide dismutase (SOD): SOD is an enzymatic antioxidant that exists in three forms in mammalian tissues and differs on their cofactor, subcellular location and tissue distribution. 1. Copper zinc superoxide dismutase (CuZnSOD) is present in the cytoplasm and organelles of almost all mammalian cells [43]. This enzyme has a molecular mass of about 32,000 kDa with two protein subunits, each containing a catalytically active copper and zinc atom. 2. Manganese superoxide dismutase (MnSOD) has a molecular mass of 40,000 kDa and is found in the mitochondria of almost all cells [44]. It consists of four protein subunits, each containing a single manganese atom. 3. Extracellular superoxide dismutase (ECSOD) is a secretory copper and zinc containing SOD which is different from CuZnSOD [45]. It is synthesized only in fibroblasts and endothelial cells and expressed on the cell surface where it binds to heparan sulfates. Following its release from heparin, it is secreted into extracellular fluids and enters into the circulation. Superoxide dismutase catalyzes the dismutation of superoxide to hydrogen peroxide:

$$O_2^{-} + O_2^{-} + 2H^{+} \rightarrow H_2O_2 + O_2. \tag{11}$$

The hydrogen peroxide can then be removed by catalase or glutathione peroxidase.

Catalase: Catalase was the first antioxidant enzyme to be characterized. It is located mostly within the peroxisomes of cells which contain most of the enzymes capable of generating hydrogen peroxide. It consists of four protein subunits, each containing a haem group and a molecule of NADPH [46]. Catalase is mostly present in liver and erythrocytes showing the greatest activities but is found in other tissues. It catalyzes the conversion of hydrogen peroxide to water and oxygen in two stages:

Stage 1: $\text{Catalase–Fe(III)} + H_2O_2 \rightarrow \text{compound I}$

Stage 2: $\text{Compound I} + H_2O_2 \rightarrow \text{catalase–Fe(III)} + 2H_2O + O_2$

Glutathione peroxidases (GPx): Glutathione peroxidase is an enzyme which is synthesized mainly in the kidney and found in almost all tissues although it is highly found in the liver [47]. Its subcellular location is usually the cytosol and mitochondria. Selenium serves as its cofactor located at the active site of the enzyme and deficiency of selenium greatly affects the activity of the enzyme [48]. Glutathione peroxidases catalyze the oxidation of reduced glutathione (GSH) decomposing hydrogen peroxide or another species such as a lipid hydroperoxide:

$$ROOH + 2GSH \rightarrow GSSG + H_2O + ROH. \quad (12)$$

The fact that GPx also acts on lipid hydroperoxides suggest it may be involved in repairing cellular damages due lipid peroxidation [49]. The activity of GPx is dependent on the constant availability of reduced glutathione which is regenerated from oxidized glutathione (GSSG).

Glutathione reductase (GRx): GRx is a flavine nucleotide dependent enzyme and has a similar tissue distribution to glutathione peroxidase [49]. The role of GRx is to generate GSH from GSSG using NADPH in order to increase the ratio of reduced to oxidized glutathione:

$$GSSG + NADPH + H^+ \rightarrow 2GSH + NADP^+. \quad (13)$$

The NADPH required by this enzyme to replenish the supply of reduced glutathione is provided by Glucose-6-phosphate dehydrogenase (G-6-PD) in the pentose phosphate pathway.

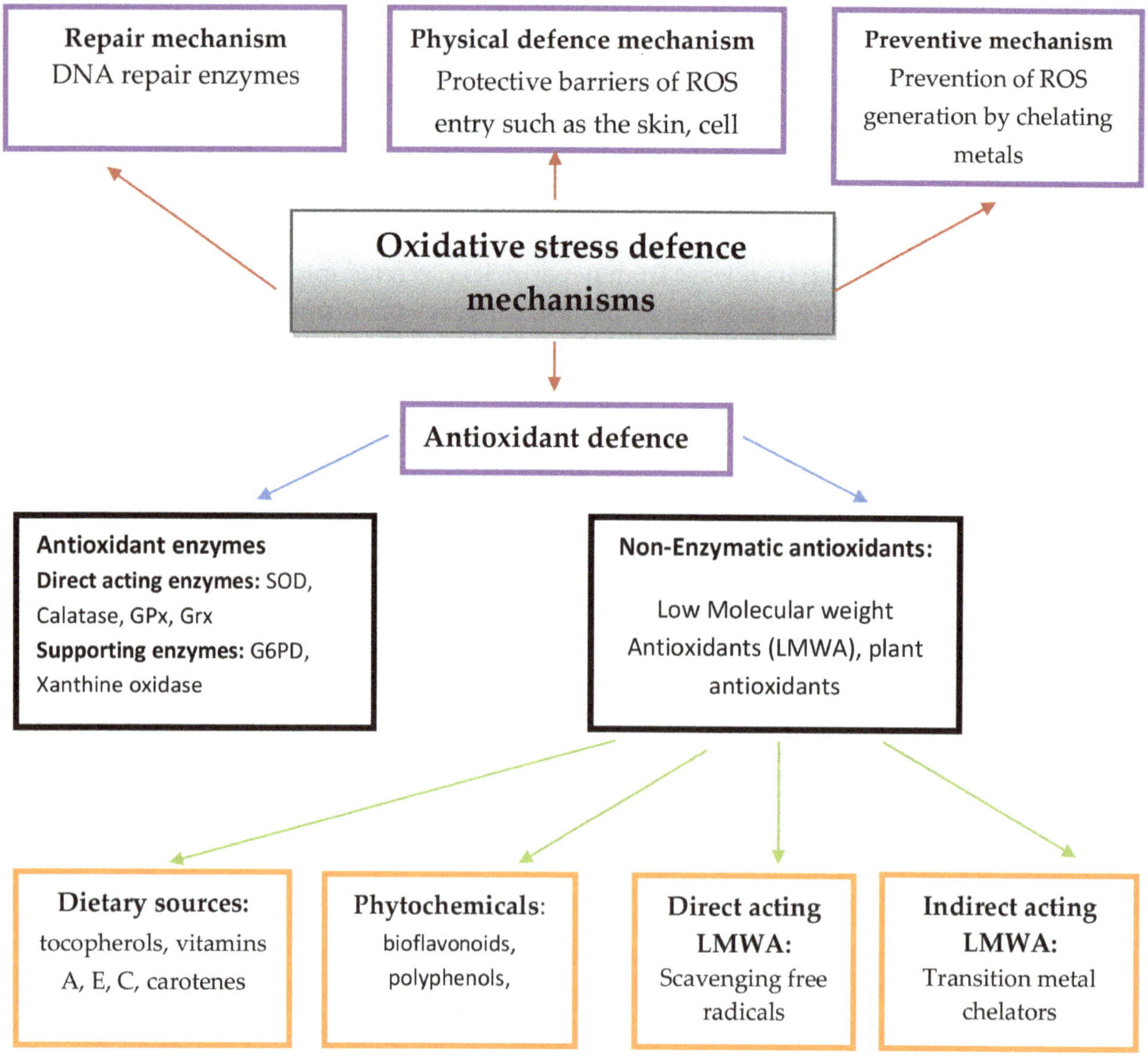

Figure 2. Oxidative stress defence mechanism.

Competing pathway that utilizes NADPH such as the aldose reductase pathway may lead to a deficiency of reduced glutathione thereby limiting the action of glutathione peroxidase.

5.2.2. Non-enzymatic antioxidants

The non-enzymatic antioxidants are usually low-molecular-weight antioxidant (LMWA) compounds capable of preventing oxidative damage either by directly interacting with ROS or indirectly by chelating metals [50]. Transition metals are directly chelated by some of this LMWA thereby preventing them from participating in metal-mediated Haber-Weiss reaction [51]. Other direct acting LMWA molecules scavenge free radicals by donating electrons to free radicals to make them stable thereby preventing attacks of biological targets. These LMWA molecules also called scavengers may be advantageous over enzymatic antioxidants as they can penetrate cellular membranes and be localized in close proximity to the biological target due to their small size. More so, these non-enzymatic antioxidants can interact together to scavenge free radicals and their scavenging activity may be synergic. Most scavengers originate from endogenous sources, such as biosynthetic processes and waste-product generation by the cell. However, the number of LMWA synthesized by the living cell or generated as waste products such as histidine dipeptides, glutathione, uric acid, lipoic acid and bilirubin is limited [52]. More so, the concentration of scavenger must be sufficiently high to compete with the biological target on the deleterious species [50]. As such, exogenous sources of non-enzymatic antioxidants especially from plant diet and phytochemicals are needed to supplement the endogenous non-enzymatic antioxidants. The oxidative stress defense mechanism in humans is summarized in **Figure 2**.

6. Plants as source of antioxidants

Plants have long been consumed as food which is rich in vitamins and other nutrients that are useful for the body. Also, various plants were used in folk medicine for various therapeutic purposes. Though these uses, the notion of plant as a source of antioxidant became more evident in recent time as oxidative stress was considered a major attribute to most diseases in humans and the antioxidant defense system in human was usually not sufficient to overcome the free radical level in the body. As such, plants have gained considerable interest as a source of antioxidants and so much research has been done to identify plants substances with antioxidant activities.

Like other humans, plants do have enzymatic and non-enzymatic antioxidant defense systems to protect them against free radicals. The enzymatic system includes catalase, SOD, glutathione peroxidase(GPx), and glutathione reductase (GRx) [7], while non-enzymatic systems consist of low molecular weight antioxidants (LMWA) such as ascorbic acid, proline, glutathione, carotenoids, flavonoids, phenolic acids, etc. and the high molecular weight antioxidants (HMWA) which are mostly secondary metabolites such as tannins [53]. The possible reason for the presence of these antioxidants in plants is that plants lack an immune system unlike animals thus, utilize the antioxidant defense system to protect them against microbial pathogens and animal herbivores. Also, these phytochemicals serve as a defense system against environmental stress.

6.1. Non-enzymatic plant antioxidants and their mode of action

Though plants have enzymatic antioxidants, it is usually difficult to isolate these enzymes for therapeutic uses in humans. Also, they are usually denatured during food processing, preparation and not sufficiently present in diets such as fruits and vegetables. On the contrary, non-enzymatic antioxidants are readily present in plants leaves, fruits and food in sufficient amounts and can easily be extracted from plants. For these reasons, this section will focus on the non-enzymatic plant antioxidants.

Glutathione: Glutathione is a low-molecular-weight, tripeptide of glutamic acid-cysteine-glycine containing a thiol. It exist as GSH in its reduced form and 2 GSH molecules can be joined via oxidation at their SH groups of the cysteine residue into a disulfide bridge to form GSSG which is the oxidized form.

GSH generally acts as a cofactor for glutathione peroxidase, thus serving as an indirect antioxidant by donating the necessary electrons for the decomposition of H_2O_2. GSH can directly scavenge ROS such as ROO•, OH• and RO• radicals as well as $^{\bullet}O_2$ and HCLO•. Upon reacting with ROS, GSH becomes a glutathione radical, which can be reconverted to its reduced form [54]. Glutathione also has other cellular functions such metabolism of ascorbic acid [55]. Also, glutathione prevents the oxidation of SH protein groups and acts as a chelating agent for copper preventing its participation in the Haber-Weiss reaction [54].

Vitamin E (α-tocopherol): Vitamin E is a lipid soluble antioxidant that functions as an efficient 'chain breaker' during lipid peroxidation in cell membranes and various lipid particles including low-density lipoprotein (LDL). Its role is to scavenge lipid peroxyl radicals (LOO•) and to terminate the lipid peroxidation chain reactions [56].

$$LOO^{\bullet} + \alpha - \text{tocopherol–OH} \rightarrow LOOH + \alpha - \text{tocopherol–}O^{\bullet}. \quad (14)$$

Also, α-tocopherol can scavenge other ROS, such as $^{\bullet}O_2$ to become tocopherolquinone and subsequently tocopherylquinone. However, it is not an efficient scavenger of OH• and alkoxyl (•OR) radicals in vivo [57]. The resultant tocopheroxyl radical in these reactions can be recycled to its active form but this radical is relatively stable in normal circumstances and insufficiently reactive to initiate lipid peroxidation itself, which makes it a good antioxidant [58].

Ascorbic acid (Vitamin C): Ascorbic acid is a water-soluble antioxidant. It also functions as a chain breaker to terminate the lipid peroxidation chain reaction. In this reaction, it donates an electron to the lipid radical (LOO•) to become ascorbate radical. Two molecules of ascorbate radicals can react rapidly to produce a molecule of ascorbate and a molecule of dehydroascorbate which do not have any scavenging activity. Dehydroascorbate can be reconverted to ascorbate by the addition of two electrons catalyzed by oxidoreductase. More so, ascorbate can react with GSH to regenerate vitamin E in cell membranes [59].

Vitamin A: Though not fully understood, vitamin A is considered as a vital antioxidant that prevents humans LDL against copper stimulated oxidation [60]. The antioxidant potential of vitamin A was first revealed by Monaghan and Schmitt who showed that vitamin A can protect lipids against rancidity [61].

Bioflavonoids: This is a group of natural benzo-γ-pyran derivatives which are widely distributed in fruits and vegetables. They are the most abundant polyphenols found to possess strong antioxidant activities in scavenging free radicals. They have generally been reported to protect against hydroxyl radical induced DNA damage [62]. Also, bioflavonoids are capable of chelating metal ions, such as copper or iron thereby preventing the generation of ROS [63]. These bioflavonoids include flavonol, flavones, flavonolols, flavan-3-ols, flavonone, anthocyanidin, isoflavone, etc.

Flavonoids: In plants, most flavonoids are attached to sugars (glycosides), although they are occasionally found as aglycones. Most flavonoids are not completely absorbed and reach the circulatory system except for some flavan-3-ols and proanthocyanidins. **Quercetin** is a flavonol, known to protect DNA from oxidative damage resulting from the attack of $^{\bullet}OH$, H_2O_2, and $O_2^{\bullet}$ on DNA oligonucleotides. However, at high concentrations of cupric ion, quercetin is reported to be a carcinogenic agent by enhancing DNA damage via ROS [64]. Therefore, it is very important to consider the concentration of the chelating metal ions such as copper or iron while evaluating the protective or degenerative effects of quercetin and other bioflavonoids. **Anthocyanidin** is a class of flavonoids with antioxidant potentials. They are effective in the inhibition of lipid oxidation due to their metal ion-chelating activity.

In general, flavonoids are oxidized by radicals, resulting in a more stable, less-reactive radical. In this reaction, flavonoids stabilize the ROS by reacting with them to become a flavonoids radical. This is achieved due to high reactive hydroxyl group of the flavonoids as shown below.

$$\text{Flavonoid(OH)} + \text{R}^{\bullet} \rightarrow \text{flavonoid(O}^{\bullet}) + \text{RH} \tag{15}$$

where $R^{\bullet}$ is a free radical and $O^{\bullet}$ is an oxygen free radical.

As reviewed from Nijveldt et al. [65], certain flavonoids can directly scavenge superoxides as well as peroxynitrite. Other flavonoids may act as antioxidants by inhibiting the activity of free radical generating enzymes such as xanthine oxidase and nitric-oxide synthase. Quercetin, rutin and silibin have shown to inhibit xanthine oxidase activity while silibin has been reported to inhibit nitric` oxide dose dependently. By scavenging radicals, flavonoids can inhibit LDL oxidation in vitro. This action protects the LDL particles and, theoretically, flavonoids may have preventive action against atherosclerosis.

Carotenoids: Carotenoids are among the common lipid soluble phytonutrients synthesized from phytoene. They include Xanthophyll (zeaxanthine, lutein) and Carotines (lycopene, b-carotene), the latter been the most abundant. Carotenoids are generally known to scavenge peroxyl radicals which are generated during the process of lipid peroxidation of cell membrane. As such, scavenging of peroxyl radicals prevents cellular lipids and membrane damage. Carotenoids are highly lipophilic and are known to play an important role in the protection of cellular membranes and lipoproteins against ROS due to their peroxyl radical scavenging activity [66]. **Lycopene** is the most potent antioxidant naturally present in many fruits and vegetables. The high number of conjugated double bonds in lycopene endows it with singlet oxygen quenching ability. Lycopene demonstrate the strongest singlet oxygen quenching ability as compared to α-tocopherol or β-carotene [67]. **β-carotene** is a naturally occurring orange-colored carotenoid, abundantly found in yellow orange fruits and in dark-green leafy vegetables [68]. Just like lycopene, β-carotene is well-known to quench singlet

Plant	In vitro antioxidant											In vivo antioxidant activity					Protective against Damage in vivo		Ref
	RP	HPS	DS	SS	AS	HS	NS	FS	TAC	TPC	TPC	GSH	CA	SOD	GRx	GPx	PCC	MDA	
Torilis leptophylla	✓	✓	✓	✓	✓	✓	–	–	✓	✓	✓	✓	–	–	–	–	–	✓	[78]
Clausena anisata	–	–	✓	–	–	–	–	✓	–	✓	✓	–	–	–	–	–	–	–	[79]
Peltophorum africanum	–	–	✓	–	–	–	–	✓	–	✓	✓	–	–	–	–	–	–	–	[79]
Zanthoxylum capense	–	–	✓	–	–	–	–	✓	–	✓	✓	–	–	–	–	–	–	–	[79]
Nypa fruticans Wurmb	✓	–	✓	–	✓	–	–	–	–	✓	✓	–	–	–	–	–	–	–	[80]
Artemisia absinthium	–	–	–	–	–	–	–	–	–	–	–	–	✓	✓	✓	✓	✓	✓	[81]
Vitex doniana	–	–	✓	–	–	–	–	–	–	–	–	–	✓	✓	–	–	–	✓	[82]
Mucuna pruriens	–	–	✓	–	–	–	–	–	–	–	–	–	✓	✓	–	–	–	✓	[82]
Schotia latifolia Jacq	✓	–	✓	–	✓	–	✓	–	–	✓	✓	–	–	–	–	–	–	–	[83]
Asphodeline Anatolica	✓	–	✓	–	✓	–	–	✓	✓	–	–	–	–	–	–	–	–	–	[84]
Ziziphus mauritiana Lam.	–	–	✓	–	–	–	✓	–	–	–	–	–	–	–	–	–	–	–	[85]
Helichrysum longifolium DC	✓	✓	✓	✓	✓	–	✓	–	✓	✓	✓	–	–	–	–	–	–	–	[86]
Strychnos henningsii Gilg	✓	✓	✓	✓	✓	–	✓	–	✓	✓	✓	✓	✓	✓	–	–	–	✓	[87]
Citrus sinensis	–	–	✓	–	–	–	–	–	–	✓	✓	–	–	–	–	–	–	–	[88]
Citrus anrantifolia	–	–	✓	–	–	–	–	–	–	✓	✓	–	–	–	–	–	–	–	[88]
Citrus limonum	–	–	✓	–	–	–	–	–	–	✓	✓	–	–	–	–	–	–	–	[88]
Acalypha manniana	–	–	✓	–	–	–	–	–	–	✓	✓	–	–	–	–	–	–	–	[89]
Chrysophyllum albidum	✓	✓	–	–	–	–	–	–	–	✓	✓	–	✓	–	–	–	–	✓	[90]
Murraya Koenigii	✓	✓	–	–	–	–	–	–	–	✓	✓	–	✓	–	–	–	–	✓	[91]

Legend: ✓ indicates present while – indicates not evaluated. RP: reducing power activity, HPS: hydrogen peroxide scavenging activity, NS: nitrogen oxide scavenging activity; FS: FRAP scavenging activity, DS: DPPH radical scavenging activity, SS: superoxide anion scavenging activity, AS: ABTS radical scavenging activity, HS: hydroxyl radical scavenging assay, TAC: total antioxidant capacity, TPC: total phenolic content, TFC: total flavonoid content, GSH: reduced glutathione, CA: catalase activity, SOD: superoxide dismutase activity, GPx: glutathione peroxidase, GRx: glutathione reductase, MDA: malondialdehyde, PCC: protein carbonyl content, Ref: references.

Table 2. Some plants with ***in vitro*** and ***in vivo*** antioxidant activities.

Oxidative stress diseases	Plant	Phytochemical	Mechanism of action	References
Cardiovascular disease	*Euterpe oleracea*	Flavonoids	*In vitro* atheroprotective effects	[92]
	Flos chrysanthemi	Flavonoids	Vasodilating effects and protected vasodilator reactivity	[93]
	Gnetum macrostachyum	Stilbenoids	Antioxidant and anti-inflammation activities	[94]
	Polyphenols	Crocin, carotenoid	protected oxidative stress-induced apoptosis of platelets	[95]
Anti-obesity	*Vaccinium floribundum* *Aristotelia chilensis*	Anthocyanins, proanthocyanidins	Limits adipogenesis and inflammatory pathways in vitro	[96]
	Grape products	Polyphenol	Antioxidant action, blocking proinflammatory cytokines	[97]
Diabetes	*Ascophyllum nodosum*	Phenolics	Antioxidant activity and anti-diabetic effect	[98]
	Chrysobalanus icaco	Polyphenolics	Strong antioxidant action and reduction of glycemia in rats	[99]
	-----------------	Curcumin	Anti-inflammatory and anti-oxidant activities	[100]
	Polyphenol	Butein	Inhibit formation of nitric oxide in vitro and protecting pancreatic β-cells against cytokine-induced toxicity	[101]
Cancer	Polyphenols	Ellagitannins and epicatechin	Anticarcinogenic properties	[102]
	Green tea, grape seeds	Polyphenols, proanthocyanidins	Protect the skin from the adverse effects of UV radiation preventing risk of skin cancers	[103]
Aging	*Elaeis guineensis leaves*	Methanol extract	High antioxidant activities and potential ability as an anti-aging agent	[104]
	Epigallocatechin gallate	Crude extract	Extended lifespan of healthy rats by reducing the damage of liver and kidney and improving age-associated inflammation and oxidative stress through inhibiting NF-β signaling	[105]
Alzheimer's disease	*Crataegus pinnatifida fruit*	Crude extract	Potential neuroprotective activity for preventing oxidative-related disorders in vitro	[106]

Oxidative stress diseases	Plant	Phytochemical	Mechanism of action	References
	Aegle marmelos	Ethyl acetate extract	Antioxidant activity as well as potential acetylcholinesterase inhibitory property	[107]
		Curcumin	Reduced levels of oxidative stress and attenuated increased acetylcholinesterase in mice	[108]

Table 3. Some plants/phytochemicals with therapeutic effects on oxidative stress-related diseases and possible mechanism of action.

oxygen with higher efficiency as compared to the α-tocopherol. More so, β-carotene can be cleaved by β-carotene-15,150-dioxygenase into the two molecules of vitamin A, another antioxidant.

Hydroxycinnamates: Hydroxycinnamic acids which include ferulic acid, caffeic acid, p-coumaric acid, sinapic acid are another category of dietary antioxidants that are known to protect LDL from oxidation and can prevent coronary heart disease and atherosclerosis [69]. In vitro studies involving human LDL as the oxidizing substrate have shown hydroxycinnamic acids to have higher antioxidant activity than hydroxybenzoic acids [70].

6.2. Plants with antioxidant properties

Several plants are known to possess antioxidant properties due to the presence of certain phytochemicals that have been shown to exhibit antioxidant activities in *in vitro* and *in vivo* studies as well as in humans. Consumption of vegetables and fruits rich in antioxidant phytochemicals has proven to increase the antioxidant capacity of serum/plasma. For example, consumption of strawberries, red wine, vitamin C or spinach in elderly women significantly increased the total antioxidant capacity of serum as well as plasma vitamin C levels [71]. Also, another study showed the plasma antioxidant capacity to significantly increase after consuming 10 servings of fruits and vegetables per day for 15 days [72]. Apart from vitamins present in these fruits and vegetables, other plant phytochemicals could be accountable for the increased total antioxidant capacity in serum as other studies have shown the presence of anthocyanins in human serum [73]. More so, apples are highly rich in phenolics and flavonoids thus polyphenols may also be accountable for total antioxidant activity in serum. As such, phytochemicals in fruits and vegetables could interact together such that their additive and synergistic effects could potentiate their antioxidant activities [74]. The pathogenesis of some chronic diseases such as cardiovascular diseases, type 2 diabetes, cancer etc. is accompanied by chronic inflammation which is mediated by the release of free radicals by inflammatory cells [75, 76]. Several antioxidant phytochemicals including resveratrol, anthocyanins, and curcumin, have been found to have anti-inflammatory action via inhibition of prostaglandin production, enzyme inhibition and nuclear factor-kB activity, as well as increase of cytokine production [77]. This section highlights on some plants which have shown to possess antioxidant activities *in vitro* and *in vivo* as well as antioxidant phytochemicals against certain oxidative stress diseases with their mode of action as summarized in **Tables 2** and **3**.

7. Conclusion

Obvious deleterious effects of free radicals as regards man's heath cannot be over emphasized. Oxidative stress due to overwhelming levels of free radicals has promoted the progression of diseases such as diabetes, cancer, cardiovascular diseases, atherosclerosis etc. and even aging. Plants phytochemicals and some vitamins have shown to possess antioxidant properties capable of scavenging free radicals, preventing cellular damages and related diseases via several mechanisms. As such, plants phytochemicals are now being considered as the most sustainable alternative source of antioxidants to supplement the endogenous oxidative stress defense system in humans. Continuous efforts are needed to characterize plants phytochemicals for their antioxidant potentials and mode of action for various therapeutic uses against oxidative stress-related diseases while regular consumption of fruits and vegetables are encouraged for the prevention of these diseases.

Author details

Godwill Azeh Engwa

Address all correspondence to: engwagodwill@gmail.com

Biochemistry, Department of Chemical Sciences, Godfrey Okoye University, Enugu Nigeria

References

[1] Young IS, Woodside JV. Antioxidant in health and diseases. Journal of Clinical Pathology. 2001;**54**:176-186

[2] Gilbert DL, editor. Perspective on the history of oxygen and life. In: Oxygen and the Living Process: An Inter-disciplinary Approach. New York: Springer Verlag; 1981. pp. 1-43

[3] Harman D. Aging, a theory based on free radical and radiation chemistry. Journal of Gerontology. 1956;**11**:298-300

[4] Harman D. The aging process. Proceedings of the National Academy of Sciences of the United States of America. 1981;**78**:7124-7128

[5] Halliwell B, Gutteridge JM. Free Radicals in Biology and Medicine. 3rd ed. Midsomer Norton, Avon, England: Oxford University Press; 1999

[6] Beckman JS, Koppenol WH. Nitric oxide, superoxide, and peroxynitite: The good, the bad and ugly. The American Journal of Physiology. 1996;**271**:C1424-C1437

[7] Baud I, Ardaillou R. Reactive oxygen species: Production and role in the kidney. The American Journal of Physiology. 1986;**251**:F765-F776

[8] Sultan S. Reviewing the protective role of antioxidants in oxidative stress caused by free radicals. Asian Pacific Journal of Health Sciences. 2014;**1**(4):401-406

[9] Fiorentino TV, Prioletta A, Zuo P, Folli F. Hyperglycemia-induced oxidative stress and its role in diabetes mellitus related cardiovascular diseases. Current Pharmaceutical Design. 2013;**19**:5695-5703

[10] Halliwell B, Gutteridge JC. Biologically relevant metal ion dependent hydroxyl radical generation—An update. FEBS Letters. 1992;**307**:108-112

[11] Becker LB, Vanden Hoek TL, Shao ZH, et al. Generation of superoxide in cardiomyocytes during ischemia before reperfusion. The American Journal of Physiology. 1999;**277**:H2240-H2246

[12] Masters CJ. Cellular signalling: The role of the peroxisome. Cellular Signalling. 1996;**8**:197-208

[13] Curnutte JT, Babior BM. Chronic granulomatous disease. Advances in Human Genetics. 1987;**16**:229-245

[14] Chance B, Sies H, Boveris A. Hydroperoxide metabolism in mammalian organs. Physiological Reviews. 1979;**59**:527-605

[15] Halliwell B, Gutteridge JC. The definition and measurement of antioxidants in biological systems. Free Radical Biology & Medicine. 1995;**18**:125-126

[16] Halliwell B, Gutteridge JMC. Role of free radicals and catalytic metal ions in human disease: An overview. Methods in Enzymology. 1990;**186**:1-85

[17] Lloyd RV, Hanna PM, Mason RP. The origin of the hydroxyl radical oxygen in the Fenton reaction. Free Radical Biology & Medicine. 1997;**22**:885-888

[18] Stohs SJ, Bagchi D. Oxidative mechanisms in the toxicity of metal ions. Free Radical Biology & Medicine. 1995;**18**:321-336

[19] Fenton HJH. The oxidation of tartaric acid in the presence of iron. Journal of the Chemical Society Proceedings. 1894;**10**:157-158

[20] Murphy MP, Packer MA, Scarlet JL, Martin SW. Peroxynitrite: A biologically significant oxidant. General Pharmacology. 1998;**31**:179-186

[21] Kohen R, Nyska A. Oxidation of biological systems: Oxidative stress phenomena, antioxidants, redox reactions, and methods for their quantification. Toxicologic Pathology. 2002;**30**(6):620-650

[22] Comporti M. Three models of free radical-induced cell injury. Chemico-Biological Interactions. 1989;**72**:1-56

[23] Meral A, Tuncel P, Surmen-Gur E, Ozbek R, Ozturk E, Gunay U. Lipid peroxidation and antioxidant status in beta-thalassemia. Pediatric Hematology and Oncology. 2000;**17**:687-693

[24] Davis KJ. Protein damage and degradation by oxygen radicals. I. General aspects. The Journal of Biological Chemistry. 1987;**262**:9895-9901

[25] Dizdaroglu M, Jaruga P, Birincioglu M, Rodriguez H. Free radical induced damage to DNA: Mechanisms and measurement. Free Radical Biology & Medicine. 2002;**32**: 1102-1115

[26] Helbock HJ, Beckman KB, Ames BN. 8-Hydroxydeoxyguanosine and 8-hydroxyguanin e as biomarkers of oxidative DNA damage. Methods in Enzymology. 1999;**300**:156-166

[27] Rahman T, Hosen I, Islam TM, Shekhar HU. Oxidative stress and human health. Advances in Bioscience and Biotechnology. 2012;**3**:997-1019

[28] Chaitanya KV, Pathan AK, Mazumdar SS, Chakravarthi GP, Parine N, Bobbarala V. Role of oxidative stress in human health: An overview. Journal of Pharmacy Research. 2010;**3**:1330-1333

[29] Vasavidevi VB, Kishor HD, Adinath NS, Rajesh DA, Raghavendra VK. Depleted nitrite and enhanced oxidative stress in urolithiasis. Indian Journal of Clinical Biochemistry. 2006;**21**:177-180

[30] Selley ML, Close DR, Stern SE. The effect of increased concentrations of homocysteine on the concentration of (E)-4-hydroxy-2-nonenal in the plasma and cerebrospinal fluid of patients with Alzheimer's disease. Neurobiology of Aging. 2002;**23**:383-388

[31] Butterfield DA, Castegna A, Lauderback CM, Drake J. Evidence that amyloid β-peptide-induced lipid peroxidation and its sequelae in Alzheimer's disease brain contribute to neuronal death. Neurobiology of Aging. 2002;**23**:655-664

[32] Linke A, Adams V, Schulze PC, Erbs S, Gielen S, et al. Antioxidative effects of exercise training in patients with chronic heart failure: Increase in radical scavenger enzyme activity in skeletal muscle. Circulation. 2005;**111**:1763-1770

[33] Polidori CM, Pratico D, Savino K, Rokach J, Stahl W, Mecocci P. Increased F2 isoprostane plasma levels in patients with congestive heart failure are correlated with antioxidant status and disease severity. Journal of Cardiac Failure. 2004;**10**:334-338

[34] De Champlain J, Wu R, Girouard H, et al. Oxidative stress in hypertension. Clinical and Experimental Hypertension. 2004;**26**:593-601

[35] Rizzo M, Kotur-Stevuljevic J, et al. Atherogenic dyslipidemia and oxidative stress. Translational Research. 2009;**153**:217-223

[36] Szabo E, Riffe ME, Steinberg SM, Birrer MJ, Linnoila RI. Altered cJUN expression: An early event in human lung carcinogenesis. Cancer Research. 1996;**56**:305-315

[37] Stewart ZA, Pietenpol JA. p53 signaling and cell cycle checkpoints. Chemical Research in Toxicology. 2001;**14**:243-263

[38] Yudoh K, Trieu NV, Nakamura H, Kayo HM, Tomohiro K, Kusuki N. Potential involvement of oxidative stress in cartilage senescence and development of osteoarthritis: Oxidative stress induces chondrocyte telomere instability and down regulation of chondrocyte function. Arthritis Research & Therapy. 2005;**7**:380-391

[39] Haydent MR, Tyagi SC. Neural redox stress and remodeling in metabolic syndrome, type 2 diabetes. Journal of the Pancreas. 2002;**3**:126-138

[40] Verzola D, Maria BB, Barbara V, Luciano O, Franco D, Francesca S, Valeria B, Maria TG, Giacomo G, Giacomo D. Oxidative stress mediates apoptotic changes induced by hyperglycemia in human tubular kidney cells. Journal of the American Society of Nephrology. 2004;**l15**:S85-S87

[41] Kohen R. Skin antioxidants: Their role in aging and in oxidative stress—new approaches for their evaluation. Biomedicine & Pharmacotherapy. 1999;**53**:181-192

[42] Atamna H, Cheung I, Ames BN. A method for detecting abasic sites in living cells: Age-dependent changes in base excision repair. Proceedings of the National Academy of Sciences of the United States of America. 2000;**97**:686-691

[43] Liou W, Chang L-Y, Geuze HJ, et al. Distribution of CuZn superoxide dismutase in rat liver. Free Radical Biology & Medicine. 1993;**14**:201-207

[44] Weisiger RA, Fridovich I. Mitochondrial superoxide dismutase: Site of synthesis and intramitochondrial location. The Journal of Biological Chemistry. 1973;**248**:4793-4796

[45] Marklund S. Human copper-containing superoxide dismutase of high molecular weight. Proceedings of the National Academy of Sciences of the United States of America. 1982;**79**:7634-7638

[46] Kirkman HN, Galiano S, Gaetani GF. The function of catalase-bound NADPH. The Journal of Biological Chemistry. 1987;**262**:660-665

[47] Roxborough HE, Mercer C, McMaster D, et al. Plasma glutathione peroxidase activity is reduced in haemodialysis patients. Nephron. 1999;**81**:278-283

[48] Nakane T, Asayama K, Kodera K, et al. Effect of selenium deficiency on cellular and extracellular glutathione peroxidases: Immunochemical detection and mRNA analysis in rat kidney and serum. Free Radical Biology & Medicine. 1998;**25**:504-511

[49] Gibson DG, Hawrylko J, McCay PB. GSH-dependent inhibition of lipid peroxidation: Properties of a potent cytosolic system which protects cell membranes. Lipids. 1985;**20**(10):704

[50] Kohen R, Gati I. Skin low molecular weight antioxidants and their role in aging and in oxidative stress. Toxicology. 2000;**148**:149-157

[51] Samuni A, Aronovitch J, Godinger D, Chevion M, Czapki G. On the cytotoxicity of vitamin C and metal ions. A site-specific Fenton mechanism. European Journal of Biochemistry. 1983;**137**:119-124

[52] Kohen R, Beit-Yannai E, Berry EM, Tirosh O. Overall low molecular weight antioxidant activity of biological fluids and tissues by cyclic voltammetry. Methods in Enzymology. 1999;**300**:285-296

[53] Deepak MK, Surendra SK, Mahabaleshwar VH, Hanhong B. Significance of antioxidant potential of plants and its relevance to therapeutic applications. International Journal of Biological Sciences. 2015;**11**(8):982-991

[54] Gul M, Kutay FZ, Temocin S, Hanninen O. Cellular and clinical implications of glutathione. Indian Journal of Experimental Biology. 2000;**38**:625-634

[55] Barhoumi R, Bowen JA, Stein LS, Echols J, Burghardt RC. Concurrent analysis of intracellular glutathione content and gap junctional intercellular communication. Cytometry. 1993;**14**:747-756

[56] Herrera E, Barbas C. Vitamin E: Action, metabolism and perspectives. Journal of Physiology and Biochemistry. 2001;**57**:43-56

[57] Niki E. Role of vitamin E as a lipid-soluble peroxyl radical scavenger: In vitro and in vivo evidence. Free Radical Biology & Medicine. 2014;**66**:3-12

[58] Morliere P, Patterson LK, Santos CM, Silva AS, Maziere J, Filipe P, Gomes A, Fernandes E, Garciah MBQ, Santusc R. The dependence of α-tocopheroxyl radical reduction by hydroxy-2,3-diarylxanthones on structure and micro-environment. Organic & Biomolecular Chemistry. 2012;**10**:2068-2076

[59] Oh C, Li M, Kim E, Park JS, Lee J, Ham SW. Antioxidant and radical scavenging activities of ascorbic acid derivatives conjugated with organogermanium. Bulletin of the Korean Chemical Society. 2010;**31**:3513-3514

[60] Livrea MA, Tesoriere L, Bongiorno A, Pintaudi AM, Ciaccio M, Riccio A. Contribution of vitamin A to the oxidation resistance of human low density lipoproteins. Free Radical Biology & Medicine. 1995;**18**:401-409

[61] Monaghan BR, Schmitt FO. The effects of carotene and of vitamin A on the oxidation of linoleic acid. The Journal of Biological Chemistry. 1932;**96**:387-395

[62] Russo A, Acquaviva R, Campisi A, Sorrenti V, Giacomo CD, Virgata G, Barcellona ML, Vanella A. Bioflavonoids as antiradicals, antioxidants and DNA cleavage protectors. Cell Biology and Toxicology. 2000;**16**:91-98

[63] De Souza RFV, de Giovani WF. Antioxidant properties of complexes of flavonoids with metal ions. Redox Report. 2004;**9**:97-104

[64] Nijveldt RJ, Els Nood V, Hoorn DEC, Boelens PG, Norren K, Leeuwen PAM. Flavonoids: A review of probable mechanisms of action and potential applications. The American Journal of Clinical Nutrition. 2001;**74**:418-425

[65] Duthie SJ, Collins AR, Duthie GG, Dobson VL. Quercetin and myricetin protect against hydrogenperoxide-induced DNA damage (strand breaks and oxidized pyrimidines) in human lymphocytes. Mutation Research. 1997;**393**:223-231

[66] Stahl W, Sies H. Antioxidant activity of carotenoids. Molecular Aspects of Medicine. 2003;**24**:345-351

[67] Erhardt JG, Meisner C, Bode JC, Bode C. Lycopene, β-carotene, and colorectal adenomas. The American Journal of Clinical Nutrition. 2003;**78**:1219-1224

[68] Rao AV, Rao LG. Carotenoids and human health. Pharmacological Research. 2007;**55**: 207-216

[69] Andreasen MF, Landbo AK, Christensen LP, Hansen A, Meyer AS. Antioxidant effects of phenolic rye (*Secale cereale* L.) extracts, monomeric hydroxycinnamates, and ferulic acid dehydrodimers on human low-density lipoproteins. Journal of Agricultural and Food Chemistry. 2001;**49**:4090-4096

[70] Natella F, Nardini M, Di Filici M, Scaccini C. Benzoic and cinnamic acid derivatives as antioxidants: Structure-activity relation. Journal of Agricultural and Food Chemistry. 1999;**47**:1453-1459

[71] Cao G, Russell RM, Lischner N, Prior RL. Serum antioxidant capacity is increased by consumption of strawberries, spinach, red wine or vitamin C in elderly women. The Journal of Nutrition. 1998;**128**:2383-2390

[72] Cao G, Booth SL, Sadowski JA, Prior RL. Increases in human plasma antioxidant capacity after consumption of controlled diets high in fruit and vegetables. The American Journal of Clinical Nutrition. 1998;**68**:1081-1087

[73] Mazza G, Kay CD, Cottrell T, Holub BJ. Absorption of anthocyanins from blueberries and serum antioxidant status in human subjects. Journal of Agricultural and Food Chemistry. 2002;**50**:7731-7737

[74] Liu RH. Health benefits of fruit and vegetables are from additive and synergistic combinations of phytochemicals. The American Journal of Clinical Nutrition. 2003;**78**:517S-520S

[75] Dahlen EM, Tengblad A, Lanne T, Clinchy B, Ernerudh J, Nystrom FH, Ostgren CJ. Abdominal obesity and low-grade systemic inflammation as markers of subclinical organ damage in type 2 diabetes. Diabetes & Metabolism. 2014;**40**:76-81

[76] Qiao L, Li X. Role of chronic inflammation in cancers of the gastrointestinal system and the liver: Where we are now. Cancer Letters. 2014;**345**:150-152

[77] Steinberg GR, Schertzer JD. AMPK promotes macrophage fatty acid oxidative metabolism to mitigate inflammation: Implications for diabetes and cardiovascular disease. Immunology and Cell Biology. 2014;**92**:340-345

[78] Saeed N, Khan MR, Shabbir M. Antioxidant activity, total phenolic and total flavonoid contents of whole plant extracts *Torilis leptophylla* L. BMC Complementary and Alternative Medicine. 2012;**12**:221

[79] Adebayo SA, Dzoyem JP, Shai LJ, Eloff JN. The anti-inflammatory and antioxidant activity of 25 plant species used traditionally to treat pain in southern African. BMC Complementary and Alternative Medicine. 2015;**15**:159

[80] Yusoff NA, Yam MF, Beh HK, Razak NA, Widyawati T, Mahmud R, Ahmad M, Asmawi MZ. Antidiabetic and antioxidant activities of *Nypa fruticans* Wurmb. vinegar sample from Malaysia. Asian Pacific Journal of Tropical Medicine. 2015;**8**(8):595-605

[81] Kharoubia O, Slimania M, Kroufb D, Seddika L, Aouesa A. Role of wormwood (*Artemisia absinthium*) extract on oxidative stress in ameliorating lead induced haematotoxicity. African Journal of Traditional, Complementary and Alternative Medicines. 2008;**5**(3):263-270

[82] Agbafor KN, Nwachukwu N. Phytochemical analysis and antioxidant property of leaf extracts of Vitex doniana and *Mucuna pruriens*. Biochemistry Research International. 2011;**2011**(459839):1-4

[83] Mbaebie BO, Edeoga HO, Afolayan AJ. Phytochemical analysis and antioxidants activities of aqueous stem bark extract of *Schotia latifolia* Jacq. Asian Pacific Journal of Tropical Medicine. 2012;**2**(2):118-124

[84] Zengin G, Aktumsek A. Investigation of antioxidant potentials of solvent extracts from different anatomical parts of Asphodeline anatolica E. Tuzlaci: An endemic plant to Turkey. African Journal of Traditional, Complementary, and Alternative Medicines. 2014;**11**(2):481-488

[85] Tagne RS, Telefo BP, Talla E, Nyemb JN, Njina SN, Asrar M, Mukhtar F, Kamdje A, Moundipa PF, Farooq DA, Choudhary MI. Bio-guided fractionation of methanol extract of *Ziziphus mauritiana* Lam. (bark) and effect of the most active fraction on cancer cell lines. Asian Pacific Journal of Tropical Medicine. 2015;**5**(4):930-935

[86] Aiyegoro OA, Okoh AI. Preliminary phytochemical screening and in vitro antioxidant activities of the aqueous extract of *Helichrysum longifolium* DC. BMC Complementary and Alternative Medicine. 2010;**10**:21

[87] Oyedemi SO, Bradley G, Afolayan AJ. In -vitro and -vivo antioxidant activities of aqueous extract of *Strychnos henningsii Gilg*. African Journal of Pharmacy and Pharmacology. 2010;**4**(2):070-078

[88] Abdur R, Ghias U, Jawad A. Phytochemical analysis and radical scavenging profile of juices of *Citrus sinensis, Citrus anrantifolia,* and *Citrus limonum*. Organic and Medicinal Chemistry Letters. 2014;**4**:5

[89] Noumedem JAK, Tamokou DJ, Teke GN, Momo RC, Kuete V, Kuiate RJ. Phytochemical analysis, antimicrobial and radical-scavenging properties of Acalypha manniana leaves. SpringerPlus. 2013;**2**:503

[90] Engwa AG, Unaegbu M, Aniakor UE, Osuji AG, Agbafor NK, Aiyegoro OA, Okoh A. Antioxidant and antidiabetic activities of the seed and leaf extracts of *Chrysophyllum albidum*. Asian Pacific Journal of Tropical Medicine. 2016;**6**(8):642-649

[91] Engwa AG, Unaegbu M, Francis OH, Obiudu IK, Ugwu FC, Agbafor NK. In vitro and in vivo antioxidant activity of aqueous and ethanol leaf extracts of *Murraya koenigii*. International Journal of Pharmacognosy and Phytochemical Research. 2016;**8**(4):551-557

[92] Costa A, Garcia-Diaz DF, Jimenez P, Silva PI. Bioactive compounds and health benefits of exotic tropical red-black berries. Journal of Functional Foods. 2013;**5**:539-549

[93] He DX, Ru XC, Wen L, Wen YC, Jiang HD, Bruce IC, Jin J, Ma X, Xia Q. Total flavonoids of Flos Chrysanthemi protect arterial endothelial cells against oxidative stress. Journal of Ethnopharmacology. 2012;**139**:68-73

[94] Kloypan C, Jeenapongsa R, Sri-in P, Chanta S, Dokpuang D, Tip-pyang S, Surapinit N. Stilbenoids from Gnetum macrostachyum attenuate human platelet aggregation and adhesion. Phytotherapy Research. 2012;**26**:1564-1568

[95] Thushara RM, Hemshekhar M, Santhosh MS, Jnaneshwari S, Nayaka SC, Naveen S, Kemparaju K, Girish KS. Crocin, a dietary additive protects platelets from oxidative stress-induced apoptosis and inhibits platelet aggregation. Molecular and Cellular Biochemistry. 2013;**373**:73-83

[96] Schreckinger ME, Wang JZ, Yousef G, Lila MA, de Mejia EG. Antioxidant capacity and in vitro inhibition of adipogenesis and inflammation by phenolic extracts of Vaccinium floribundum and *Aristotelia chilensis*. Journal of Agricultural and Food Chemistry. 2010;**58**:8966-8976

[97] Chuang CC, McIntosh MK. Potential mechanisms by which polyphenol-rich grapes prevent obesity-mediated inflammation and metabolic diseases. Annual Review of Nutrition. 2011;**31**:155-176

[98] Apostolidis E, Karayannakidis PD, Kwon YI, Lee CM, Seeram NP. Seasonal variation of phenolic antioxidant-mediated alpha-glucosidase inhibition of *Ascophyllum nodosum*. Plant Food for Human Nutrition. 2011;**66**:313-319

[99] Barbosa A, Silveira D, de Menezes I, Neto J, Bitencurt J, Estavam CD, de Lima A, Thomazzi SM, Guimaraes AG, Quintans LJ, et al. Antidiabetic effect of the *Chrysobalanus icaco* L. aqueous extract in rats. Journal of Medicinal Food. 2013;**16**:538-543

[100] Meng B, Li J, Cao H. Antioxidant and antiinflammatory activities of curcumin on diabetes mellitus and its complications. Current Pharmaceutical Design. 2013;**19**:2101-2113

[101] Jeong GS, Lee DS, Song MY, Park BH, Kang DG, Lee HS, Kwon KB, Kim YC. Butein from *Rhus verniciflua* protects pancreatic beta cells against cytokine-induced toxicity mediated by inhibition of nitric oxide formation. Biological & Pharmaceutical Bulletin. 2011;**34**:97-102

[102] Cordero-Herrera I, Martin MA, Bravo L, Goya L, Ramos S. Epicatechin gallate induces cell death via p53 activation and stimulation of p38 and JNK in human colon cancer SW480 cells. Nutrition and Cancer. 2013;**65**:718-728

[103] Nichols JA, Katiyar SK. Skin photoprotection by natural polyphenols: Antiinflammatory, antioxidant and DNA repair mechanisms. Archives of Dermatological Research. 2010;**302**:71-83

[104] Soundararajan V, Sreenivasan S. Antioxidant activity of *Elaeis guineensis* leaf extract: An alternative nutraceutical approach in impeding aging. APCBEE Procedia. 2012;**2**:153-159

[105] Niu YC, Na LX, Feng RN, Gong LY, Zhao Y, Li Q, Li Y, Sun CH. The phytochemical, EGCG, extends lifespan by reducing liver and kidney function damage and improving age-associated inflammation and oxidative stress in healthy rats. Aging Cell. 2013;**12**:1041-1049

[106] Chang CL, Chen HS, Shen YC, Lai GH, Lin PK, Wang CM. Phytochemical composition, antioxidant activity and neuroprotective effect of *Crataegus pinnatifida* fruit. South African Journal of Botany. 2013;**88**:432-437

[107] Asaduzzaman M, Uddin MJ, Kader MA, Alam A, Rahman AA, Rashid M, Kato K, Tanaka T, Takeda M, Sadik G. In vitro acetylcholinesterase inhibitory activity and the antioxidant properties of *Aegle marmelos* leaf extract: Implications for the treatment of Alzheimer's disease. Psychogeriatrics. 2014;**14**:1-10

[108] Rinwa P, Kumar A. Piperine potentiates the protective effects of curcumin against chronic unpredictable stress-induced cognitive impairment and oxidative damage in mice. Brain Research. 2012;**1488**:38-50

12

Introduction to Phytochemicals: Secondary Metabolites from Plants with Active Principles for Pharmacological Importance

Nadia Mendoza and Eleazar M. Escamilla Silva

Abstract

Phytochemicals are substances produced mainly by plants, and these substances have biological activity. In the pharmaceutical industry, plants represent the main source to obtain various active ingredients. They exhibit pharmacological effects applicable to the treatment of bacterial and fungal infections and also chronic-degenerative diseases such as diabetes and cancer. However, the next step in science is to find new ways to obtain it. In this chapter, we discuss about the main groups of phytochemicals, in addition to presenting two case studies. One of the most important secondary metabolites is currently Taxol, which is a natural compound of the taxoid family and is also known for its antitumor activity against cancer located in breasts, lungs, and prostate and is also effective with Kaposi's sarcoma. Our case studies will be about Taxol, extracted from an unexplored plant species, and the production of Taxol by its endophytic fungi.

Keywords: phytochemicals, biosynthesis, alkaloids, flavonoids, taxoids, Taxol, *Taxodium mucronatum*

1. Introduction

In the history of humanity, plants have always been present as a source of health. The knowledge of the various healing properties of plants has been transmitted in an empirical way. However, over time, man has been interested in knowing where the properties of plants come from. In the process of knowledge generation, man has developed many methodologies to know the structures of organic compounds responsible for the healing properties of plants. This is the birth of phytochemistry that is defined as the science responsible for the study of the compounds contained in plants. In this field, various techniques have been developed, ranging from the preparation of the plant tissue sample to sophisticated techniques for the elucidation of organic structures. The search for new products for the pharmaceutical and agrochemical industries is an ongoing process that requires continual optimization [1]. Previously, the screening of 10,000 natural products resulted in one commercial product. In the advent of combinatorial chemistry, this relationship changed. Presently, the screening of 100,000 structures day^{-1} from combinatorial chemistry together with the natural products screened yields less than one commercial product year^{-1} (F. Hansske, pers. comm.). Its development takes approximately 12 years and costs ~$350 M [2]. Considering that 6 out of 20 of the most commonly prescribed medications are of fungal origin [3] and only ~5% of the fungi have been described [4], fungi offer an enormous potential for new products.

Endophytic fungi, a polyphyletic group of highly diverse, primarily ascomycetous fungi defined functionally by their occurrence within asymptomatic tissues of plants, are found in aboveground tissues of liverworts, hornworts, mosses, lycophytes, equisetopsids, ferns, and seed plants from the arctic to the tropics, and from agricultural fields to the most biotically diverse tropical forests. Their cryptic lifestyle, ubiquity and richness within individual plants, coupled with emerging evidence of their often overlooked ecological importance, have inspired growing enthusiasm regarding these little known fungi over the past four decades. In particular, David Hawksworth's much discussed estimates of fungal diversity at a global scale [4, 5] engendered tremendous enthusiasm for understanding endophyte diversity. Comprising interactions that range from mutualism to antagonism, fungal symbioses with plants are key determinants of biomass, nutrient cycling and ecosystem productivity in terrestrial habitats from the poles to the equator [6, 7]. Most plant-associated fungi catalogued to date have been recognized because of the fruitbodies they produce in association with their hosts (e.g., plant pathogens, mycorrhizal fungi). Yet plants in all major lineages, including liverworts, mosses, seed free vascular plants, conifers, and angiosperms, also form cryptic symbioses with fungi that penetrate and persist within healthy aboveground tissues such as leaves. Foliar fungal endophytes (i.e., endophylls or mycophyllas) are a fundamental but frequently overlooked aspect of plant biology: all plant species surveyed thus far harbor one or more endophytic symbionts in their photosynthetic tissues [8]. Plants live in association with microorganisms with different levels of interaction. This assumption stimulates insights on plant microbiome, intended as the collective genome of microorganisms living in contact with plants [9], and new concepts in plant evolution have been developed considering a basic role of the associated fungal endophytes [10]. Regarded as an underexplored niche of chemo diversity [11], endophytic fungi have a recognized ability to produce bioactive compounds which may play a role in plant protection against pathogens and pests [12, 13]. Colonization by endophytes may offer significant benefits to their host plants by producing various metabolites that protect against pathogen attack, promote plant (or vegetative) growth, improve crop yields, show herbicide activity and induce resistance. Fungal natural products are currently used in agriculture as active ingredients of different bioformulates [14] and several endophytes are known to have anti-insect properties [15]. Although bioinsecticides currently occupy only a small amount of the market, these compounds are very interesting and their use is constantly increasing [16].

In 1991, researchers began studying the microbial endophytes of the Northwest Pacific yew tree *Taxus brevifolia*, in search for a fungus or bacterium that could produce paclitaxel in de novo fashion [17]. At that time, there were few reports describing the chemistry of plant endophytes, although there was a rich literature cataloguing the secondary metabolism of plant pathogenic fungi and bacteria. Phytotoxins, secondary metabolites produced by plant pathogenic microorganisms, have been studied for almost a century as virulence factors and the initiators of diseases in susceptible plants. Three well-known examples are the host-specific toxins produced by three different *Cochliobolus* species, all of which caused severe blight diseases of economically important crops [18]. *C. carbonum* (*Helminthosporium carbonum*) produces host-specific HC-toxin, which causes Northern leaf blight of maize and inhibits maize histone deacetylase [18]. *C. heterostrophus* (H. maydis) produces T-toxin which caused Southern Corn Leaf Blight, one of the worst plant disease epidemics in modern history, and which was especially virulent toward maize carrying Texas male sterile cytoplasm [18]. *C. victoriae* produces victorin which caused a devastating epidemic in the Victoria race of oats that was developed by plant breeders in an effort to produce oats that were resistant to crown rust [18].

Plant endophytes are subtler, however, rarely causing problems and coexisting with their hosts under most circumstances. Hirsch and Braun provided an inclusive and widely accepted definition of endophytes: "microbes that colonize living, internal tissues of plants without causing any immediate, overt negative effects" [19, 20]. They are generally nonpathogenic in nature, but may produce secondary metabolites that enable them to survive in the competitive world of plant interstitial space without harming their host. Microorganisms in most ecosystems establish and define their ecological niches by their ability to control fellow microbes with only their cell walls or membranes and chemical arsenals to defend them. But these chemical arsenals have provided many of the important chemotherapeutics used to date. The potent antifungal agent griseofulvin is of fungal origin [21] and both the antibiotic streptomycin [21] and the anticancer agent calicheamycin are produced by actinomycetes [22].

Plant endophytes, however, received less attention until the discovery of a Taxol-producing fungus in the bark and needles of the Northwest Pacific yew tree. In 2011, we published a review of cytotoxic or anticancer compounds produced by plant endophytes [23]. Over 100 compounds with demonstrated cytotoxicity or anticancer activity had been isolated from endophytic fungi—including several compounds originally isolated from higher plants [8]. Less than 10% of these compounds were isolated from coniferous species [24]. Our own work with the fungal endophytes of conifers has shown them to be rich producers of bioactive secondary metabolites.

Two reasons led us to start this research project: produce secondary metabolites of pharmaceutical application to reduce a type of cancer and reduce the cutting of trees and apply biotechnology to produce taxanes by endophytic microorganisms. The main aim of this book chapter is to present case studies of isolation, characterization and application of secondary metabolites: Taxoles.

2. Metabolism

Metabolism is a set of chemical reactions carried out by the cells of living beings, to synthesize complex substances from simpler ones, or to degrade complexes and obtain simple ones [25]. Plants, autotrophic organisms, have two metabolisms, the primary metabolism present in

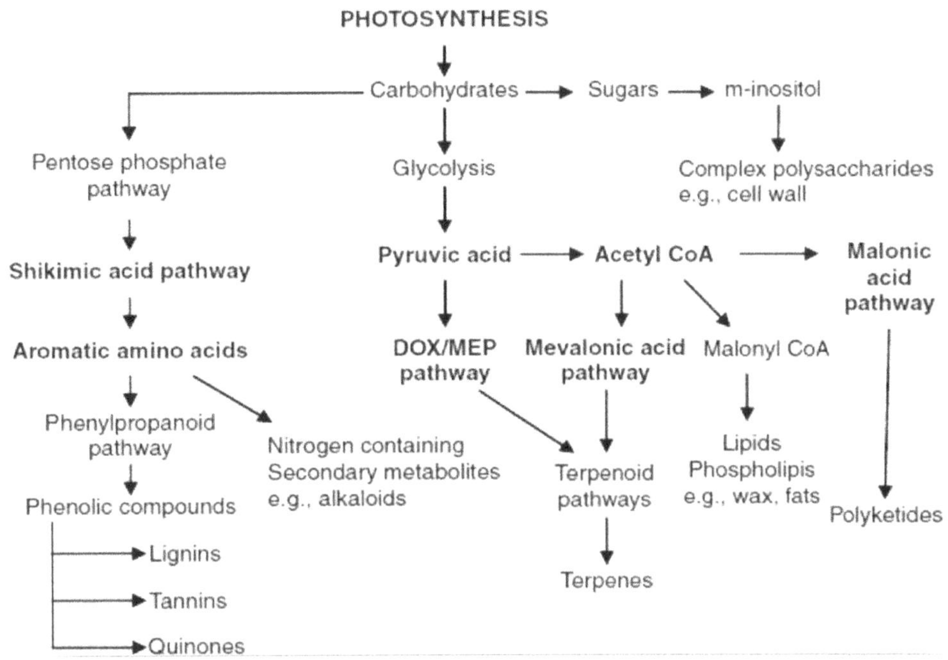

Figure 1. The metabolism of plants.

all living beings and a secondary metabolism that allows them to produce and accumulate compounds of diverse chemical nature (**Figure 1**).

Most of the carbon, nitrogen and energy ends up in common molecules to all the cells, which are necessary for their functioning and the organisms they belong [26]. These are amino acids, nucleotides, sugars and lipids, present in all plants and performing the same functions. They are called primary metabolites.

Plants allocate a significant amount of assimilated carbon and energy to the synthesis of a wide variety of organic molecules, that do not seem to have a direct function in photosynthetic, respiratory processes, nutrient assimilation, solute transport or protein synthesis, carbohydrates or lipids, and which are called secondary metabolites (also called by-products, natural products) [27].

Secondary metabolites are characteristic of superior plants. The essential characteristic of the superior plants is that they possess flower and, consequently, seeds. Its reproductive mechanism is different from that of the inferior ones. They are also called spermatophytes because their reproductive organs are visible and they are subdivided into gymnosperms and angiosperms.

Natural products have biological properties, and they are characterized by their different uses and applications as medicines, insecticides, herbicides, perfumes or dyes, among others. The biosynthesis of secondary metabolites is usually restricted to specific stages of plant development and periods of stress [25]. Some plant cells produce important secondary metabolites of the interactions of the plant with the environment (protection against predators, pathogens or environmental stress) or some related to the reproductive mechanism of the plant (attraction of insects for the promotion of pollination) (**Figure 2**).

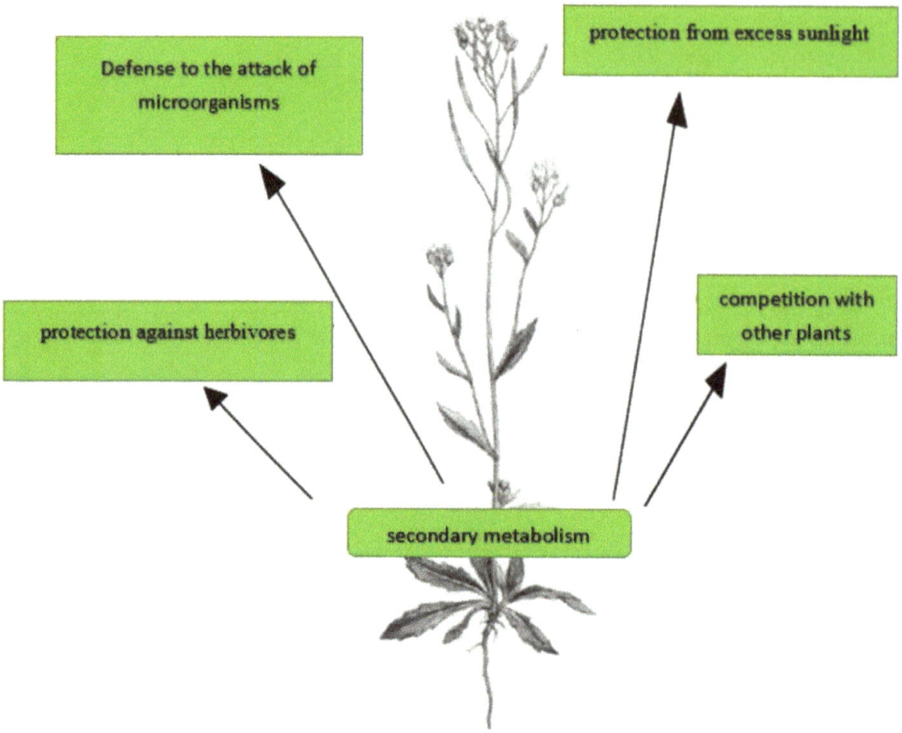

Figure 2. Production of secondary metabolites.

3. Phytochemistry

The discipline whose main objective is the study of the chemical constituents of plants is Phytochemistry. The study of such compounds includes: their chemical structures, metabolism (biosynthesis and degradation), natural distribution, biological function, extraction and qualitative-quantitative evaluation. Before starting, any phytochemical analysis is important to have an adequate preparation of our plant material. A practical and simple way of stabilization is by heat treatment, applied, for example, in an oven at a reference temperature of 60°C until the samples reach constant weight; this way, we will make sure that our compounds will be in the optimal conditions to be analyzed.

Phytochemical research of a plant includes several aspects:

- Extraction of the compounds to be analyzed from a sample or specimen.
- Separation and isolation of them.
- Identification and/or characterization of the isolated compounds.
- Investigation of the biosynthetic routes of a certain molecule.
- Determination or quantitative assessment.

In the extraction and purification of organic compounds through the use of solvents, usually follows certain rules based on structural analogies between the substance to be extracted and the solvent that will be used for that purpose.

Chromatography	Thin-layer chromatography (TLC)
	Gas chromatography (GC)
	High-resolution liquid chromatography (HPLC)
	Capillary liquid chromatography (u-LC)
Electrophoresis	Thin-layer electrophoresis (TLE)
	Isotachophoresis (ITP) (electrophoresis at uniform speed)
	Capillary electrophoresis (CE)
Spectroscopic techniques	UV spectroscopy
	Infrared spectroscopy (IR)
	Near infrared spectroscopy (NIR)
	Nuclear magnetic resonance spectroscopy (NMR)
	Mass spectroscopy (MS)

Table 1. Separation and identification techniques.

The polarity of the compounds is another element to be taken into account, when considering the solubility of a solute in a given solvent. Thus, strongly polar solvents dissolve ionic or highly polar solutes, while low-polar solvents do not efficiently dissolve ionic solutes but do dissolve low-polarity solutes.

The extraction of the vegetal material is done consecutively using solvents, from a low polarity until reaching the water, which is the most polar solvent.

The obtained extracts can be clarified by filtration through celite with a vacuum pump and then concentrated under reduced pressure. This is generally carried out in a rotary evaporator, in which the solutions are concentrated until a volume reduction is achieved, at temperatures between 30 and 50°C. The concentrated extracts must be stored refrigerated.

In the separation and identification of natural products, different techniques for isolation and identification have been developed, in **Table 1** is a summary of the main techniques.

4. Families of phytochemicals

To establish an ordering, these compounds will be classified considering some characteristics like: their biosynthetic origin, the common structural characteristics and the solubility properties.

Some large groups of secondary metabolites are:

- Nitrogen and sulfur compounds, characterized by possessing nitrogen and/or sulfur in their structure, of solubility and diverse biosynthetic origin, but mostly derived from amino acids. Example of these compounds are the cyanogenic glycosides are nitrogen compounds, which are not toxic by themselves but degrade when the plant is crushed releasing toxic volatile substances such as hydrogen cyanide (HCN). An example is the amygdalin (**Figure 3**), found in the seeds of almond, apricot, cherry or peach.

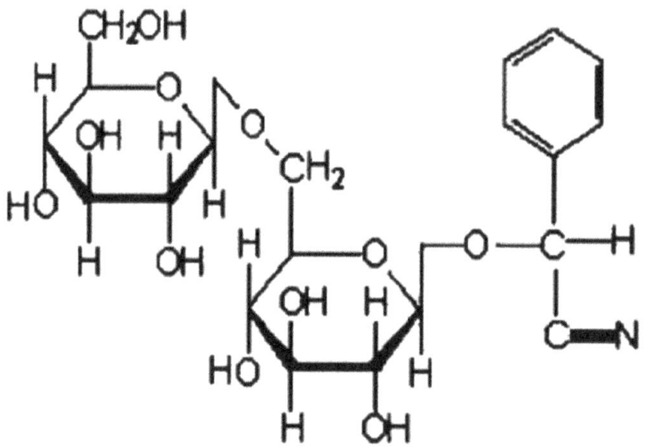

Figure 3. Structure of the amygdalin.

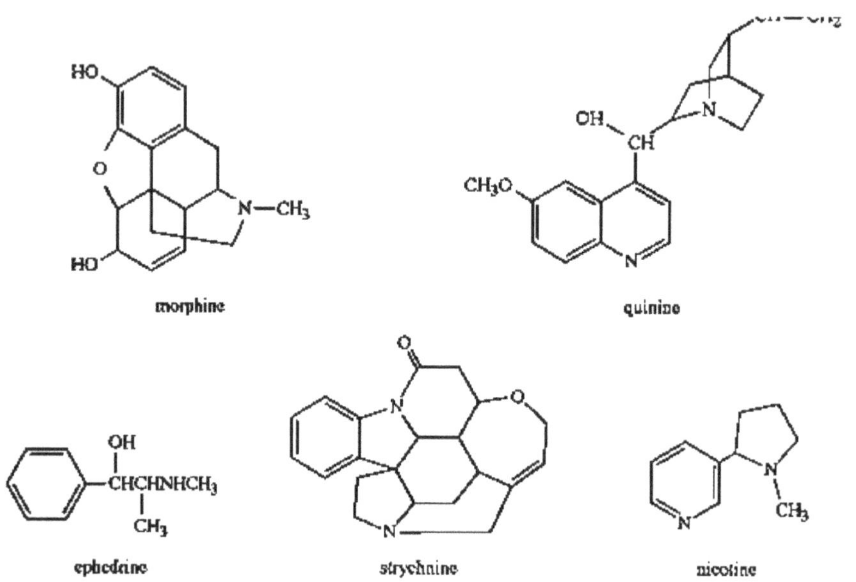

Figure 4. Alkaloid structures.

Other natural nitrogenated products with an important biological activity are alkaloids; some examples of alkaloids are in **Figure 4**. Alkaloids are a large family of more than 15,000 secondary metabolites that have these three characteristics in common: they are soluble in water, contain at least one nitrogen atom in the molecule and exhibit biological activity. The majority of them are heterocyclic although some are aliphatic (noncyclic) nitrogen compounds such as mescaline or colchicine, for example [28].

- Phenolic compounds, with at least one hydroxyl group attached to one or more aromatic rings in its chemical structure, most of which are water-soluble and biosynthetically derived from shikimic acid.
- Terpenoids, with the isoprene molecule as a structural unit, liposoluble, and biosynthetically associated to the mevalonic acid pathway or to the glyceraldehyde phosphate-pyruvic

Isoprene units n	Carbon atoms n	Name	Example
1	5	Hemi-terpenes	isoprene
2	10	Mono-terpenes	thymol
3	15	Sesqui-terpenes	δ-cadinene
4	20	Di-terpenes	taxol
6	30	Tri-terpenes	β-amyrin
8	40	Tetra-terpenes	β-carotene
9 – 30,000	> 40	Poly-terpenes	rubber

Table 2. Classification of terpenoids.

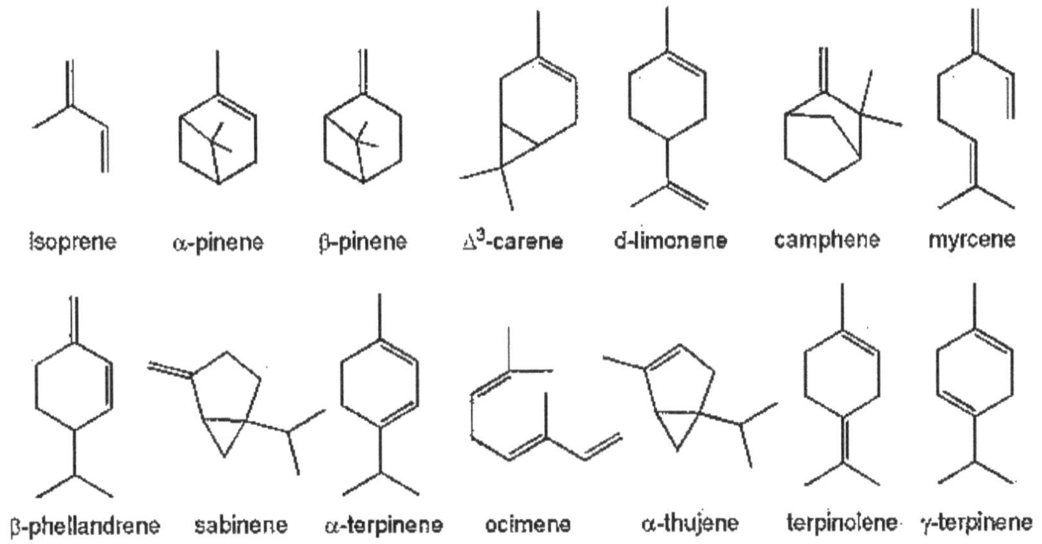

Figure 5. Examples of terpenoid structures.

acid pathway, depending on the class of terpenoids in question [29]. **Table 2** shows the classification of the terpenoids, with respect to the number of isoprene units they contain, as well as an example of each type of terpenoid and **Figure 5** shows some structures of terpenoids.

5. Case 1. Exploring new ways: Taxol

5.1. Taxol

Among the metabolites with greater interest are the toxoids, these are secondary metabolites that are synthesized by the *Taxus* spp. They are found in the foliage and bark of this tree. The main taxoid of pharmacological interest is Taxol; a polyoxygenated diterpene alkaloid approved by the Office of the Administration of Drugs and Foods. This taxoid is used in the treatment of breast, ovarian, lung and Kaposi's sarcoma related to HIV. Hence, the importance of knowing everything related to the production of this powerful medicine.

5.2. Biosynthesis of Taxol

Several studies have been conducted on the biosynthesis of taxoids, especially Taxol. In **Figure 6**, it is one of the biosynthetic routes for the production of Taxol. Biosynthesis is a process that requires knowing the mainly enzymatic reactions that involve the construction of the skeleton and the addition of various oxygen and acyl functional groups. The central skeleton of the Taxol molecule is a taxane ring of isoprenoid nature and is derived from geranylgeranyl diphosphate (GGPP). What is the common precursor of 20 carbon atoms isoprenoids (diterpenes), among which compounds such as carotenoids can be found. The phytol chain of chlorophylls or gibberellins participates in the growth and development of plants. However, all of them are formed in the same way precursors, isopentenyl diphosphate (IPP) and dimethylalyl diphosphate (DMAPP) are formed. However, and despite the studies carried out, no biosynthetic route of Taxol has been reached. In **Figure 2**, there is one of the different proposed schemes for Taxol biosynthesis.

5.3. Research carried out

Several researches have been developed with the aim of finding new sources to obtain Taxol. But it has only been isolated from trees of the *Taxus* species. **Table 3** shows the percentage of yield obtained from the Taxol extractions of the different species of the *Taxus* spp., as well as the analysis of the different parts of the species.

Based on the previous table of contents, another taxonomic species was investigated such as *Taxodium mucronatum*. The *Taxodium mucronatum* belongs to the Cupressacea which is a gymnosperm. They are large trees over 25 m in height and 1.5 m in diameter from the trunk at chest height. Its leaves are small, elongated and grouped in twigs, in autumn the leaves turn reddish and fall.

The new shoots appear in spring. They can be distinguished at a distance by their dense foliage and their hanging branches, and they are always close to the water or in places with shallow water table (**Figure 7**).

They are distributed from Texas (USA) to Guatemala, but its presence is larger in Mexico. Best known as Ahuehuete tree, which comes from Nahuatl "atl" which means water and "huehuetl" which means old or grandfather, so the whole meaning is "old" of the water" [29–31]. The reason to choose this species, in addition to being abundant from North America to South America, this tree species has many similar characteristics to the species of *Taxus*, which makes it a potential source of Taxol.

The plant material from *Taxodium mucronatum* was collected by members of the Biotechnology laboratory of the Technological Institute of Celaya, from the community of Chamacuaro located on the outskirts of the municipality of Salvatierra in the state of Guanajuato, on the banks of the Lerma river. We proceeded to separate the plant material (branches, fruits and leaves), then dried under pressure and room temperature.

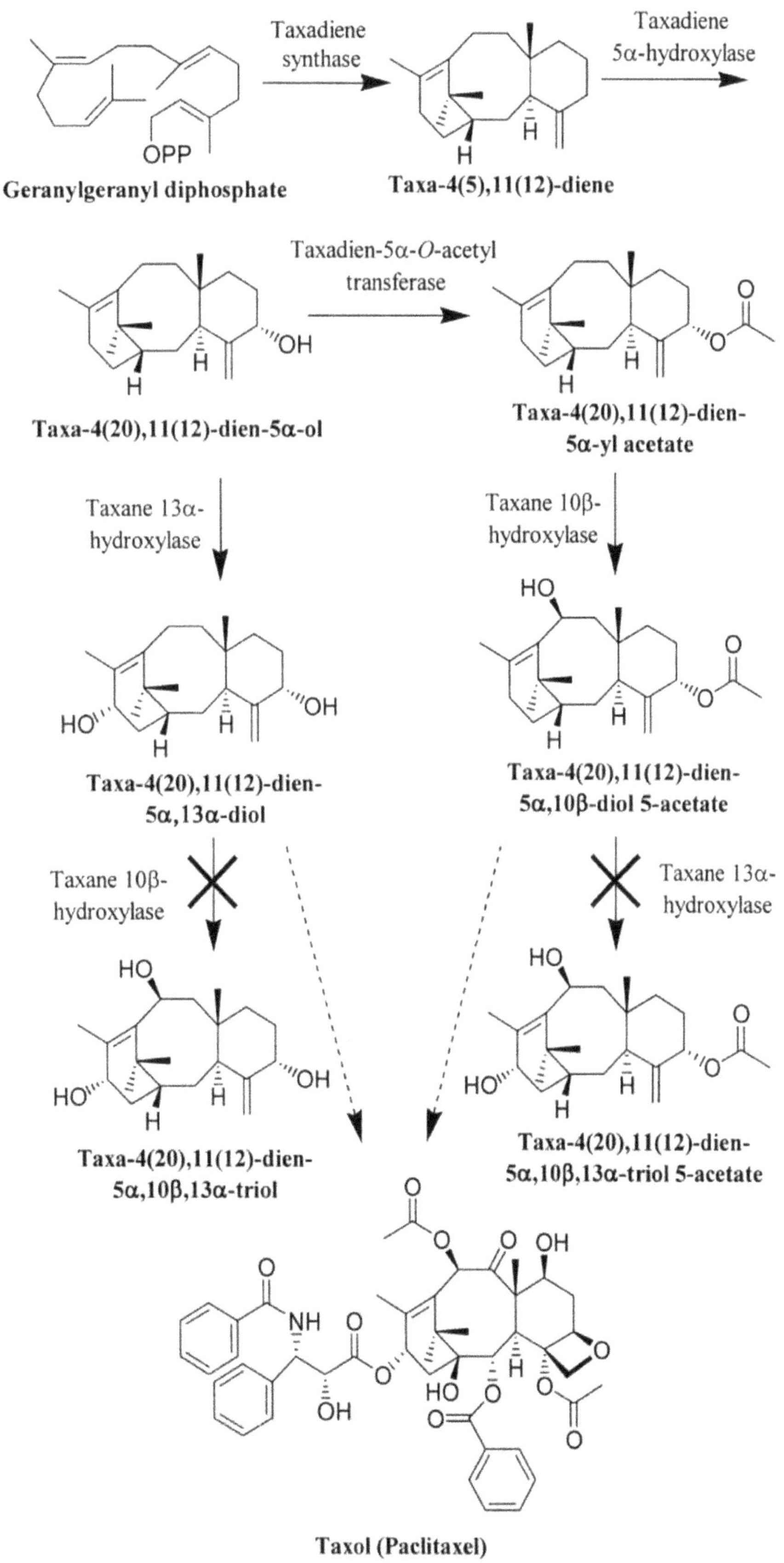

Figure 6. Taxol biosynthetic pathway.

Species of *Taxus*	Trivial name	Part of the tree	Taxol (% of dry weight)	Year
T. brevifolia	Yew of the pacific	Cortex	0.0075–0.01	1986
T. brevifolia	Yew of the pacific	Leaves	0.0081	1992
T. wallichiana	Yew of the Himalayas	Cortex	0.0108	1981
T. baccata	European yew	Cortex	0.0165	1984
T. baccata	European yew	Leaves	0.0088	1992
T. cuspidata	Japanese shuffle	Leaves	0.0077	1992
T. media	Yew of Sumatra	Leaves	0.0056	1992
T. floridiana	Florida yew	Leaves	0.006	1992
T. globosa	Mexican Tejo	Cortex	0.0085	2000
T. globosa	Mexican Tejo	Leaves	0.013	2000
T. globosa	Mexican Tejo	Stem	0.0064	2000
T. globosa	Mexican Tejo	Sheet	0.0121	2003

Table 3. Obtaining Taxol from the different species of ***Taxus*** [6].

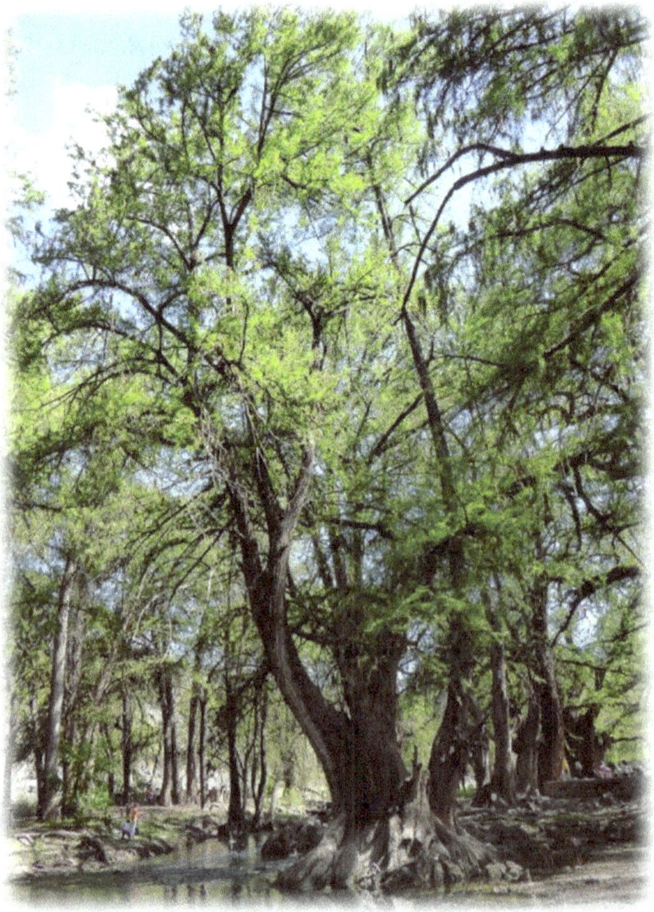

Figure 7. *Taxodium mucronatum.*

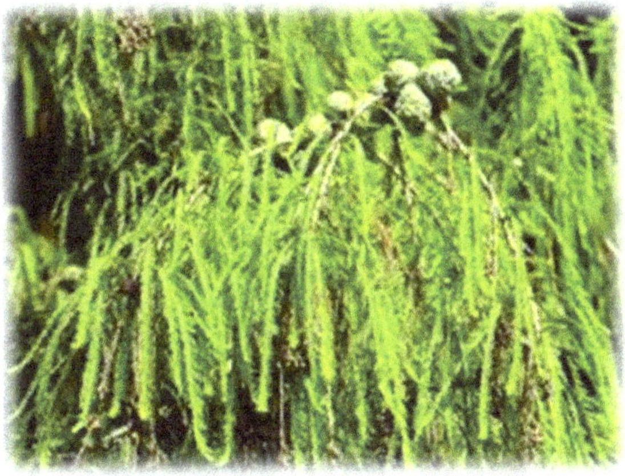

Figure 8. Fruits and leaves of *Taxodium mucronatum*.

They were used 300 g of dry leaves of *Taxodium mucronatum*. Milled with methanol, which were later packed for extraction in a glass column, where methanol was passed until the material was used up.

The study was also carried out with fruit, for which 467 g of fresh fruits of *Taxodium muncronatum* (**Figure 8**) were milled with methanol, which were subsequently packed for extraction in a glass column, where methanol was passed until the material was exhausted. The extractives were evaporated at reduced pressure in a rotary rotator at a temperature of 50°C.

5.4. Column chromatography

Column chromatography was used to separate the compounds. For this purpose, 1 g of sample was taken as a result of the rotations of the extracts and placed in a column (measures 20 cm long, 3 cm in diameter), prepacked with 30 g suspended in hexane. Silica gel was used to complete the separation of the components of the sample.

Three solutions were prepared at different proportions of hexane and ethyl acetate. The first solution containing 40 ml of hexane plus 10 ml of ethyl acetate, the second 20 ml of hexane plus 20 ml of ethyl acetate, and the third 10 ml of hexane plus 40 ml of ethyl acetate. To pack the column, 30 g silica gel were mixed with 100 ml of hexane, then poured into the column. Hexane is passed through the column to have a uniform packing. Then it was proceeded to repeat this operation several times to achieve a homogeneous packing. 3 ml of hexane was left on the surface of the silica, and then the sample was prepared. It is homogenized with 2 g of silica and rotavapor for a few minutes to evaporate solvent residues, and is added little by little to the column, leaving at least 1 ml of hexane remaining on the surface. Elute with the prepared solutions. Collect in a flask each fraction of the column (different color layers), evaporate each of the fractions in a rotavapor under reduced pressure and at a temperature of 50°C. Seven fractions of each of the columns were obtained for both the fruits and leaves. These were analyzed by thin-layer chromatography and HPLC.

5.5. Thin-layer chromatography

The technique of column chromatography helps us to know if the fractions recovered from the column chromatography are pure, otherwise it tells us how many components we

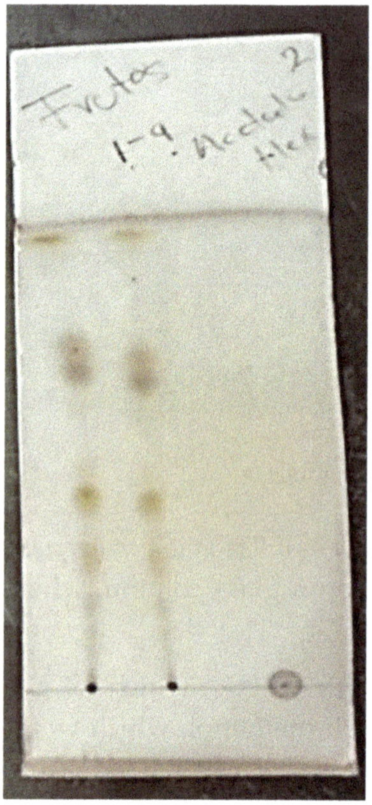

Figure 9. Chromatographic plates of the fruit extract.

have in these fractions. Column chromatography also helps us to know the polarity of our compounds present in the sample, and therefore it is necessary to make several different solvent systems, this is vitally important because the good or bad purification of our compounds will depend on it. For thin-layer chromatography, the following components were used: A stationary phase: Silica gel 60F 254 Merk 0.25 mm thick, with a ceric sulfate developer solution, and the following solvent systems were tested: chloroform-methanol (7:3) (9:1) (1:9) (5:5), hexane-ethyl acetate (9:1) (5:5) (1:9), methanol-acetone (4:6) (9:1) (3:9), chloroform-ethyl acetate (3:7), methanol-hexane (3:7), chloroform-acetone (9:1), and ternary systems were also tested: ethyl acetate-chloroform-methanol (2:7:1), acetone-chloroform-methanol (2:7:1).

In **Figure 9**, the separation of components of the fruit extract is observed, where at least six components are distinguished, the solvent mixture was hexane/ethyl acetate in a 9:1 ratio. **Figure 10** shows the results for the leaf extract, where at least three main components are identified.

In **Figure 11**, other plates are shown chromatography's with a different mixture of solvents, without success in the separation of components. Observing the results of the chromatography, we know that most of our compounds have an intermediate polarity, this based on our solvent system that is the best for the separation of compounds. Another interesting fact about our results is that we have several compounds with very similar characteristics, this is deductible because although you can see spots individually (each corresponding to a different compound) they are too close together.

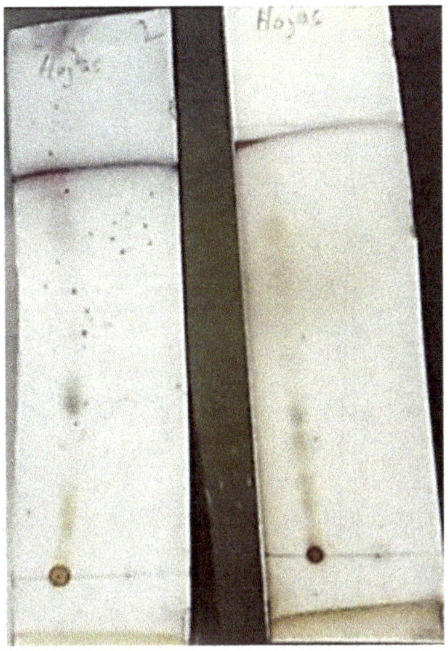

Figure 10. Chromatographic plates of the leaf extract.

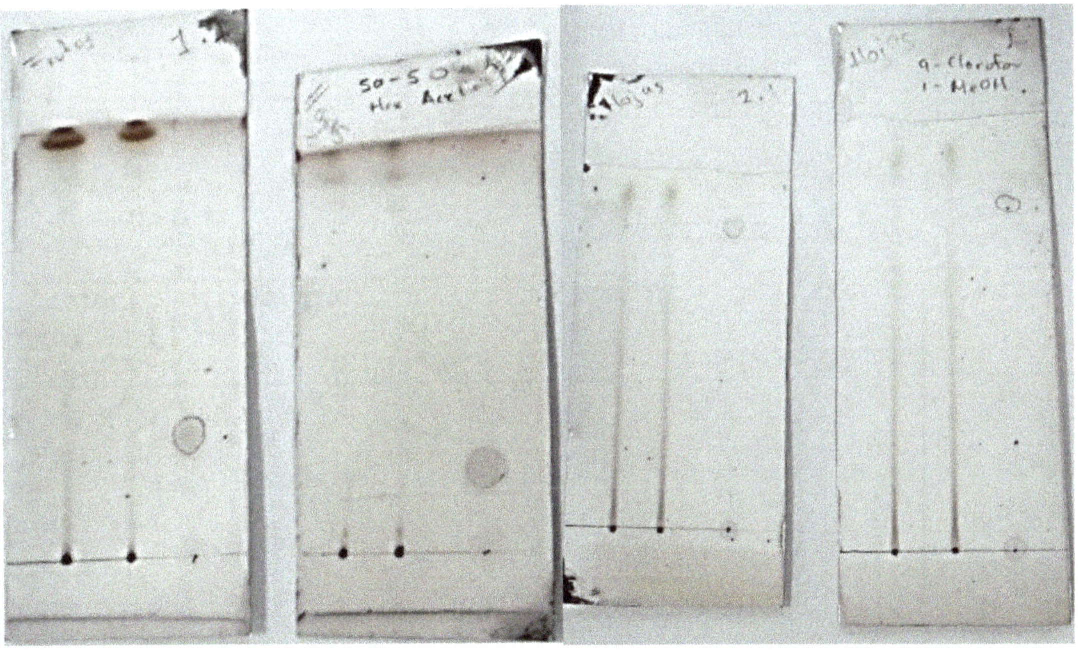

Figure 11. Chromatographic plates with other solvent mixtures.

5.6. High-resolution liquid chromatography

The identification of compounds is a task for liquid chromatography of high resolution, as long as our sample meets the necessary characteristics. The extracts obtained by means of column chromatography were analyzed by means of HPLC, in a Varian chromatograph with a C18 column an isocratic development acetonitrile-water was made 70:30 at a rate of 1 ml/min, and the injection volume was 20 μl. The identification of Taxol, in this case our metabolite of interest, was carried out by means of an external standard from the *Taxus brevifolia* (**Figure 12**), a retention time of 4.65 min is observed.

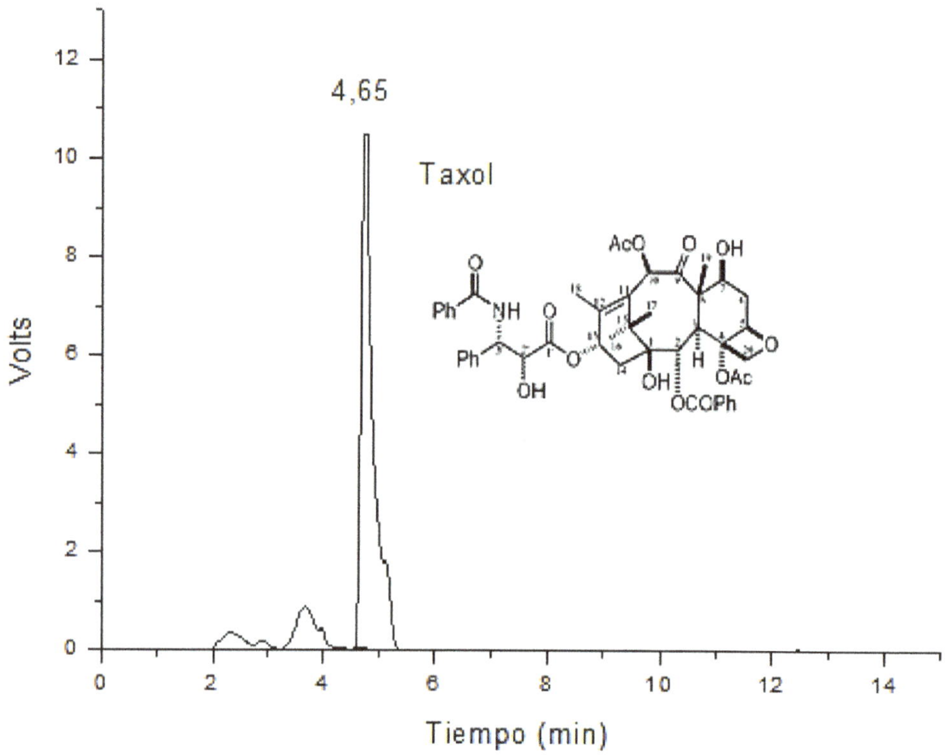

Figure 12. Taxol standard.

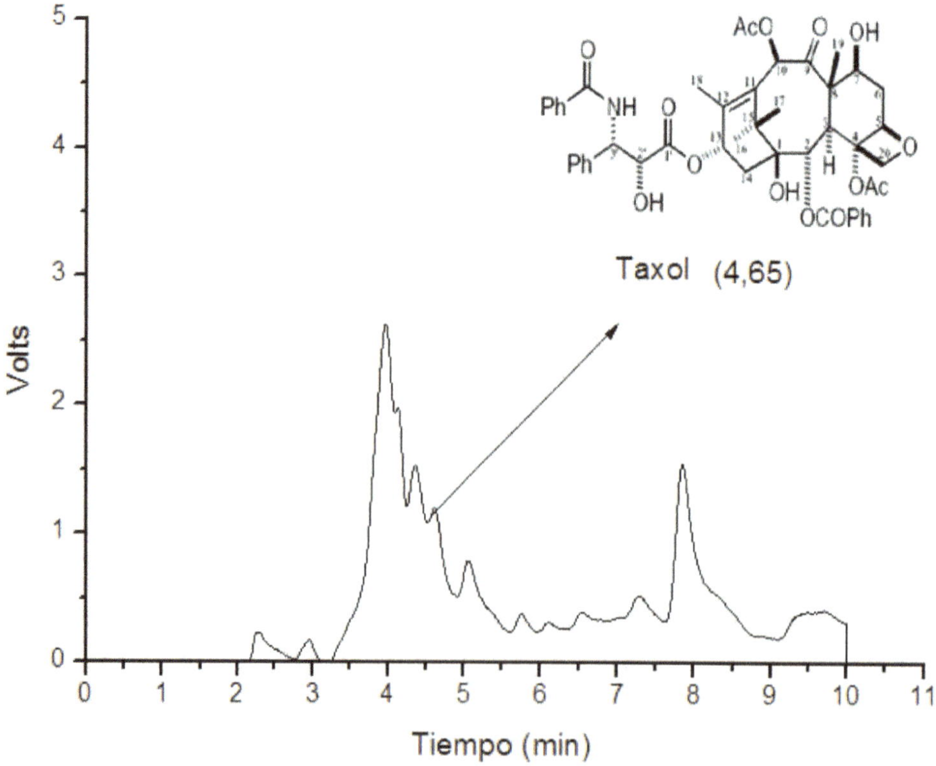

Figure 13. Fraction 4 of the preparative column of silica with leaf extract of *Taxodium mucronatum*.

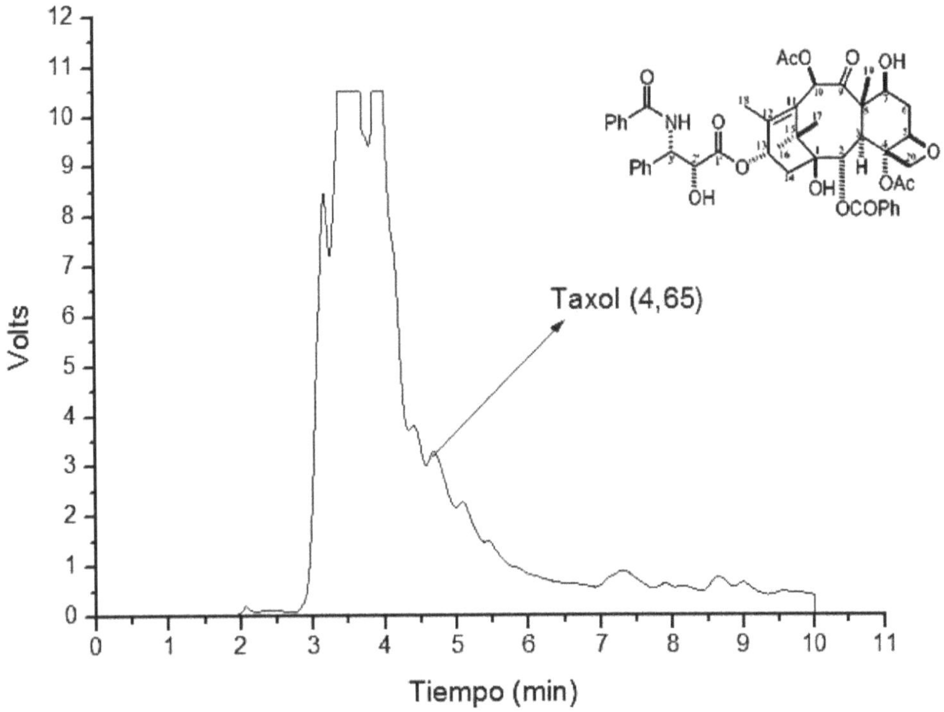

Figure 14. Fraction 5 of the silica preparative column with leaf extract of *Taxodium mucronatum*.

In **Figure 13**, it is the chromatogram of the analysis of fraction 4 of the column of silica gel of 1 g of the leaf extract of *Taxodium mucronatum*, in it a peak is observed with the same retention time with the standard which indicates us Taxol inside the leaves. Observing the distance that exists between the signals that are close to the retention time characteristic of Taxol, one of these signals could also be about a mixture of taxoids. **Figure 14**, corresponding to fraction 5 of the extract of the leaves shows a characteristic retention time of Taxol, but as in fraction 4, it also presents signals with times very close to the retention time of Taxol, which is why we can also deduce that there is presence of other taxoids.

6. Case study 2: alternative for obtaining natural products

Secondary metabolites can also be produced by endophytic fungi, and this feature has opened the door to new research. Some of the most important advantages of this find are that no plant species will be threatened. The process for the production of natural products can be industrialized. Therefore, the following research is about the production of Taxol by means of endophytic fungi of *Taxodium mucronatum*.

The main source of obtaining Taxol until now is the extraction of trees of the genus *Taxus* (Tejo); however, it is estimated that the amount of purified Taxol required to treat only 500 patients with cancer is 1 kg, equivalent to the performance of near of 10 tons of bark or the felling of 700 trees. Therefore, the next step for science is to find new ways to obtain this drug. Some of the sources to obtain this medicine, are the semi-synthesis, from other Taxanes being the most used the 10-Deacetilbaccatina III obtained from the leaves of *Taxus*, the disadvantage that this method has, is the low yield and the high cost; by total synthesis of plant cell cultures of *Taxus* and cultures of microorganisms such as fungi and bacteria (**Table 4**). The production

Isolation source	Fungus	Concentration (μg/L)	Year
T. brevifolia	*T. andrene*	0.024–0.025	1993
T. wallaiciana	*Pestalotiopsis. Microespora*	60–70	1996
T. baccata	*Monochaetia* sp.	0.102	1996
T. baccata	*Fusarium lateritium*	0.13	1996
T. cuspidata	*Alternaria* sp.	0.157	1996
T. cuspidata	*Pestalotiopsis. Microespora*	0.268	1996
T. wallaiciana	*Pestalotiopsis. Microespora*	0.5	1996
T. Sumatrana	*Phitomyces* sp.	0.095	1996
T. baccata	*Pestalotia bicilia*	1.081	1996
Wollemia nobilis	*P. guepinii*	0.481	1997
	Pestalotiopsis. Microespora	1.487	1998

Table 4. Production of Taxol by endophytic fungi [32].

of Taxol, by means of microorganisms, represents a potential source of Taxol; due to its multiple advantages among them that no plant species is affected, the process is reproducible and controllable, which is important for its industrial scaling.

For this reason, the main purpose of this project is to isolate and select strains of endophyte microorganisms capable of producing Taxol and also develop a biotechnological process that allows the production.

The proceeding of isolating the fungi associated with *Taxodium mucronatum* was made by getting a collection of samples of microorganisms than was carried out in test tubes with nutritious broth, at room temperature. A short and deep cut was made in the bark of the selected tree; in the cut with an applicator, three samples were taken. Later in the laboratory, the preparation of five culture media was made: Czapeck medium, Sabourod, PDA, YPD, Agar Plate count; microorganisms were seeded from each in tubes in five different culture media. This was realized with the purpose of observing in which agar these microorganisms grow better and make a cellular differentiation.

Then proceeded to cultivate the fungi; using 2 ml of saline containing the contents of a fungal Petri dish in 250 ml of PDA were inoculated and incubated in a shaker at 250 rpm and 27°C for 7 days. After this time, the culture broths were filtered to remove the biomass, and extractions of each Erlenmeyer flask were carried out with ethyl acetate. The organic phase was separated and dried with anhydrous sodium sulfate and filtered; then the organic phase was evaporated in a rotatory evaporator until the solvent was removed at 50°C and in vacuum. The extract was resuspended in 1 ml of acetonitrile HPLC grade with 0.01% acetic acid to avoid esterification of Taxol and was placed in Bakelite tubes and kept in refrigeration at 4°C for future analysis.

6.1. High-resolution liquid chromatography

All the extracts were analyzed in HPLC, in a Varian chromatograph 8090 mod. (USA) with a C18 column under isocratic conditions and in an 80:20 acetonitrile-water mixture at a flow rate of 1 ml/min, the injection volume was 20 μl. The identification of Taxol was carried out

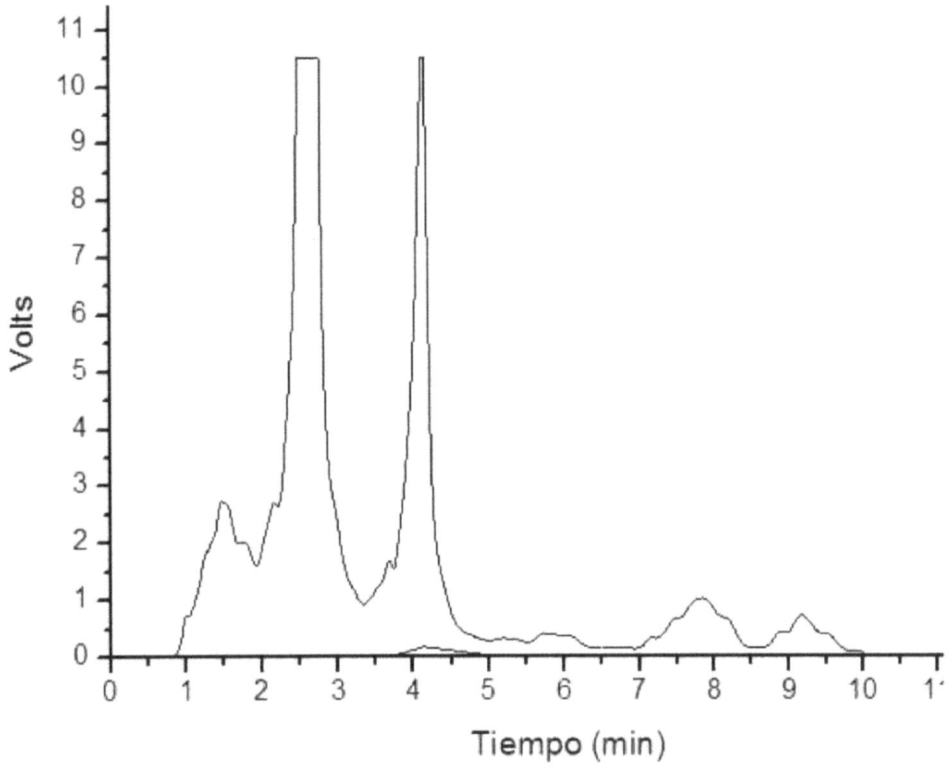

Figure 15. Chromatogram of the culture extract of strain 1.

by means of a Taxol standard of sigma Aldrich (Toluca, México) from *Taxus brevifolia* which presented a retention time of 4.65 min.

Figure 12 shows the chromatogram corresponding to the Taxol standard of Sigma Aldrich from *Taxus brevifolia*. **Figure 15** is the chromatogram corresponding to strain 1, and this strain is matter of interest because it produces very few natural products, although it does not show any time characteristic of Taxol. Therefore, the purification process would be easier and identify these products. **Figure 16** shows the chromatogram corresponding to strain 17, in which we observe a signal with the same retention time as the characteristic signal of Taxol.

Based on our chromatogram of the extract of strain 17 and identifying Taxol in our extract, we conducted another experiment in which we enriched our culture medium using brown sugar, which contains different types of salts as well as different carbon sources (sucrose, glucose, etc.). In the chromatogram of **Figure 17**, we observe the effect of enrichment of the medium, our corresponding to Taxol increases its area and volume; however, the rest of our compounds also increase significantly. The result of Taxol production was confirmed by adding 0.5 ml of standard as internal control To 0.5 ml of sample **Figure 18**.

In the identification of the Taxol-producing endophytic fungus, lacto phenol blue staining was performed for its microscopic morphological structure. **Figure 19** shows the endophytic fungus with Taxol production capacity, in the image, the growth in petri box and its microscopic view is appreciated.

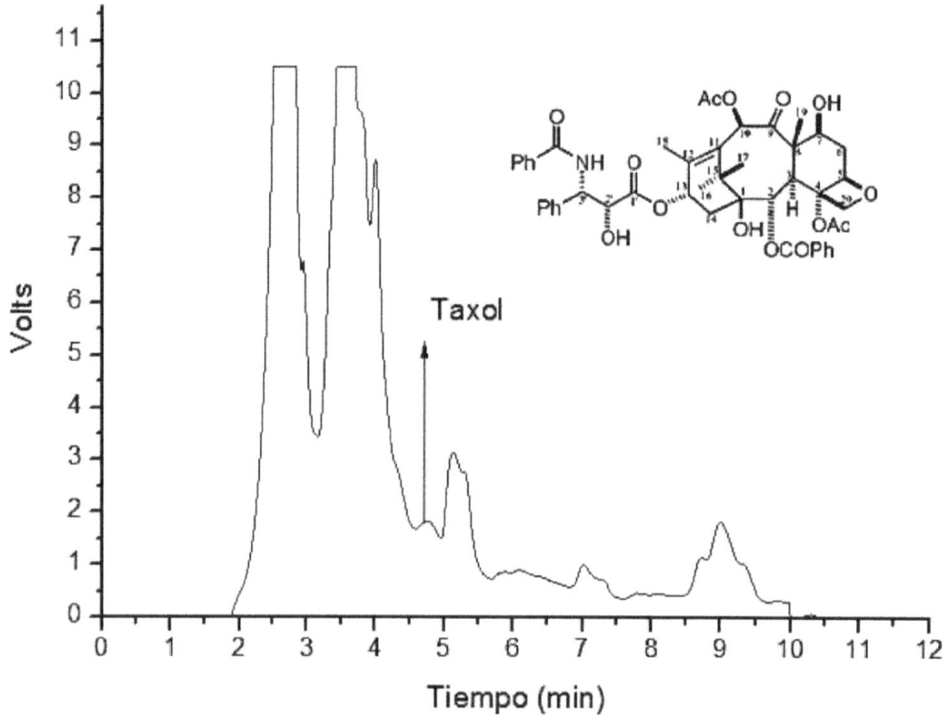

Figure 16. Chromatogram of the culture extract of strain 17 in potato broth.

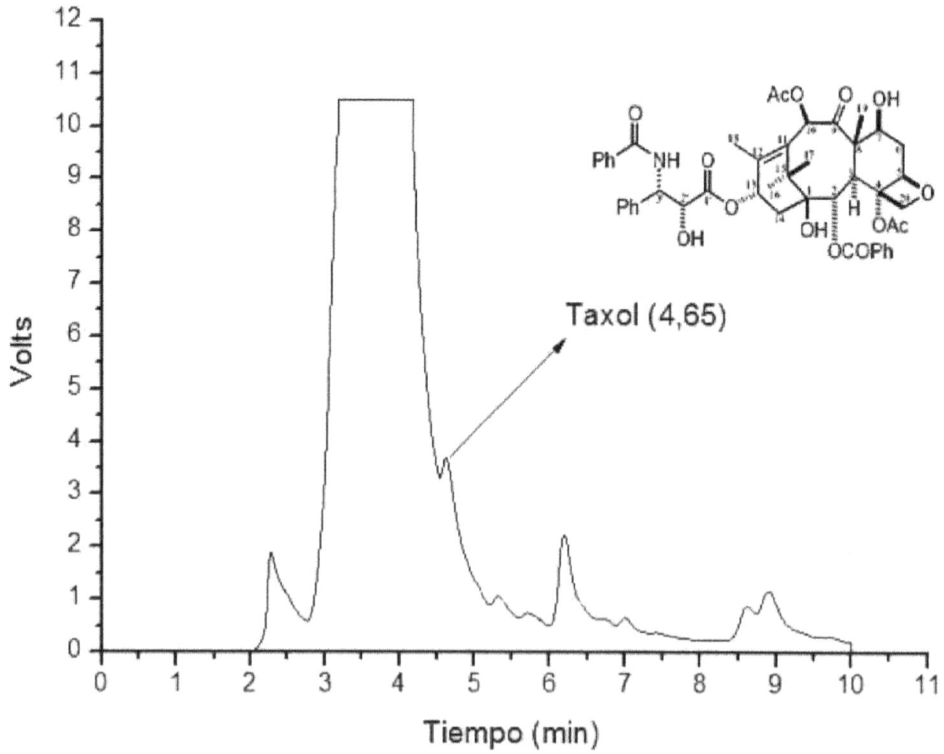

Figure 17. Chromatogram of extract of strain 17.

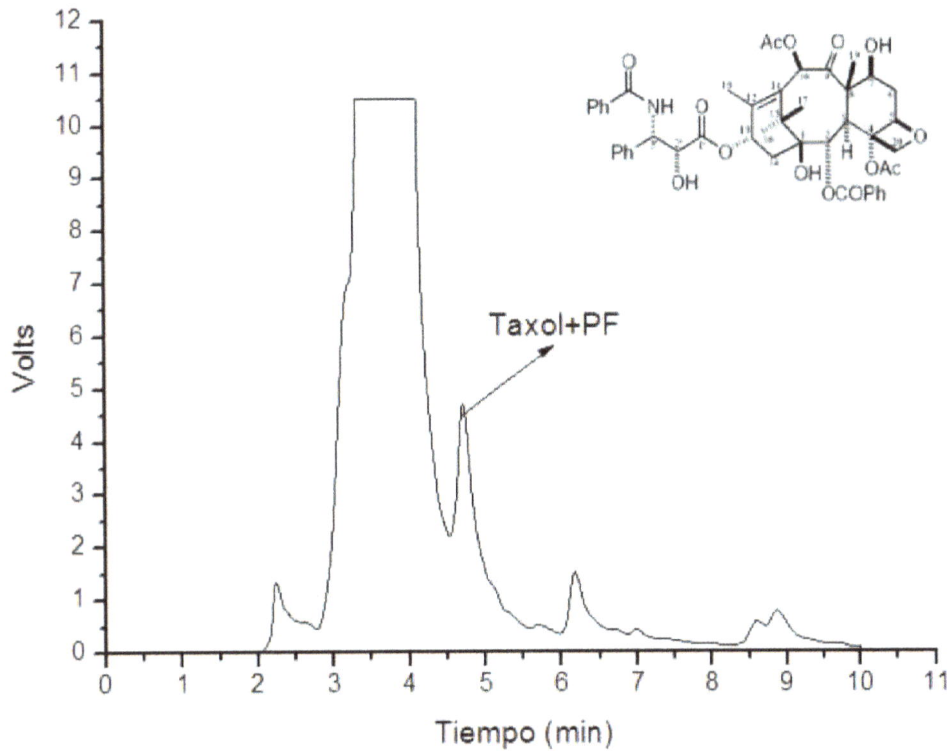

Figure 18. Chromatography of the extract of strain 17 with the addition of 0.5 ml of standard.

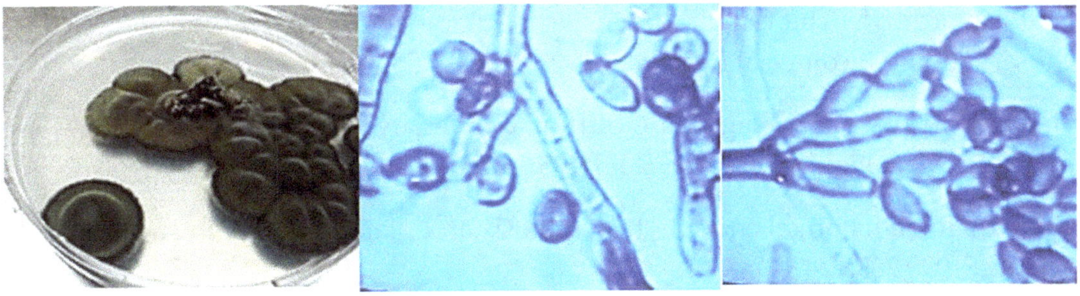

Figure 19. Image of the Taxol producing endophytic fungus.

7. Conclusion

Natural products (secondary metabolites) are important sources for the cure against many of the diseases that humans are currently fighting. However, it is necessary to conduct research whose objective is the production of natural products through biotechnological routes, protecting plant species. One of the clear examples is Taxol, which can be obtained through its endophytic fungi; the production of Taxol was achieved by the submerged fermentation of one of the native strains of *Taxodium mucronatum*, identifying it by means of high-resolution chromatography. In the production of Taxol by fermentation it is possible that the processes must be sought by which other secondary metabolites can be obtained for conservation of plant species. As is the case of Taxol, there are other substances that can be obtained by fermentative routes, always protecting our plant species.

Author details

Nadia Mendoza and Eleazar M. Escamilla Silva*

*Address all correspondence to: eleazar@iqcelaya.itc.mx

Department of Chemical Engineering, Technological Institute of Celaya, Celaya, Guanajuato, Mexico

References

[1] Dreyfuss MM, Chapela IH. Potential of fungi in the discovery of novel, low-molecular weight pharmaceuticals. In: Gullo VP, editor. The Discovery of Natural Products with Therapeutic Potential. Stoneham, MA: Butterworth-Heinemann; 1994

[2] Barengo N, Sieber TN, Holdenrieder O. Diversity of endophytic mycobiota in leaves and twigs of pubescent birch (*Betula pubescens*). Sydowia. 2000;**52**:305-320

[3] Gloer JB. Applications of fungal ecology in the search for new bioactive natural products. In DT Wicklow, BE Soderstrom, editors. The Mycota. Environmental and Microbial Relationships. Vol. IV. New York: Springer-Verlag; 1997

[4] Hawksworth DL. The fungal dimension of biodiversity: Magnitude, significance, and conservation. Mycological Research. 1991;**95**:641-655

[5] Hawksworth DL. The magnitude of fungal diversity: The 1.5 million species estimate revisited. Mycological Research. 2001;**105**:1422-1432

[6] Clay K, Holah J. Fungal endophyte symbiosis and plant diversity in successional fields. Science. 1999;**285**:1742-1744

[7] Gilbert GS. Evolutionary ecology of plant diseases in natural ecosystems. Annual Review of Phytopathology. 2002;**40**:13-43

[8] Stone JK, Bacon CW, White JF Jr. An overview of endophytic microbes: Endophytism defined. In: Bacon CW, White JF, editors. Microbial Endophytes. New York, NY, USA: Marcel Dekker; 2000. pp. 3-29

[9] Schlaeppi K, Bulgarelli D, Schulz B, Haas S, Junker C, Andrée N, Schobert M. The plant microbiome at work. Molecular Plant-Microbe Interactions. 2015;**28**:212-217

[10] Schulz B, Haas S, Junker C, Andrée N, Schobert M. Fungal endophytes are involved in multiple balanced antagonisms. Current Science. 2015;**109**:39-45, 2015

[11] Hardoim PR, van Overbeek LS, Berg G, Pirttilä AM, Compant S, Campisano A, Döring M, Sessitsch A. The hidden world within plants: Ecological and evolutionary considerations for defining functioning of microbial endophytes. Microbiology and Molecular Biology Reviews. 2015;**79**:293-320

[12] Kusari S, Singh S, Jayabaskaran C. Biotechnological potential of plant-associated endophytic fungi: Hope versus hype. Trends in Biotechnology. 2014;**32**:297-303

[13] Nicoletti R, Fiorentino A. Plant bioactive metabolites and drugs produced by endophytic fungi of Spermatophyta. Agriculture. 2015;**5**:918-970

[14] Gouda S, Das G, Sen SK, Shin HS, Patra JK. Endophytes: A treasure house of bioactive compounds of medicinal importance. Frontiers in Microbiology. 2016;**7**:1538. DOI: 10.3389/fmicb.2016.01538

[15] Copping LG, Duke SO. Natural products that have been used commercially as crop protection agents. Pest Management Science. 2007;**63**:524-554

[16] Barelli L, Moonjely S, Behie SW, Bidochka MJ. Fungi with multifunctional lifestyles: Endophytic insect pathogenic fungi. Plant Molecular Biology. 2016;**90**:657-664

[17] Guo B, Wang Y, Sun X, Tang K. Bioactive natural products from endophytes: A review. Applied Biochemistry and Microbiology. 2008;**44**:136-142

[18] Stierle A, Strobel G, Stierle D. Taxol and taxane production by Taxomyces andreanae an endophytic fungus of Pacific yew. Science. 1993;**260**:214-216

[19] Kimura M, Anzai H, Yamaguchi I. Microbial toxins in plant-pathogen interactions: Biosynthesis, resistance mechanisms, and significance. Journal of General and Applied Microbiology. 2001;**47**:149-160

[20] http://masters.agron.iastate.edu/classes/514/lesson06/6.2.1.html

[21] Hirsch GU, Braun U. Communities of parasitic microfungi. In: Winterhoff W, editor. Handbook of Vegetation Science: Fungi in Vegetation Science. Vol. 19. Dordrecht: Klu wer Academic; 1992. pp 225-250

[22] Grove JF, MacMillan J, Mulholland TPC, Rogers MAT. Griseofulvin. Part IV. Structure. Journal of the Chemical Society. 1952;**762**:3977-3987 Resumed

[23] Schatz A, Bugie E, Waksman S. Streptomycin: A substance exhibiting antibiotic activity against Gram-positive and Gram-negative bacteria. Proceedings of the Society for Experimental and Biological Medicine. 1944;**55**:66-69

[24] Maiese WM, Lechevalier MP, Lechevalier HA, Korshalla J, Kuck N, Fantini A, Wildey MJ, Thomas J, Greenstein M. Calicheamicins, a novel family of antitumor antibiotics: Taxonomy, fermentation and biological properties. Journal of Antibiotics. 1989;**42**:558-563

[25] Ávalos A, Elena G. Metabolismo secundario de plantas. Reduca. 2009;**2**(3):119-145

[26] Stewart JJP et al. Capítulo II. Revista Cubana de Cardiología y Cirugía Cardiovascular. 2014;**22**(1):61-104

[27] Sepúlveda-jiménez G. Sepúlveda Jiménez, Gabriela; Porta Ducoing, Helena; Rocha Sosa, Mario. Rev Mex Fitopatol. 2003;**21**(3):355-363

[28] Rodriguez-Garcia A, Hosseini S, Martinez-Chapa SO, Cordell GA. Multi-target activities of selected alkaloids and terpenoids. Mini-Review in Organic Chemistry. 2017;**14**(4)

[29] Bonkanka CX. Evolución farmacológica de terpenos y flavonoides de origen vegetal. 2007

[30] José Villanueva Díaz, Vicenta Constante García, Julián Cerano Paredes, Juan Estrada Ávalos y Miriam M. Tostado Plascencia; Impact of dams on *Taxodium mucronatum* Ten. In the san pedro-mezquital river, durango; Rev. Mex. Cien. For. **18**(4):44-56

[31] Retana-Ramos A, Escamilla Silva EM, Calderon J, Rodriguez B. 8β-hydroxypimar-15-en-19-oic acid from taxodium mucronatum. Phytochemistry. 1984;**23**(6):1329-1330

[32] Rivera-Orduña FN, Suarez-Sanchez RA, Flores-Bustamante ZR, Gracida-Rodriguez JN, Flores-Cotera LB. Diversity of endophytic fungi of *Taxus globosa* (Mexican yew). Fungal Diversity. 2011;**47**(1):65-74

Permissions

All chapters in this book were first published in PSARDP, by InTech Open; hereby published with permission under the Creative Commons Attribution License or equivalent. Every chapter published in this book has been scrutinized by our experts. Their significance has been extensively debated. The topics covered herein carry significant findings which will fuel the growth of the discipline. They may even be implemented as practical applications or may be referred to as a beginning point for another development.

The contributors of this book come from diverse backgrounds, making this book a truly international effort. This book will bring forth new frontiers with its revolutionizing research information and detailed analysis of the nascent developments around the world.

We would like to thank all the contributing authors for lending their expertise to make the book truly unique. They have played a crucial role in the development of this book. Without their invaluable contributions this book wouldn't have been possible. They have made vital efforts to compile up to date information on the varied aspects of this subject to make this book a valuable addition to the collection of many professionals and students.

This book was conceptualized with the vision of imparting up-to-date information and advanced data in this field. To ensure the same, a matchless editorial board was set up. Every individual on the board went through rigorous rounds of assessment to prove their worth. After which they invested a large part of their time researching and compiling the most relevant data for our readers.

The editorial board has been involved in producing this book since its inception. They have spent rigorous hours researching and exploring the diverse topics which have resulted in the successful publishing of this book. They have passed on their knowledge of decades through this book. To expedite this challenging task, the publisher supported the team at every step. A small team of assistant editors was also appointed to further simplify the editing procedure and attain best results for the readers.

Apart from the editorial board, the designing team has also invested a significant amount of their time in understanding the subject and creating the most relevant covers. They scrutinized every image to scout for the most suitable representation of the subject and create an appropriate cover for the book.

The publishing team has been an ardent support to the editorial, designing and production team. Their endless efforts to recruit the best for this project, has resulted in the accomplishment of this book. They are a veteran in the field of academics and their pool of knowledge is as vast as their experience in printing. Their expertise and guidance has proved useful at every step. Their uncompromising quality standards have made this book an exceptional effort. Their encouragement from time to time has been an inspiration for everyone.

The publisher and the editorial board hope that this book will prove to be a valuable piece of knowledge for researchers, students, practitioners and scholars across the globe.

List of Contributors

Muhammad Shahzad Aslam and Humayun Riaz
Rashid Latif College of Pharmacy, Lahore, Pakistan

Muhammad Syarhabil Ahmad
School of Bioprocess Engineering, Universiti Malaysia Perlis, Arau, Perlis, Malaysia

Syed Atif Raza and Osama Javed
University College of Pharmacy, University of the Punjab, Lahore, Pakistan

Shahzad Hussain
National Institute of Health, Islamabad, Pakistan

Omer Salman Qureshi
Department of Pharmacy, University of the Lahore, Pakistan

Povydysh Maria
Saint-Petersburg State Chemical-Pharmaceutical Academy, Ministry of Healthcare of the Russian Federation, St. Petersburg, Russia

Zainab Hamzah
Department Chemical Engineering, Faculty of Engineering Technology (FETech), Universiti Malaysia Perlis, Padang Besar, Perlis, Malaysia

Sechene Stanley Gololo
Department of Biochemistry, School of Science and Technology, Sefako Makgatho Health Sciences University, Pretoria, South Africa

Vasil Pirgozliev, Stephen C. Mansbridge and Paul Rose
The National Institute of Poultry Husbandry, Harper Adams University, England

David Bravo
Pancosma S.A., Geneva, Switzerland

Salem Alghamdi, Hussein Migdadi, Muhammad Khan, Ehab H. El-Harty and Muhammad Afzal
Legume Research Group, Plant Production Department, Faculty of Food and Agricultural Sciences, King Saud University, Riyadh, Saudi Arabia

Megahed Ammar
Rice Research and Training Center, Kafr El Sheikh, Egypt

Muhammad Farooq
Legume Research Group, Plant Production Department, Faculty of Food and Agricultural Sciences, King Saud University, Riyadh, Saudi Arabia
Department of Agronomy, University of Agriculture, Faisalabad, Pakistan
Department of Crop Sciences, College of Agricultural and Marine Sciences, Sultan Qaboos University, Al-Khoud, Oman

Md Asaduzzaman
Department of Agriculture, Faculty of Life and Environmental Science, Shimane University, Matsue, Shimane, Japan
Olericulture Division, Horticulture Research Center, Bangladesh Agricultural Research Institute, Gazipur, Bangladesh

Toshiki Asao
Department of Agriculture, Faculty of Life and Environmental Science, Shimane University, Matsue, Shimane, Japan

Vishal Ganessingh, Raeesah Sahibdeen and Rohanie Maharaj
Biosciences, Agriculture and Food Technologies (BAFT), ECIAF Campus, the University of Trinidad and Tobago, Trinidad & Tobago

Zorița M. Diaconeasa, Alexandra D. Frond, Ioana Ştirbu, Dumitrița Rugină and Carmen Socaciu
University of Agricultural Sciences and Veterinary Medicine, Cluj-Napoca, Romania

Ana-Alexandra Sorescu and Rodica-Mariana Ion
The National Research and Development Institute for Chemistry and Petrochemistry—ICECHIM, Evaluation and Conservation of Cultural Heritage, Bucharest, Romania
Materials Engineering Doctoral School, Valahia University, Târgoviște, Romania

Alexandrina Nuta
The National Research and Development Institute for Chemistry and Petrochemistry—ICECHIM, Evaluation and Conservation of Cultural Heritage, Bucharest, Romania
The Romanian Academy, "Stefan S. Nicolau" Institute of Virology, Bucharest, Romania

Lorena Iancu
The National Research and Development Institute for Chemistry and Petrochemistry—ICECHIM, Evaluation and Conservation of Cultural Heritage, Bucharest, Romania

Krishna N. Patel and Kalpeshkumar B. Ishnava
Ashok and Rita Patel Institute of Integrated Study and Research in Biotechnology and Allied Sciences, New Vallabh Vidyanagar, India

Godwill Azeh Engwa
Biochemistry, Department of Chemical Sciences, Godfrey Okoye University, Enugu Nigeria

Nadia Mendoza and Eleazar M. Escamilla Silva
Department of Chemical Engineering, Technological Institute of Celaya, Celaya, Guanajuato, Mexico

Index

www.ingramcontent.com/pod-product-compliance
Lightning Source LLC
LaVergne TN
LVHW060607210926
848485LV00005B/1384